Plastic Materialities

Plastic Materialities

POLITICS, LEGALITY, AND METAMORPHOSIS
IN THE WORK OF CATHERINE MALABOU

BRENNA BHANDAR AND
JONATHAN GOLDBERG-HILLER, EDITORS

Duke University Press ■ *Durham and London* ■ 2015

© 2015 Duke University Press
All rights reserved

Typeset in Chaparral by Westchester
Publishing Services

Library of Congress Cataloging-in-Publication Data
Plastic materialities : politics, legality, and
metamorphosis in the work of Catherine
Malabou / Brenna Bhandar and Jonathan
Goldberg-Hiller, eds.
pages cm
Includes bibliographical references and index.
ISBN 978-0-8223-5845-9 (hardcover : alk. paper)
ISBN 978-0-8223-5857-2 (pbk. : alk. paper)
1. Malabou, Catherine. 2. Philosophy of mind. 3.
Adaptability (Psychology) 4. Brain—
Philosophy. I. Bhandar, Brenna
II. Goldberg-Hiller, Jonathan
BD418.3.P53 2015
194—dc23
2014036269
ISBN 978-0-8223-7573-9 (e-book)

Cover art: Greg Dunn, *Two Pyramidals*, 2010
(detail). Enamel on composition gold; 18"x 24".
Courtesy of the artist.

CONTENTS

Acknowledgments, vii

Introduction. Staging Encounters, 1
Brenna Bhandar and Jonathan Goldberg-Hiller

1 ■ Will Sovereignty Ever Be Deconstructed?, 35
Catherine Malabou

2 ■ Whither Materialism? Althusser/Darwin, 47
Catherine Malabou

3 ■ From the Overman to the Posthuman:
How Many Ends?, 61
Catherine Malabou

4 ■ Autoplasticity, 73
Alain Pottage

5 ■ Plasticity, Capital, and the Dialectic, 91
Alberto Toscano

6 ■ Plasticity and the Cerebral Unconscious: New Wounds,
New Violences, New Politics, 111
Catherine Kellogg

7 ■ "Go Wonder": Plasticity, Dissemination,
and (the Mirage of) Revolution, 133
Silvana Carotenuto

8 ■ Insects, War, Plastic Life, 159
Renisa Mawani

9 ■ Zones of Justice: A Philopoetic Engagement, 189
Michael J. Shapiro

10 ■ Law, Sovereignty, and Recognition, 209
Brenna Bhandar and Jonathan Goldberg-Hiller

11 ■ Something Darkly This Way Comes: The Horror of Plasticity in an Age of Control, 233
Jairus Grove

12 ■ The Touring Machine (Flesh Thought Inside Out), 265
Fred Moten

13 ■ Interview with Catherine Malabou, 287

Bibliography, 301

Contributors, 325

Index, 329

ACKNOWLEDGMENTS

The making of this book has been a collaboration of many who have contributed time, money, and passion. We thank the authors for their scholarly engagements that led to these chapters. In addition, we would like to acknowledge the contributions of Denise Ferreira da Silva and Bradley Bryan, who participated in a seminar with the other authors from which this book emerged. That seminar, held in London, was funded by the National Science Foundation of the United States, with contributions from Queen Mary University of London, and the University of Hawai'i at Mānoa. We deeply thank these institutions for their generosity and their trust. Courtney Berger and Ken Wissoker of Duke University Press have earned our sincere gratitude for their support, advice, and encouragement. We sincerely thank the anonymous readers of this manuscript who offered intellectual guidance. Finally, we thank Catherine Malabou, who met our ideas for this project with early enthusiasm and enduring friendship.

INTRODUCTION

Staging Encounters

Brenna Bhandar and Jonathan Goldberg-Hiller

Catherine Malabou's philosophical thought stages a new and restless encounter with form and so transforms the possibilities of philosophy for thinking contemporary politics, law, and justice. In a series of books, most of which have been recently translated into English, she has pioneered a distinctive mode of reading the Continental philosophical tradition, revealing a new materialism that survives and brings to restored relevance Hegel, Heidegger, Derrida, Irigaray, Deleuze, Foucault, and Freud, among others. Traversing the philosophical groundwork of these thinkers, Malabou uncovers and exposes elements of their work that metabolize and metamorphosize concepts and logics that otherwise appear to be unmoving, if not static. The restless form that survives philosophical critique, which she explores with her signature concept of *plasticity*, has its material counterparts in socioeconomic structures such as neoliberal capitalism, the science of neurobiology, the theory and practice of psychoanalysis, the experience and expression of subjectivity and identity, and the political organization of sovereignty. Oriented firmly against the naturalization of these enterprises, Malabou asks us instead to see each institution engaged with a kind of immanent thought that materially grounds its potential metamorphoses. The form of thought today, she argues, is ontologically plastic; self-transformation is built into our bodies, it suffuses our possible readings of philosophy, and it promises us new perspectives on political and social change.

Decades after a Continental turn away from structuralism, Malabou's scholarship invites us to imagine what we might gain by reconceptualizing form and bringing it back into philosophical and political grammar. In this new metamorphic structuralism,[1] might we find an emergent legal form more attuned to justice? Might the constant alteration of social identity and sexuality that has animated so much contemporary politics provide a more robust ethical basis for social policy than the political languages of recognition and equality have hitherto provided? Can the rapid changes in form, and form's almost explosive reversals, tell us more about the psychoanalytic subject than eros and the persistence of the libidinal economy of drives has revealed? "Form is the metamorphizable but immovable barrier of thought,"[2] Malabou has argued, and in different ways, this collection of essays tests the explosive potential of this plastic frontier as it asks these questions.

If the point, Marx once reminded us, is not only to interpret the world but ultimately to change it,[3] in which ways might we grasp Malabou's central concept of plasticity to facilitate political praxis? In the making of this volume, we asked the authors to liberally but critically explore the economic, psychoanalytic, and sociocultural dynamics that Malabou has also identified as her political field. All the authors share concerns regarding the limits and potentials of contemporary neoliberal economics and the reconfiguration of sovereign power that engender techniques of accumulation and dispossession relying upon the flexibility of labor, the porosity of national borders to flows of capital but not working bodies, and juridical apparatuses that riddle the rule of law with exception.[4] This neoliberal flexibility is accompanied by forms of violence that reinscribe colonial relations of subjection. What intellectual directions might Malabou's thinking about change, metamorphosis, and destructive plasticity provide in our attempts to disrupt these structures? How might we use her work to reconceive the philosophical foundations of a globalized capitalism, as Alberto Toscano asks in this volume? What philosophical resources might her thought provide in our excavation of the originary, foundational subject that is constituted through racial-scientific knowledges, this subject that persists, stubbornly refusing to vacate its sovereign place in the ontological *grundnorms* of a Western episteme, as Fred Moten queries? Does the plasticity of being offer a means to deconstruct the anthropocentrism of our episteme, as Renisa Mawani asks? Do forms of law and justice exhibit a plasticity that harbors the promise of newly relational, perhaps even emancipatory, political practices, as Michael J. Shapiro pursues? These questions are articulated in and throughout the essays in this volume and structure the primary concerns elaborated in this introductory chapter: form, materialism, and subjectivity.

FORM BEYOND METAPHYSICS: METAMORPHOSIS

Form is a concept that has had uneven histories within and among various disciplines. In the dialectical tradition, form is an energy—for Fredric Jameson, the "jumping of a spark between two poles, the coming into contact of two unequal terms, of two apparently unrelated modes of being"[5]—which at various times has illuminated the connection between law and political economy,[6] narrative and historical representation,[7] identity and colonialism,[8] among other unions. Yet in these accounts form often represents structural antinomies that ethically must be transcended or eliminated. In many of the human sciences, particularly in North America, form has also been depicted in irresolvable tension with historical, empirical, and behavioral disciplines whose pragmatic spirit sought to undo a nineteenth-century concern for the aridity and purity of metaphysical thought.[9] The influence of poststructuralist thought has also submerged the (often Sausseurian) attention to form[10] or deterritorialized it to scrub its connections with dialectical thought.[11] Form has perhaps endured longest within cultural studies and political theory that have emphasized a post–Kantian concern for aesthetics and its formal dependence on a distance or gap between the subject and its political or artistic objects.[12]

Thinking instead through the scientific (and materially *with* the) neurological synaptic gap, Malabou seeks to philosophically recover form by grasping it as always already in restless motion. She is foremost a philosopher of change: a thinker of the concept of transformation as it contaminates the dialectical logic of Hegel, the destructive reason of Heidegger, the deconstructive philosophy of Derrida; the potential for and realization of transformation that inheres in the bios and the biological; the destructive, annihilating force of change that contours the psychic life of those who have suffered neurological trauma. We have most often turned to narrative to reveal the potential of metamorphic change: a story told by Ovid or Hegel or Kafka,[13] a cinematic trick. The symbolic image of a hybrid—a centaur or minotaur—that can disclose the spatial and visual character of immanent change cannot work as well, suggesting that plasticity's potential exceeds the aesthetic bounds of the eponymous plastic arts. As Caroline Bynum notes: "Unlike hybridity there is, to be sure, a certain twoness in metamorphosis; the transformation goes from one being to another, and the relative weight or presence of the two entities suggests where we are in the story. At the beginning and end, where there is no trace of the otherness from which and to which the process is going, there is no metamorphosis; there is metamorphosis only in between. Nonetheless metamorphosis is about process, mutation, story—a constant series of replacement-changes, . . . little deaths."[14]

Seizing a fragile point of access, an ironic process of giving weight to that which is weightless within a philosophical oeuvre that she calls the "fantastic," Malabou seeks to make these little deaths again visible as form and, hence, accessible to philosophy and politics beyond the aesthetic register.[15] However, just as the form of the synaptic gap gains its neuroscientific significance through its weightless potentials (to fire or not, to rearrange its circuits of influence), so does it demonstrate the fantastic philosophical potentials between biology and history, determinism and freedom.[16] As Malabou writes in *The Heidegger Change*, "simultaneously a mode of visibility and manifestation, the fantastic . . . designates . . . the phenomenality of ontico-ontological transformations—those of man, god, language, etc.—which unveil the originary mutability of being while revealing at the same time that being is perhaps nothing . . . but its mutability."[17]

If, in Malabou's words, "to behold essence is to witness change,"[18] how can we know the value of this mutability? Commodities also change and exchange, in formal ways that Marx once similarly called metamorphic and fantastic.[19] Scientific truths and technology likewise persistently transform themselves, as do many aspects of law, democracy, and identity. How can we grasp what is radical and new, that which promises an alternative to capitalism, to sovereign power, to the influence of the norm, especially where capitalism, sovereignty, and governance constantly reinvent themselves? What can we secure when all that is solid melts into air? Malabou answers that there is form and then there is *form* and we must philosophically distinguish the two. One reformulates its elements in an infinitely flexible, malleable, or elastic manner akin to "hypercapitalism," adding only a supplement to metaphysics,[20] while the other demonstrates that "form can cross the line."[21] This other is the plasticity of form, that character of metamorphosis (repeated throughout her work as the tripartite motif of plasticity: the giving, receiving and exploding of form) that is simultaneously resistant to and open to change and capable of annihilating itself. "If form cannot cross the line, then there is no alterity for metaphysics. In a sense, there is no alterity at all. I'm laying my bets for the meaning of my work on the success of the first term of this alternative. In other words, I believe in the future not of the other of form but of the other form, a form that no longer corresponds to its traditional concept.[22]

Where form crosses this line, the line in turn becomes form. This transubstantiation is, for Malabou, "precisely the other of the idea—a nonideal form that is at once both the condition and the result of change"; form, still, because it is a product of "creative minds giving form to the line; the form of a life that is from here out revolutionized, reversed, and opened in its middle."[23] As her phrasing suggests, crossing the line is a spatial metaphor with a complex shape, but it is also clear that such intricacies—the reversals, the simultaneity of cause and result—draw as well on new temporalities and their contributions to new forms of self-perception. In Malabou's early book *The Future of Hegel*, she reads time such that there is both a future of Hegel and a future for Hegel, a time of plasticity in which temporal forms are themselves placed in motion.

> It is not a matter of examining the relations between past, present and the conventional sense of the future presented in the discussions of time in Hegel's different versions of the *Philosophy of Nature*. Rather, these texts themselves demand that we renounce the "well-known" definition of time. The possibility that one temporal determination, the future, can be thought differently, beyond its initial, simple status as a moment of time, from "that which is now to come," makes it immediately clear that time for Hegel cannot be reduced to an ordered relation between moments. By "plasticity" we mean first of all the excess of the future over the future; while "temporality," as it figures in speculative philosophy, will mean the excess of time over time.[24]

As this quote makes clear, Malabou reads the Hegelian subject as anticipatory and thus riven by distinctive notions of time: the first a classical teleological sense connoting necessity; another as the modern time of representation that does not move forward.[25] In this philosophical register, Malabou shows how reading is itself a plastic enterprise, a constant renewal and transformation of the Hegelian text. "Reading Hegel amounts to finding oneself in two times at once: the process that unfolds is both retrospective and prospective. In the present time in which reading takes place, the reader is drawn to a double expectation: waiting for what is to come (according to a linear and representational thinking), while presupposing that the outcome has already arrived (by virtue of the teleological ruse)."[26] These distinct senses of time establish gaps within which contemporary forms of thought and subjectivity continue to strive. "[The Hegelian] discourse—where . . . times meet and intersect—is beholden to the very thing it is trying to describe: that speculative suppleness which is neither passion nor passivity, but plasticity."[27]

Working within these gaps, Malabou presents us with a mode of reading Hegel's thought that demonstrates its capacity for transformation. In subsequent work she has originated a reading of Heidegger that emphasizes a similar mobility. Concentrating on elements of Heidegger's thought that have hitherto not received very much attention, particularly his ethics and the instabilities of *Dasein*, Malabou has uncovered the insistent presence of the triad *Wandel* (change), *Wandlung* (transformation) and *Verwandlung* (metamorphosis) in his philosophy. This is a triangulation that exposes, in her view, the "transformative rupture" that Heideggerian destruction presents, "the moment by which thinking henceforth 'prepares its own transformation.'"[28]

Malabou's attention to the excesses of temporality and futurity, according to Derrida, has "inscribed a mutation, or even better, an absolute heterogeneity between the two senses or meanings of the same word, between the two concepts, and the two concepts of time, and the two concepts of the future."[29] Similar mutations drawn from temporal complexity emerge as well in Malabou's work on mourning and history in Freud and Nietzsche, where she argues for a mourning of the impossible;[30] on the complex and nonlinear meaning of generations in the biology of the crocus and the reflective poetry of Apollinaire and anthropology of Lévi-Strauss;[31] and on the genetic stem cell manipulation that advances life by reactivating once lost functions and, in returning to the past, allowing for the recovery of a new pathway.[32] Temporality is also the theme of "From the Overman to the Posthuman," her third chapter in this book, where she asks whether it will be possible to cease our revenge against time. In these varied sites, plasticity is revealed as an immanent characteristic of life and its apprehension.

Malabou suggests that disruptive temporalities emerge in the form of the accident, an idea central to her notion of destructive plasticity. Destructive plasticity challenges the easily assimilable idea of a reparative or positive plasticity that responds to life's "vagaries and difficulties, or simply the natural unfolding of circumstance, appear[ing] as the marks and wrinkles of a continuous, almost logical, process of fulfillment that leads ultimately to death. In time, one eventually becomes who one is; one becomes only who one is."[33] Instead, destructive plasticity cuts this time from its mooring; a stroke or other brain trauma instantly makes one "a stranger to the one before,"[34] suffering because of the lack of suffering: "an indifference to pain, impassivity, forgetting, the loss of symbolic reference points."[35] Yanked out of the familiar times of life, destructive plasticity, like Freud's death drive, reveals the "power of change without redemption, without teleology, without any meaning other than strangeness."[36] Deleuze, too, addressed the accident, but he sees it as an aspect of everyday occurrence, opposed to the ideal Event.[37] Malabou pushes against Deleuze's reading, in which the accidental is recuperated as form stripped of its ideal essence, a limit to true metamorphic possibilities. Rather than the philosophical conservatism of metaphysical form, Malabou suggests, the accident reveals that form is not the problem; it is rather that form is thought separately from essence.

> The critique of metaphysics does not want to recognize that in fact, despite what it claims loud and clear, metaphysics constantly instigates the dissociation of essence and form, or form and the formal, as if one could always rid oneself of form, as if, in the evening, form could be left hanging like a garment on the chair of being or essence. In metaphysics, form can always change, but the nature of being persists. It is this that is debatable—not the concept of form itself, which it is absurd to pretend to do without.[38]

Destructive plasticity, initiated by the accident, reveals the challenge to philosophy: to acknowledge it as "a law that is simultaneously logical and biological, but a law that does not allow us to anticipate its instances."[39]

In endless and creative motion to recover a new path, plasticity flourishes in the excesses of philosophical reason, promising an antidote to what Malabou has diagnosed as the growing contemporary sense of ideological and metaphysical closure. Malabou describes this closure as the "contradictory couple" of saturation and vacancy. Saturation captures the social, theoretical, and figurative meanings of a rapidly globalizing future in which no event can be marginal, a condition heralding the end of speculative philosophy and of other vital tasks. This simplification of the world that Hegel first described revels in the sense of vacancy—that there is "nothing left to do"—but it paradoxically reveals the promise of novelty, "a promise that there are forms of life which must be invented."[40] Plasticity is what designates the possibility of this promise, and it serves as a creative response to the contemporary experience of closure. Where plasticity emerges—within the biological and psychological maintenance of organisms, within the social and political institutions that maintain contemporary life, and within philosophical thought—and under what conditions it can be read occupies much of Malabou's work grounded in her autobiographical inquiries into the transformations of her own subjectivity in her philosophical and professional encounters, her own attempts to grasp herself.[41]

Malabou's reaction against closure is shared with much post–1968 French philosophy, notably the work of Gilles Deleuze and the scholarly lines of flight he inspired, as well as the return to Spinoza, Bergson, and Nietzsche that infuses much of the work of the New Materialists.[42] But where Hegel's dialectical system and the atemporal and static notions of form that it traditionally generated have often been pictured as the totalizing and conceptually fecund foils against which a new vibrant materialism is oriented,[43] Malabou creatively reads Hegel as open to the surprise of such a vitalist future. This has consequences for transformative readings of French philosophical traditions, as well as a fundamental recuperation of the subject, endlessly deconstructed or shunned in much French poststructuralist thought[44] and now invited to cognize her own subjectivity as plastic and transformative. What potentials does this dialectic within a new materialism bring?

NEW MATERIALISMS

Exploring the materialist dimension in Malabou's work is central to understanding her philosophical project and situates her in conversation with contemporary political concerns about the linkages among capitalism, democracy, and the fashioning of political subjects. Malabou's materialism is rooted in an attempt to rethink the relationship between neuroscience and philosophical conceptualizations of consciousness and the self. In *What Should We Do with Our Brain?* she asks whether neoliberalism's reliance upon and cultivation of flexibility as one of its key organizing concepts and drivers is equivocal with a neuronal plasticity that provides a biological justification for contemporary modes of alienation and exploitation.

Malabou interrogates historically predominant concepts of the brain (e.g., Henri Bergson's idea that the brain functions like a telephone exchange and later analogies to the computer) and explains how neuroscientific explanations of the brain's inherent plasticity reveal each individual's inherent capacity to remake herself. She argues that this shift in the way in which we understand the brain and, in turn, ourselves has the capacity to alter our current alienation from our consciousness that results from modeling our brains as rigid, mechanical entities that are entirely genetically determined, even where our neurological circuits are understood to be decentralized and diffuse. By relating our knowledge of our brains to consciousness, Malabou reveals what is at stake in embracing our own neuroplasticity. If we understand how our brains have been interpellated (as structurally rigid entities overdetermined by genetics or as docile facilitators of the capitalist mode of production) and if we instead embrace our brains as plastic ("as something modifiable, 'formable,' and formative at the same time"),[45] it then becomes possible to change our relationship to history through a different relationship to the self. The neuroscientifically aware subject, gaining consciousness of her own plastic potentialities, "produces the conditions for a new world of questioning,"[46] a new capacity for revolt. "To talk about the plasticity of the brain means to see in it not only the creator and receiver of form but also an agency of disobedience to every constituted form, a refusal to submit to a model."[47]

Our brains are unruly; biology can break the symbolic realm into which our thinking is plunged. The vital importance of this insurgent biological materialism, for Malabou, is the need to escape the endless cycle of capitalism's absorption of its own critique into what Luc Boltanski and Eve Chiapello have called the "spirit of capitalism" capable of reengineering its production of value. If a critique of capitalism such as environmentalism can be digested into "green" commodities, if globalized circuits of production continually engulf other modes of production, and if capitalism "now includes, as its condition of possibility, the deconstruction of presence, nomadism or deterritorialisation,"[48] then there is no real "outside" and no transcendental position from which to launch a critique of capitalism. Even Marxism, Malabou suggests, belongs, paradoxically, to the "voracious monster" of capitalism.[49]

> I think if we continue today to affirm the priority of the symbolic, political criticism has no chance to escape its assimilation by the capitalist system. The similarity of thought and capital lies precisely in the production of surplus value. The symbolic supplement is the equivalent of the theory of profit. The two surpluses unite in the possibility of fetishism. Boltanski's right. The "spirit" as it is thought as

surplus (surplus of meaning, excess of ideology) forms the hyphen, the indistinguishability between capitalism and criticism because it is the mark of their synonymy. Surplus value—meaning and economic value—is precisely what constitutes the spirit of capitalism. In this sense, the symbolic is the best ally of capital.[50]

This symbolic closure sets up the problem that plasticity seeks to resolve. Can philosophy break the priority of the symbolic with a concept such as plasticity? Is plasticity sufficiently material so that it can effectively grasp a robust notion of the historical? Malabou suggests that developing a consciousness of our individual brain plasticity may allow us to think "a multiplicity of interactions in which the participants exercise transformative effects on one another through the demands of recognition, of non-domination, and of liberty...."[51] By associating plasticity with the rupturing and refiguring of the symbolic, Malabou critiques a neuronal ideology that relies on a reflexive relationship between neoliberal forms of capitalism and brain plasticity: "The mental is not the wise appendix of the neuronal. And the brain is not the natural ideal of globalized economic, political, and social organization; it is the locus of an organic tension that is the basis of our history and our critical activity."[52]

In light of a sordid history of the convergence of biology and economics, including the scientific racism and sexism of social Darwinism and sociobiology[53] and more recently the convergence of consumer choice and biology in the field of neuroeconomics,[54] the denaturalization of the relationship between biology and the social-cultural traits of neoliberal capitalism is an important intervention into the language utilized to describe and structure contemporary forms of labor exploitation, managerialism, and consumerism. However, in reinventing the way we understand and think the brain and, accordingly, our critical capacities and understanding of history, a question arises as to whether the absence of engagement with dialectical materialism retains a concept of consciousness that appears untouched by Marx's crucial interventions into Hegelian idealism. There is a parallel within psychoanalysis as well. Lacan's notion of the Real, which exceeds and escapes the symbolic realm of the law, is, as Fredric Jameson has argued, "simply History itself," a history that takes us directly to the problems posed by Marx.[55]

Malabou begins *What Should We Do with Our Brain?* with a reference to Marx's famous statement from *The 18th Brumaire of Louis Bonaparte*. However, Malabou renders Marx's words as follows: "humans make their own history, but they do not know that they make it . . ."⁵⁶ One common translation of Marx's statement reads, "Men make their own history, but they do not make it just as they please; they do not make it under circumstances chosen by themselves, but under circumstances directly encountered, given, and transmitted from the past."⁵⁷

This slippage between knowing and making history draws attention to a fundamental difference between a historical materialist understanding of political subjectivity and of its relationship to history and Malabou's materialism. While Marx invokes a consciousness about historicity, as Malabou points out, he does this in order to reveal how the political and economic conditions in which humans act, live, labor, and revolt are ones that constrain and deracinate the rich and potentially explosive germ that lies in revolutionary movements. In what ways can neuronal plasticity dispel the symbolic weight of the past, what Marx poetically called the "tradition of all the dead generations [that] weighs like a nightmare on the brain on the living?"⁵⁸ What would it take for a critique of neuronal ideology to account for the material conditions of alienation that not only work to disorient and disembody consciousness of one's potential as a political agent of change and transformation but rely on actual, structural relations of exploitation (of labor) and dispossession (of land and resources)?

This raises another query that is taken up in more detail in the consideration of subjectivity. To note this briefly here, however, the role of habit and repetition, learning and memory, in the formation of individual human brains⁵⁹ points to the ways in which class, race, gender, and sexuality materially render the neuronal subject. How do social relations of inequality affect a political potentiality based in a "nervous circuit [that] is never fixed" but rather is constituted by and through synapses that are "reinforced or weakened as a function of experience,"⁶⁰ as a result of particular histories?

Beginning with faint echoes of Marx, *What Should We Do with Our Brain?* ends with a turn to Hegel. Exploring the relationship between the brain and the mind, neuronal plasticity has the potential to create new forms of consciousness through the recognition of its essentially unmodelable, or deconstructed, nature. The plasticity of the Hegelian dialectic shows the transformation of the mind's natural existence (in her idiom, the brain; in his, the "natural soul"), into its historical and speculative being. "If there can be a transition from nature to thought, this is because the nature of thought contradicts itself."⁶¹ And thus Malabou's materialism is one that focuses on consciousness, which is material insofar as it refers to the matter of the brain but appears to remain ideal in that it does not confront the materialist critique rendered by Marx. "A reasonable materialism, in my view, would posit that the natural contradicts itself and that thought is the fruit of this contradiction. One pertinent way of envisaging the "mind-body problem" consists in taking into account the dialectical tension that at once binds and opposes naturalness and intentionality, and in taking an interest in them as inhabiting the living core of a complex reality. Plasticity, rethought philosophically, could be the name of this *entre-deux*."[62]

The idea of a "reasonable materialism" is a significant philosophical problem today, and it animates several contributions to this volume. Malabou insists that we must critique neuroscience that converges with political economy, making a strong claim that the epistemology of neuroscience must be tempered by a primary ontological commitment. When the brain's plastic potential becomes an object of value—as have so many biological materials today[63]—science itself has no neutral ground on which to fix reality. As Alexander Galloway recently argued, to ask Malabou's political question—which he rephrases as "What should we do so that thinking does not purely and simply coincide with the spirit of capitalism?"[64]—requires that we affirm the "aligned" ontological commitments of materialism espousing that "everything should be rooted in material life and history, not in abstraction, logical necessity, universality, essence, pure form, spirit, or idea. . . . The true poverty of [realism is] its inability to recognize that the highest order of the absolute, the totality itself, is found in the material history of mankind. To touch the absolute is precisely to think this correlation, not so much to explain it away, but to show that thought itself is the correlation as such, and thus to think the material is to spread one's thoughts across the mind of history."[65]

Toscano's and Pottage's chapters in this volume amplify some of these concerns while taking particular aim at Malabou's reliance on philosophy as a key to exposing the potential of a new, neuroscientific materialism. We discuss Pottage's chapter in the next section and consider Toscano's contribution here. Toscano interrogates the logics of capital, social forms, and forces that push philosophy outside of itself, a condition of being under capital "which implies the *expatriation* of philosophy." Malabou is right, he argues, to urge us to rethink the dialectic of contemporary social forms. But if we are to understand the hold that neoliberal models take on the potential of neuroplasticity and thereby to criticize the limits arbitrarily imposed on this discourse by scientists, philosophers, journalists and others,[66] then we must build a critique that is immanent and dialectical but not beholden to capital. Toscano thus brings that old materialist, Marx, back into play in the new materialism of Malabou. Marx's critique was that the essence and history of philosophy could not meaningfully be its own object, that philosophy fought "phrases" only with "phrases," "in no way combatting the real existing world."[67] In what ways, Toscano asks, is Malabou's attempt to recover a philosophical concept of transformation capable of doing more than turning phrase or analogical model against the real existing world of capital that she targets?

Toscano points out that Malabou's efforts to examine the articulation of exchangeability as a capitalist and metaphysical principle is at the heart of her interrogation of Heidegger, risking a conceptual anchor in the Western philosophical "originary" rather than the real relations of economic exchange. One element of this philosophical risk for Toscano is apparent in Malabou's emphasis upon changes to capitalism's "spirit," following Boltanski and Chiapello, a concern skeptical of the impact that a new "motor scheme" heralded by plasticity may bring to critical analysis and practice. Stepping away from historical materialist analysis and taking perspective from neuroplasticity risks seeing too much ideological consistency within actually existing capitalism and a nondialectical perspective forced by an analogical and ultimately philosophical lens. Malabou's rejoinder and her affirmation of the need to incorporate Marxism only with Derridean deconstruction and Heideggerian destruction can be read in the interview that concludes this volume. Another alternative based in the materialism of Althusser can be found in chapter 2, "Whither Materialism? Althusser/Darwin."

SUBJECTIVITY, JUSTICE, AND THE END OF SOVEREIGNTY

If the age of grammar is being replaced by an age of plasticity, as Malabou suggests, what might it mean to see oneself today in neuronal terms? The decentering of the subject within poststructuralist theory, perhaps expressed most ardently by Deleuze and Guattari as the subject's "becoming" and its potential "nomadism" open to its own reconstruction, has its analogue in the neuroscientific recognition that the mind is located "everywhere and nowhere" in the brain and that brains are not just replete with genetically organized neurons but are, in the end, grown through movement, action, and accident. Brains express the very histories of embodiment, and to see oneself in this history is to recognize the political ambivalence of emancipation and control that embodiment establishes.[68] The potential for political ruptures—of inequality, exploitation, and alienation—that a transformative subjectivity might enact raises a more specific question, namely one of justice that lingers in any discussion of political metamorphosis.

New sexualities illustrate one aspect of this issue. The proliferation of new sexual identities since the 1970s has emerged hand in glove with new political demands. Some gay and lesbian identities have been voiced as matters of biological diversity, subjects realizing their true essences and on these grounds demanding rights and recognition. Yet from some quarters the granting of recognition for gay rights, such as same-sex marriage, as well as the recognition of an economic niche for sexual citizenship,[69] has been argued to be another straitjacket,[70] a homonormativism[71] that is ultimately unable to escape the discursive and juridical power over the body. What happens in the name of sexual freedom when the elimination of one norm, strictly heterosexual marriage, becomes another: sexual constancy regulated through marriage?[72] Queer theoretical alternatives have turned away from law, premising liberation on the basis of deconstructing biological essentialism and the norms for bodily comportment.[73] They demonstrate that sexuality and gender, as much as sex itself, are not naturally given "but rather an ideological norm whose function is to regulate and control behavior and identity codes."[74] Malabou's insistence on a materiality to subjectivity raises important questions of justice here. If there is no biological essence, there are no "women" in whose name feminist struggles for justice are waged and no sexual differences to liberate. "Antiessentialism destroys any claims by theory to displace the traditional limits of theory, to exist as a space of the feminine, to separate from the beehive, to be anything other than another cell in the honeycomb."[75]

Malabou has argued that the recovery of valid political struggle involves rejecting the current understanding of essence, which is, on the one hand, naturally given and therefore easily regulated and, on the other hand, merely the effect of extant norms. In order to plastically apprehend essence, Malabou proposes a concept of essence based on neuroscience: ontological and biological yet without presence.

> We must rethink the relation of philosophy and science today, not in order to isolate a "feminine" contingent that would be, for example, the mechanics of fluids, but rather to show, always according to the hypothesis of an originary transformability of presence and nature, that *the place of sex has moved*. . . . Today, the brain is becoming the place of affects, passions and drives, delocalizing "sexuality" from the central, etiological role—both psychic and genital—with which Freud endowed it. This does not mean that gender identity is only developed by neurons, but that the space of play between (anatomic) sex and gender, between the so-called "biological essence" and "cultural construction" of identity, has profoundly changed meaning. . . . To construct one's identity is a process that can only be a development of an original biological malleability, a first transformability. If sex were not plastic, there would be no gender. If something were not offered for transformation in the natural and anatomical determination of sex, then identity construction would not be possible.[76]

This type of deconstructed essence locates within metamorphosis and transformation a form of resistance—with potentialities, Malabou suggests, for political transformation.

Malabou has explored the relationship between subjectivity and resistance in other areas as well. In *Plasticity at the Dusk of Writing*, she has conceptualized her own intellectual autobiography through her encounters with the philosophy of plasticity. "I am just trying to show how a being, in its fragile and finite mutability, can experience the materiality of existence and transform its ontological meaning. The impossibility means first of all the impossibility of fleeing oneself. It is within the very frame of this impossibility that I propose a philosophical change of perspective that focuses on closure as its principal object."[77] Malabou's rejection of fleeing from oneself brings to the fore a substance of the self—whether autobiographical, psychoanalytic, or biological—where a material resistance to flexibility can be activated.

AESTHETICS AND THE MATERIAL SUBJECT

Michael J. Shapiro's chapter in this volume demonstrates that this materialism may also be significant at the aesthetic level. Shapiro analyzes Mathias Énard's novel *Zone* (2010), written over five hundred pages as a single sentence, by reading philosophical and literary concepts against its distinctive flowing grammar in order to reveal a discursive relief through which subjectivity is formed. Between the literary concepts of Bakhtin, which stress a narratological plasticity in the changing form of the novel as it strives to interrogate the mutable life world, and the philosophical concepts of Malabou lie the possibilities of what Shapiro calls an aesthetic subjectivity and a conceptual persona capable of self-fashioning and releasing passions signaling new appraisals of the world. The mix of genres is essential to Shapiro's plastic reading of the novel, a technique that he notes to be evident in Malabou's and Bakhtin's own oeuvres. "Political discernment derives from the mixing of idioms," he argues.

Shapiro emphasizes the significance of archives for the novel's emplotment; they also model the novel's own form: it too becomes an archive. Utilizing Foucault's concept of the *dispositif*, Shapiro unfolds what a *"justice dispositif"* might be composed of: a "heterogeneous amalgam" of different narrative forms, of a protagonist's journeys both symbolic and territorial, of the desire to map both a philosophical and literary plasticity. The political potential of plasticity resides, for Shapiro, in the archive. The complex temporality of an archive is plastic "inasmuch as although aspects of the past shape it, the very form of the record keeping in turn reshapes the way the past is understood." Shapiro's reading builds the archive as a new material basis on which to conceive the political potential of plasticity, as it alters the number and kinds of voices included in what he calls "zones of justice." While archives are textual and ideological, they are also sites of reading the self for literary characters and readers, both revealed as aesthetic subjects. Shapiro shows that aesthetic subjectivity can be understood as material, and he demonstrates that this subject has a radical plastic potential to escape ideological formation in encounters with the archive.

Silvana Carotenuto's chapter also explores the aesthetic dimensions of plasticity by reading philosophically the work of Zoulikha Bouabdellah, a Maghrebian artist, who has herself grappled with the concept of plasticity in an effort to artistically come to grips with the revolutionary potentials of the Arab Spring. Examining Bouabdellah's paintings and the writing she has produced about her work leads Carotenuto to ask to what degree Malabou's philosophy has fully metabolized Derrida's deconstruction and whether his critique of the Hegelian dialectic, in signature concepts such as dissemination and the persistence of writing, might signal resistance to the motor scheme of plasticity. In exposing philosophy again to its own death, Carotenuto argues, Malabou hinges plasticity on a form of mourning. Derrida, however, is interested less in the transformation of the philosophical system than in its "'deferment'— dis-location, dis-adherence, post-ponement—capable of bringing 'elsewhere'/*ailleurs* all instances of vital affirmation and their surviving ghosts." Paper may be shinking, Derrida has argued,[78] but it remains spectral in its withdrawal, revealing that "the modes of its appropriation are not disappearing": it explains the foundation of our anxieties over risks to identity theft in a digital age and what moves attention to Maghrebian immigrants and other *sans-papiers*. Carotenuto argues that these remnants show that paper can "continue to provoke the permanent desire of transgressing it" as well as force a swerve around a plastic reading, provoking instead a retrospective interpretation that is "the anterior future of the past resources of paper itself."

Carotenuto applies this Derridean temporality to her analysis of Bouabdellah's experimental art, which appears, in several ways, to confront Malabou's assumption that *"Writing will never abolish form. The trace will never pierce the figure."*[79] Bouabdellah's art, she shows, juxtaposes writing of various forms with image in an effort to reconnect figurative representation and nonrepresentation, not only in the finished pieces, but also in her philosophical musings on the aesthetics that she constructs. By piercing the surface of her sculptural and painted figures through probing, cutting, scraping, filing, sewing, shredding, stitching, and other techniques, she strives to see herself on the other side of her art. This offers, in Carotenuto's words, "a 'chance' to 'chance.'" And in so doing, she remains plastically and deconstructively open to the difference that the revolutionary future can bring.

PSYCHOANALYSIS AND MATERIALISM

If the psychoanalytic subject can be thought of as an intervention into the stories we tell ourselves,[80] Malabou's interrogation of psychoanalysis is framed by the question of its adequacy to comprehend a materialist basis for subjectivity beyond its aesthetic concepts of plasticity and, by extension, its competence to critique contemporary subjectivity in the interest of therapeutic healing. Freud's theory of the indestructability of the psyche and the fluidity of the libido—its ability to shape itself in cathexis but detach from and move on to various objects throughout life—represent the giving and receiving of form that characterizes two aspects of plasticity. So too does the psychic process of mourning (and its historical counterpart of memorialization) that seeks to balance forgetting and detachment with preservation of the lost object.[81] Malabou's criticism of Freud's psychoanalytic model stems from his inability to incorporate the death drive—that which lies beyond the pleasure principle—into his concept of psychoanalytic plasticity.

Freud's failure, according to Malabou, results from an inability to model the simultaneity of life and death that characterizes the "time of materiality" in which we must live. While the life drive—eros—creates forms, the death drive destroys them. While Freud argues that the organism fashions or forms its own death, this is not plastic but only elastic—an oscillation between the impossibility of preserving a form and a rigid attachment to a form, a form ultimately constituted only by the life drives. Freud's attachment to elasticity is insufficiently materialist, in Malabou's thinking, because it cannot escape the limitations of an aesthetic frame. Freud's models for the death drive retain this aesthetic presence, while plasticity demands a form of resistance.

If aesthetics is a dimension of plasticity's ability to receive and donate form, destructive plasticity seems to hint at another scale of relief, a more complicated "fold" within discourse.[82] Destructive plasticity, in the form of the disassembly of neural circuits preparatory to reassembly, is part of neurological functioning, but so are traumatic accidents and the diseases of aging that seemingly destroy the self and overthrow the sovereignty of the brain.[83] Unlike the aesthetic gaps in which the self synaptically forms itself, destructive plasticity "enables the appearance or formation of alterity where the other is absolutely lacking. Plasticity is the form of alterity when no transcendence, flight or escape is left. The only other that exists in this circumstance is being other to the self."[84] The radical metamorphosis that results from destructive plasticity is the *real* form of being; it is "well and truly the fabrication of a new person, a novel form of life, without anything in common with a preceding form."[85] Malabou's recent work on destructive plasticity suggests that aesthetic models of the interstitial gap between temporal modes, philosophical traditions, and psychoanalytic drives of life and death are thus insufficient to escape the ideological deformations and power over the subject, the closure against which plasticity is levered. This is significant for the therapeutic potentials of psychoanalysis. "To be flexible is to receive a form or impression, to be able to fold oneself, to take the fold, not to give it. To be docile, to not explode. Indeed, what flexibility lacks is the resource of giving form, the power to create, to invent or even to erase an impression, the power to style. Flexibility is plasticity minus its genius."[86]

Malabou's rereading of psychoanalysis links this materialist notion of form's spontaneous transformation—its genius—to reconceptualizing Freud's death drive. If the death drive is understood in aesthetic terms by Freud, Malabou's substitution of cerebrality for the sexuality in which the Freudian psychoanalytic subject is conceived is designed to account for a radical otherness; it "allows for the possibility of a disastrous event that plays no role in an affective conflict supposed to precede it."[87] This is not, she argues, a head-on attack on Freud but rather a rethinking of the psychic event. For Freud, the psychic event is always tied to love; the death drive remains formless and thus devoid of plasticity, represented, at best, by sadomasochism, another form of love.[88] The promise of cerebrality, of thinking the subject from the perspective of trauma beyond the pleasure principle, is to place the subject "beyond the will to know."[89] The traumatic vacancy of the brain-damaged subject with no reference to her past is indistinguishable from the trauma of natural catastrophe, sensory deprivation, or torture in the modern penal institution. The new wounded, as she calls these sufferers, signal a new age of violence that has superseded the reparative possibilities of psychoanalysis.

Catherine Kellogg's chapter argues against too quickly closing the case file on Freud's and, subsequently, Lacan's and Žižek's materiality of the subject. For Lacan, she argues, who overtook Freud's reticence to fully theorize the pleasure in death, this "fold" beyond the pleasure principle is not death but jouissance, the surplus of pleasure beyond pleasure. Jouissance threatens the loss of the symbolic, potentially collapsing the distance between the "real" and its symbolization. The resultant anxiety is, in this perspective, less fear of the loss of an object than dread over the failure of the order of symbolization in which the subject is constituted. "The conflict in anxiety is not a matter of conscious or unconscious thought, but rather a matter of the *discontinuity between the real of the organism and the imaginary unity of the body*." In this manner, Kellogg argues, the Lacanian subject has already survived a death, making Lacan's subject Malabou's object but without a conceptual detour through neuroscience.

If Malabou emphasizes the destructive possibility of the loss of subjecthood, what might we lose, asks Kellogg, were we to ignore the loss already encountered within psychoanalysis? The answer to this profound question seems to hinge on what ontological meaning can be derived from the kinds of loss that Malabou emphasizes as the central questions for subjectivity today and on how well the psychoanalytic story serves its plastic promise of repair. Malabou writes, "Destructive plasticity deploys its work starting from the exhaustion of possibilities, when all virtuality has left long ago, when the child in the adult is erased, when cohesion is destroyed, family spirit vanished, friendship lost, links dissipated in the ever more intense cold of a barren life. . . . The history of being itself consists perhaps of nothing but a series of accidents which, in every era and without hope of return, dangerously disfigure the meaning of essence."[90] An accidental essence stripped of the child within: how do we tell these stories of ourselves, psychoanalytic or not?

BEYOND LAW AND SOVEREIGNTY

While Malabou's work remains for the most part firmly registered in the discipline of philosophy, explicitly political concerns about recognition, sexual equality, sovereign power, and neoliberal forms of capitalism run throughout her ouevre.[91] As a philosopher of transformation, she continually thinks against ontological, epistemological, and material closures that she confronts in her deconstruction of the thought of Hegel, Heidegger, Derrida, and Freud and, more recently, in her work on Foucault and Agamben. Many of these political concerns are shared by scholars engaged in the field of critical legal theory. Here, we ask what intellectual resources and directions might the thought of plasticity offer contemporary theories of law, justice and politics.

Influenced by Marxist theory, early Anglo–American critical legal scholars sought to denaturalize and expose the relationship between law and politics in liberal societies. Examining the ways in which law structures capitalist relations of exploitation and ownership, critical legal scholarship cast its attention to the role played by law in maintaining capitalist hegemony.[92] With growing attention to the work of Foucault and Derrida, critical legal theory shed its preoccupations with Marxist theory in order to consider the way in which law is constituted through diverse and multiple forms of power (political, economic, and social), as well as law's politically productive limits. Understanding law as text in a deconstructive sense brought with it rich analyses of the minor jurisprudences embedded within law, as well as legal studies of literature, visuality, travel writings, and other genres.[93]

The other recent major innovation in critical legal theory stemmed from identifying the co-constitutive relationship between the emergence of modern law and colonialism.[94] This field of inquiry has focused on the politics of law in colonial settler societies and their contemporary formations, including the nature of sovereign power in colonial and imperial contexts.[95] In the United States, critical race theory emerged in the 1980s to explore the racial dimension of legal forms and introduced groundbreaking shifts in legal pedagogy and forms of writing that reflect marginalized histories and experiences normally invisibilized within law's purview.[96] This brief overview would be incomplete, of course, without mention of feminist legal theory and the more emergent field of queer legal theory, which place gender and sexuality at the forefront of a very diverse range of work that extends from legal reform and policy analysis to philosophical critiques of the hetero-phallogocentrism of the law.[97]

Despite the vast differences among these fields of inquiry, the preoccupation with justice—as political objective, ethical matter, aesthetic concern, philosophical concept, or a combination thereof—persists across the domain of critical legal theory. This attention to justice appears in many guises; one manifestation of it appears as a consideration of that which is inescapable when one enters the juridical frame.[98] It is a consideration that cuts across philosophical, political and legal terrains and goes to the fundamental question of who and what are cognizable as legal subjects. This is the question of recognition.

This is one concern that Bhandar and Goldberg-Hiller, in their chapter in this volume, consider in light of colonial encounters. Where law has been deployed as both the agent of civilization (particularly in its reformation of "unruly" sexualities, as well as its codification of individual property rights) and as the mode through which indigenous peoples are encouraged to press for political relief (sometimes embraced as "reconciliation"), the problem of recognition is made stark. Is the form of recognition that stems from the conquest of land and power capable of achieving justice in light of continuing settler power?

While Malabou identifies recognition explicitly as a political concern in *What Should We Do with Our Brain?*, her rethinking of the Hegelian dialectic exposes the plasticity inherent in the temporal dimensions of his philosophy and offers a space for rethinking the limits of legal-political recognition. In *The Future of Hegel: Plasticity, Temporality and Dialectic*, Malabou uncovers the plasticity in Hegel's dialectical logic that breaks with the reception of Hegel's thought as effecting ontological closure. She does this, as previously mentioned, by contesting the idea that there is a mechanical inevitability to this formulation of the dialectical logic and the emergence of the subject who arrives at the end point of a long struggle for recognition. Her argument for a "future" time that exists within Hegelian thought rethinks the subject "as a structure of anticipation, and, by the same token, a structure of temporalization."[99] In other words, the Hegelian subject is in some sense structured by its capacity to temporalize itself. Bhandar and Goldberg-Hiller suggest that this temporalization may not be sufficiently plastic for indigenous justice, particularly because settler colonial states exploit this temporal divergence, limiting the demands that indigenous peoples can legally make for future consideration to concerns of an imagined past. While such a past is creatively incorporated into many aspects of contemporary indigenous identities and practices, the law has, in numerous ways, precluded political demands on the legal impossibility of this ontology.

Malabou has also explored the corporeal aspects of Hegelian recognition in a piece, jointly written with Judith Butler, entitled *Sois mon corps*, or "You Be My Body for Me: Body, Shape, and Plasticity in Hegel's *Phenomenology of Spirit*."[100] In this dialogue, Butler and Malabou locate the body smuggled into Hegel's argument about self-consciousness. Dispossessed of itself, the imperative to "be my body for me" is both a plea and command issued by the subject, who refuses the violent ontoepistemic closure of recognition through the simple fact of *being*. Bhandar and Goldberg-Hiller conclude that indigenous ontologies that figure the body in ways distinctive from Western assumptions may be useful sites to consider this plastic potential.

Malabou's recent work applies these ontological questions of justice to the critique of sovereignty and its relationship to political and biological life. In chapter 1 in this volume, "Will Sovereignty Ever Be Deconstructed?," Malabou interrogates Foucault's assertion that we must develop a political philosophy "that isn't erected around the problem of sovereignty." Malabou begins with the assertion that despite the critical interventions of Foucault, Agamben, and Derrida, this has not yet happened. In other words, the king's head has yet to be finally severed.

Malabou argues that Foucault's notion of the biopolitical—that dispositif remaining after the removal of sovereign power—operates as a critique of sovereign power in that it both challenges the latter's very structure and also hides behind the traditional ideological mask of sovereignty.[101] Biopower, by "inaugurating the reign of the norm," ultimately retreats behind the "old figure of the law." Thus, she sets as her task to deconstruct this deconstructive tool, the biopolitical, "to unveil it and resist its ideological tendency."

The reinstantiation of the partition between the biological and the symbolic occurs with its exposure to a logic of sacrifice. Malabou argues that whether one considers Agamben's notion of bare life, Foucault's concern for biological materials, such as blood, that become abstracted into symbolic value, or the place of the empty signifier in the structural anthropology of Lévi-Strauss, there remains a body who, structurally, is exposed to death through sacrifice. This sacrificial impulse urgently needs to be challenged, Malabou claims, and she seeks to identify resources for political resistance to this logic of the exposure to death in the biological body. Malabou observes that many juridical and political formations, such as the nation, rely on this kinship between the symbolic and the biological. Consider, for instance, the nationalist politics of "blood and belonging" that fuse an ethnoracialist discourse of biological unity with the transcendent and abstract concept of the nation.[102]

Malabou's provocative engagement with Foucault, Agamben, and Derrida opens up several avenues of inquiry about the juridical, sovereign forms of power and political resistance. One question is about the place of law in her theorization of biological resistance to sovereign forms of power. If what are at stake in this engagement with Foucault's theory of the biopolitical are popular sovereignty and democracy, the question arises as to what form law and juridical power might take if the partition between the symbolic and the biological were to be truly deconstructed. Might this open a space for a form of immanent critique of the law and sovereign juridical power?

Peering into this space, the notion of destructive plasticity presents us with a queer notion of law, one governed more by its own self-displacement than sovereign self-mastery. Thinking in the idiom of identity, destruction (in the sense of destructive plasticity) properly belongs to the species of accident:

> Destruction remains an accident while really, to make a pun that suggests that the accident is a property of the species, destruction should be seen as a species of accident, so that the ability to transform oneself under the effect of destruction is a possibility, an existential structure. This structural status of the identity of the accident

does not, however, reduce the chance of it happening, does not annul the contingency of its occurrence, which remains absolutely unpredictable in all instances. This is why recognizing the ontology of the accident is a philosophically difficult task: it must be acknowledged as a law that is simultaneously logical and biological, but a law that does not allow us to anticipate its instances. Here is a law that is surprised by its own instances. In principle, destruction does not respond to its own necessity, and when it occurs, does not comfort its own possibility. Strictly speaking, destruction does not come to pass.[103]

This radical contingency that is imported into the "law" of a destructive plasticity opens space for thinking of conceptual structures that tug the biological reality of being from under the symbolic realm governed by the thought of sovereignty.

Alain Pottage's chapter, "Autoplasticity," challenges Malabou's contention that the symbolic and the biological are necessarily preserved in the work of Foucault, implying that sovereignty may have to find another avenue of deconstruction. The emergence of epigenetics, on which much of Malabou's scientific and philosophical reflections rely, Pottage argues, demonstrates a communicative process that is itself plastic. Pottage relies upon Niklas Luhmann's "systems" theory of autopoiesis, which was developed from biological studies of organism and environment[104] in order to cast skepticism on the possibility or need for direct access to the biological itself.

Epigenetics, thought poietically and biologically, raises questions about the nature of the relative environment. As a metabolic process, its contexts include both the cellular tissue and the organismic system. This reveals, as Pottage shows, that environments are correlative to an organism and, simultaneously, functional and mobile. Understood philosophically, poiesis demonstrates that there is no such thing as an objective environment for living systems or for social systems. Luhmann argued that this was true for all systems of communication, with the consequence of radically deontologizing all objects. As Pottage demonstrates, this radical position is true of Foucault's work on "ethopoiesis" as well.

Ethopoiesis, one of the "techniques of the self," is a means of discriminating knowledge that would enhance the right character of a self from that which would not, unfolding the character of the self from the horizon, or environment, of the world. Techniques such as meditation and memorization were Stoical versions of ethopoiesis, and writing made the self absorb these techniques into the constitution of the self. Foucault's self, Pottage claims, is not ontic but poietic: the self consists in making.

The consequence is subversive. Malabou's critique of Foucault in chapter 1 accounts for ethopoiesis, but she claims that in the final accounting, Foucault remains committed to a division between the symbolic and the biological body, making power always a less vital issue than the body. Yet from Luhmann's autopoietic perspective, one that would ultimately "environmentalize" biology, biopower is rendered evanescent. "If life, nature, or biology are no longer ontic or universal realms, but dimensions whose sense and configuration are dependent on the fashioning of the self that is correlative to the environment, then there is no such thing as 'life itself,'" Pottage writes.

Pottage's argument is addressed to Malabou's arguments about sovereignty and biopolitics, but it has interesting implications for Malabou's own practices of self-reflection and autobiography, as well as for the question of what may emerge beyond an age of plasticity. Malabou has argued that plasticity is itself plastic, susceptible to its own destruction, a consequence of our own communicative potentials and our attention to other ways of organizing our environments.

The question of whether these environments are always human are raised by Renisa Mawani in "Insects, War, Plastic Life." Malabou's efforts to deconstruct the divide between biology and history is an opportunity, Mawani claims, to think the human/nonhuman divide that has passed without question among many critics of biopolitics. Insects constitute an interesting subject for plasticity, Mawani shows: they are metamorphic and often complexly social creatures, designated as both expendable and killable by humans yet conscriptable into human military functions. Insects are also a trope for humans who themselves are seen as expendable, particularly in colonial contexts. What might we gain from exploding the species differentiation that persists in biopolitical conceptions of life and death?

Mawani's chapter asks us to think of the contemporary global closure, which Malabou sees as the condition of the age of plasticity, as also a moment "produced through uneven circuits and circulations of power. Thus, the 'ontological combustion' of plasticity harbors the potential to explode its own possibility, reinforcing existing geopolitical divides while also producing new ones that ultimately constrain and even eliminate itineraries for emancipatory politics."[105] These geopolitical divides are, in the end, colonial, and their environments are increasingly diffuse and manipulated by nonhuman agents. Insects, as Mawani shows, may be trained to sniff chemicals, detect explosives, and observe enemies in the "war on terror." They have become a dispositif incorporated into other discourses and technologies of global security. Plasticity that runs through all forms of life emerges, then, as deeply ambivalent: both liberatory and subjectifying. Extending Bergson's notion of vitalism beyond the human, Mawani identifies this plasticity as political vitality. In the context of contemporary geopolitics, this implies that plasticity may also be generative of dystopic worlds "always already situated within uneven distributions of life and death."

Jairus Grove's chapter exposes the dystopic fears of neuroscience; he both historicizes Malabou's work on neuronal plasticity and draws out some of the political risks of destructive plasticity. Grove explores the double fold inherent in Malabou's "adventurous" neuronal materialism, which is the epistemological and philosophical challenge posed by Malabou's assertion that we are constituted as and by our brains. Grove explores how this double fold raises troubling questions for settled philosophical separations of the brain as mere noumena from the human capacity for thought. The notion that the brain is not under the absolute command of the faculties of the individual human actor challenges Kantian, neo–Arendtian, and other humanist traditions that "see the recourse to the brain as the death of man." Grove, dispensing with these enfeebled humanists and their attachment to a human (and humanity) who never existed anyway, attempts to push Malabou's concept of destructive plasticity to new limits.

By situating Malabou's work on neuronal plasticity alongside the work of cyberneticists and other writers, Grove explores how neuronal plasticity is at the heart of scientific and literary experimentation involving the brain and human systems. Taking up mid-twentieth-century concerns with control, security and the capacity for understanding and transforming the cognitive behavior of individuals and populations, Grove engages the political context and concerns of a generation of scientists. Ultimately, he argues that Malabou's concept of destructive plasticity invites us to confront the "horrors" of political plasticity and that lesions, decay, dementia, Alzheimer's, and shock therapy reflect life's indifference to radical change that leaves no trace of what preceded it. He argues that "decay and catastrophe" are sovereign, not the human subject. Any attempt to think of life's relation to the political, then, must necessarily acknowledge a mode of change that *forgets* the loss of form and its symbolic points of reference and thus appears to us an entirely un- if not posthuman mode of alienation.

In *Changing Difference*, Malabou also searches for a posthuman alterity, looking beyond ontology, even where ontological difference is pluralized, as it is by Derrida and Levinas.[106] Alterity is incalculable, she argues, but locatable in the "flesh of difference."[107] The notion of flesh exceeds an ontological register plagued by myths of origin and originary exclusions; it falls outside the two domains of the biopolitical: the technological manipulation of things and signs (linguistics and science) and Foucauldian technologies of domination and the self. These two spheres are identified by Fred Moten, in chapter 12, as ones that the field of black studies takes responsibility "for forging an understanding between." Moten renders a critique that obliquely touches that of Malabou, although he points to something she omits: spaces not of opening but of collapse amid spheres otherwise bifurcated. Moten writes that the double edge of the constitution of techniques of self-care, of self-concern, exhibit a "kind of anoriginal potential that is often constrained to submit to what it generates, to what represents or gives accounts—where giving an account is a taking stock of oneself that is inseparable from a taking stock of one's things."

Moten's chapter questions the political adequacy of a plasticity conceived within the gap between brain and society without recognition of the ways in which the deconstruction of a centralized executive in the brain is reconstructed in the privileged position of neural matter. Doesn't the emphasis on the brain, he asks, reinscribe the executive? "Isn't the deconstruction of biopolitical deconstruction still a sovereign operation? Isn't the brain . . . where the sovereign now resides?" Moten's concern is not only for the political models of sovereignty condensed in the model of brain function but also for the genealogy of brain science that has always imagined a particular (white, male, European) privilege of rationality. However much it shares the significance of affect to interrogate the symmetry of brain and self, Moten's argument rubs against the inventive freedom of Shapiro's post–Kantian aesthetic subject as it aims for an alternative biological reference to neuroplasticity. For him, the flesh that exceeds the brain and the self must become the locus of any biological imagination of resistance to the biopolitical and its symbolic structures. This is a subjectivity designed for those historically denied the symbolism of the brain.

In the chapters that follow, Malabou's interlocutors are sandwiched between three original chapters by Catherine Malabou and an interview in which she reengages some of the themes and considers criticisms brought out by the writers of the chapters within. Malabou has written of her own philosophical reading that she seeks to find "a childhood to come in the text.... Childhood is an age that does not belong to either metaphysics or to its superseding and that, just like 'metamorphosis,' is both before and after history, mythic and ultrahistorical at the same time."[108] The reader is invited to take this same spirit of a plastic reading that the authors published here have applied to Malabou's own texts.

INTRODUCTION TO MALABOU CHAPTERS

Chapters 1 through 3 are written by Catherine Malabou; originally prepared as lectures, they offer multiple perspectives on the relationship of plasticity to politics and law. In "Will Sovereignty Ever Be Deconstructed?," Malabou asks whether the critique of sovereignty begun by Foucault, Agamben, and Derrida might unwittingly have resuscitated sovereignty instead. Her argument focuses on the symbolic potential of biology, which theories of biopolitics have relegated to a political veil for sovereign power. What would happen, Malabou inquires, if we read the biological not just as a concealment for the normative basis of biopower but as its own plastic symbolic system? Might we then, finally, be in a position to orient our political theories beyond any vestiges of sovereignty?

In her chapter, "Whither Materialism? Althusser/Darwin," Malabou asks us to consider another materialism, one that is contingent or aleatory and glimpsed in the philosophy of Althusser and the biology of Darwin, as grounds for a new politics. Rather than the conservative force of social Darwinism and sociobiology, two uses of the biological that see the function of social selection as the reproduction of order, Malabou urges us to embrace a new balance between variation and selection that a plastic reading of this new materialism can provide.

Chapter 3, "From the Overman to the Posthuman: How Many Ends?," raises important questions for legal and political theory. If our own universal conception of the human subsumes and erases particular differences, might our critical engagements with the category of the human merely reproduce the concept in its essential form? Might this repetition of the human—seen in such issues as human rights, which have been extended to encompass women's rights and gay rights, among others originally excluded from the category—be its essence, Malabou asks? And if so, might law and our ideas of justice be little more than symbols of this repetition? If one promise of plasticity is repair, how should we now reorient ourselves and our legal notions to prevent repeating violence in the name of the human?

NOTES

1. Malabou writes about this structuralism, "By 'structure of philosophy,' I mean the form of philosophy after its destruction and deconstruction. This means that structure is not a starting point here but rather an outcome. Structure is the order and organization of philosophy once the concepts of order and organization have themselves been deconstructed. In other words, the structure of philosophy is metamorphosized metaphysics." Malabou, *Plasticity at the Dusk*, 51; italics in the original. See also Martinon, *On Futurity*.

2. Malabou, *Plasticity at the Dusk*, 49.

3. Marx, "Concerning Feuerbach," 423 (Thesis XI).

4. See Weizman, *Hollow Land*; Sassen, *De-facto Transnationalizing*; Ong, *Neoliberalism as Exception*.

5. Jameson, *Marxism and Form*, 4.

6. Pashukanis, *Law and Marxism*; Balbus, "Commodity Form," 571.

7. White, *Content of the Form*.

8. Fanon, *Black Skin, White Masks*; Wolfe, *Settler Colonialism*.

9. White, "Revolt against Formalism," 131–52; Purcell, *Crisis of Democratic Theory*.

10. Derrida, "Form and Meaning," 155–73.

11. Deleuze, *Difference and Repetition*.

12. Kant, *Critique of Judgement*; Gasché, *Idea of Form*; Rancière, *Disagreement*; Panagia, *Political Life of Sensation*.

13. See Malabou, *Ontology of the Accident*, 1.

14. Bynum, *Metamorphosis and Identity*, 30. See also Paul Ricoeur's compatible arguments about the necessity of narrative to the comprehension of time. Ricoeur, *Time and Narrative*.

15. Malabou understands this process of becoming fantastically visible to reveal what she has called *ontological transformability*. Malabou, *Heidegger Change*, 269. As one of her translators, Peter Skafish, has observed, her language reaches to but not within the aesthetic. She uses "a poetic style rich

enough to evoke a vivid picture of transformation but unobtrusive enough to not make the image seem like an artifact of language." Malabou, *Heidegger Change*, xiv.

16. See chapter 8.

17. Malabou, *Heidegger Change*, 11.

18. Malabou, *Heidegger Change*, 16.

19. "The commodity form, is nothing but the definite social relation between men themselves which assumes here, for them, the fantastic form of a relation between things." *Marx, Capital*, 165. Marx liberally uses the term metamorphosis when discussing the commodity.

20. The visibility of ontological transformation in this form of form "does not allow for the . . . supersession [of metaphysics], and modern technology simply closes the loop of a generalized equivalence where everything is of equal value . . . and everything possible—every manipulation, bargain, direction, and ideological advance." Malabou, *Heidegger Change*, 272.

21. Malabou, *Heidegger Change*, 193.

22. Malabou, *Plasticity at the Dusk*, 50.

23. Malabou, *Heidegger Change*, 279.

24. Malabou, *Future of Hegel*, 6.

25. Malabou, *Future of Hegel*, 19, 192.

26. Malabou, *Future of Hegel*, 17.

27. Malabou, *Future of Hegel*, 20.

28. Malabou, *Heidegger Change*, 9.

29. Derrida, "Preface," xxxi.

30. Malabou writes, "The world thus bears the mourning of that which has not arrived, the worse trace or what is unaccomplished in the actual event. But as the non-event has precisely never taken place, and is by definition not historical, its mourning cannot exist in the order of idealization. The mourning of the possible, in the double sense of the genitive, can only be the conservation of the possible itself which does not reify it in an image or a phantasm. Thus conserved, the possible remains forever possible, and to this extent the not having happened is also the resource for that which can arrive, the resource of all faith in the future, of all confidence in another becoming of the world." Malabou, "History and the Process of Mourning," 20.

31. Malabou, "Following Generation," 19–33.

32. Malabou writes, "Cette plasticité implique donc la possibilité d'un retour en arrière, d'un effacement de la marque, de la différence, de la spécialisation, effacement dont il faut, paradoxalement, retrouver la piste. Il s'agit de retrouver la trace du processus même d'effacement de la trace." ["This plasticity implies the possibility of turning back, the deletion of the mark of difference, of specialization, a deletion that requires, paradoxically, the need to rediscover

the path. It is a question of recovering the trace of the same process of erasing the trace."] Malabou, "Les Régénérés," 537.

33. Malabou, *Ontology of the Accident*, 1.
34. Malabou, *Ontology of the Accident*, 18.
35. Malabou, *Ontology of the Accident*, 18.
36. Malabou, *Ontology of the Accident*, 24.
37. Deleuze writes, "Events are ideal. Novalis sometimes says that there are two courses of events, one of them ideal, the other real and imperfect—for example, ideal Protestantism and real Lutheranism. The distinction however is not between two sorts of events; rather, it is between the event, which is ideal by nature, and its spatio-temporal realization in a state of affairs. The distinction is between *event* and *accident* . . . [an effort to] thwart all dogmatic confusion between event and essence, and also every empiricist confusion between event and accident." Deleuze, *Logic of Sense*, 53–54.
38. Malabou, *Ontology of the Accident*, 17.
39. Malabou, *Ontology of the Accident*, 30.
40. Malabou, *The Future of Hegel*, 192.
41. Malabou, *Changing Difference*; Malabou, *Plasticity at the Dusk*.
42. Coole and Frost, *New Materialisms*; Bennett, *Vibrant Matter*; Thacker, *After Life*.
43. See Deleuze, *Nietzsche and Philosophy*; Deleuze, *Difference and Repetition*. But see also the rejoinders in Malabou, "Who's Afraid?," 114–38; Malabou, "Eternal Return," 21–29.
44. Nancy, "Introduction," 1–8.
45. Malabou, *What Should We Do?*, 5.
46. Malabou, *What Should We Do?*, 54.
47. Malabou, *What Should We Do?*, 6.
48. Malabou, "Préface," 23.
49. Malabou, "Préface," 20, 22.
50. Malabou, "Préface," 26, 27.
51. Malabou, *What Should We Do?*, 31.
52. Malabou, *What Should We Do?*, 81.
53. Gould, *Mismeasure of Man*.
54. Glimcher, *Foundations*; see also the critique of Fine, "Development as Zombieconomics," 885–904; Fine and Milonakis, *Economic Imperialism*.
55. Jameson writes, "Nonetheless, it is not terribly difficult to say what is meant by the Real in Lacan. It is simply History itself: and if for psychoanalysis the history in question here is obviously enough the history of the subject, the resonance of the word suggests that a confrontation between this particular materialism and the historical materialism of Marx can no longer be postponed." Jameson, "Imaginary and Symbolic," 384.

56. Marx originally wrote, in German, "Die Menschen machen ihre eigene Geschichte, aber sie machen sie nicht aus freien Stücken, nicht unter selbstgewählten, sondern unter unmittelbar vorgefundenen, gegebenen und überlieferten Umständen." The usual translation in French is "Les hommes font leur propre histoire, mais ils ne la font pas arbitrairement, dans les conditions choisies par eux, mais dans des conditions directement données et héritées du passé." Malabou's rendition in French is "Les hommes font leur propre histoire mais ne savent pas qui'ils la font." Here, she substitutes *savoir*, "to know," for *faire*, "to make." Malabou's language is drawn from phrasing popularized by Raymond Aron: "les hommes font leur histoire, mais ils ne savent pas l'histoire qu'ils font" (Aron, *Introduction*, 168; see also Mahoney, *Liberal Political Science*, 131).

57. Marx, *Eighteenth Brumaire*, 10.

58. Marx, *Eighteenth Brumaire*, 10.

59. Malabou, *What Should We Do?*, 24.

60. Malabou, *What Should We Do?*, 24.

61. Malabou, *What Should We Do?*, 81.

62. Malabou, *What Should We Do?*, 82.

63. Pitts-Taylor, "Plastic Brain," 635–652; see also Rajan, *Biocapital*; Waldby, *Visible Human Project*.

64. Galloway, "Poverty of Philosophy," 364.

65. Galloway, "Poverty of Philosophy," 366.

66. Rand, "Organism," 353.

67. Marx and Engels write in *The German Ideology*, "The most recent of [the Young Hegelians] have found the correct expression for their activity when they declare they are only fighting against 'phrases.' They forget, however, that they themselves are opposing nothing but phrases to these phrases, and that they are in no way combating the real existing world when they are combating solely the phrases of this world." Marx and Engels, *Karl Marx, Frederick Engels*, 30.

68. On embodiment and plasticity, see Papadopoulos, "Imaginary of Plasticity," 432–56. See also Watson, "Neurobiology of Sorcery," 23–45.

69. Evans, *Sexual Citizenship*; Hennessy, *Profit and Pleasure*.

70. Warner, *Trouble with Normal*.

71. Halberstam, "What's That Smell?," 313–33.

72. Franke, "Domesticated Liberty," 1399–426.

73. Butler, *Gender Trouble*.

74. Malabou, *Changing Difference*, 1.

75. Malabou, *Changing Difference*, 104.

76. Malabou, *Changing Difference*, 137, 138.

77. Malabou, *Plasticity at the Dusk*, 81.

78. Derrida and Reader, "Paper or Myself."

79. Malabou, *Plasticity at the Dusk*, 49; italics in original.

80. Felman, "Beyond Oedipus," 1021–53.

81. Malabou, "Plasticity and Elasticity," 85.

82. The idea of a fold within discourse is attributed to Jean-Francois Lyotard, *Discourse, Figure*. Malabou addresses this concept in *Plasticity at the Dusk*, 56; "Eye at the Edge," 16–25.

83. Malabou, *Ontology of the Accident*, 39–54.

84. Malabou, *Ontology of the Accident*, 11.

85. Malabou, *Ontology of the Accident*, 18.

86. Malabou, *What Should We Do with Our Brain?*, 39.

87. Malabou, *New Wounded*, 189–202.

88. Malabou, *New Wounded*, 205.

89. Malabou, *New Wounded*.

90. Malabou, *Ontology of the Accident*, 89–91.

91. See esp. Emmanuelli and Malabou, *La Grande Exclusion*.

92. Fine et al., *Capitalism and the Rule of Law*; Thompson, *Whigs and Hunters*; Feinman and Gabel, "Contract Law as Ideology," 373.

93. Goodrich, *Law in the Courts of Love*; Haldar, *Law, Orientalism*; Dore, "Law's Literature," 17–28.

94. Fitzpatrick's *Mythology of Modern Law* was a seminal text, if not *the* seminal text, in the field of postcolonial legal theory.

95. Fitzpatrick, *Mythology of Modern Law*; Darian-Smith and Fitzpatrick, *Laws of the Postcolonial*; Anghie, *Imperialism*; Borrows, "Frozen Rights," 37–64.

96. Lawrence, "The Id," 317; Matsuda, *Where Is Your Body?*; Crenshaw, "Demarginalizing," 139.

97. Davies, "Queer Property," 327–52; Cooper, *Sexing the City*; Herman, *Antigay Agenda*.

98. Butler, *Undoing Gender*.

99. Malabou, *Future of Hegel*, 130.

100. Butler and Malabou, *Sois mon corps*; Malabou and Butler, "You Be My Body."

101. Malabou, ch. 1, 36.

102. Balibar and Wallerstein, *Race, Nation, Class*; Butler and Spivak, *Who Sings the Nation-State?*

103. Malabou, *Ontology of the Accident*, 18.

104. Luhmann, *Social Systems*.

105. Mawani, ch. 8, 161.

106. Malabou, *Changing Difference*, 36.

107. Malabou, *Changing Difference*, 36.

108. Malabou, *Plasticity at the Dusk*, 54.

CHAPTER 1

Will Sovereignty Ever Be Deconstructed?

Catherine Malabou

In "Truth and Power," an interview from 1977, Michel Foucault declares: "What we need . . . is a political philosophy that isn't erected around the problem of sovereignty, nor therefore around the problems of law and prohibition. We need to cut off the King's head: in political theory that has still to be done."[1]

Why does Foucault affirm this persistence of kingship in contemporary political theory? Hasn't the passage from royal to democratic or popular sovereignty already been accomplished for a long time in the West? According to Foucault, this passage hasn't changed the very structure of sovereignty, which is always attached—whatever the polity it characterizes—to monarchy—that is, with a system of power having a single center and in which the law is the only expression of authority. This model is, according to Foucault, that of Hobbes's *Leviathan*. To cut off the king's head means that we "abandon the model of Leviathan, that model of artificial man who is at once an automaton, a fabricated man, but also a unitary man who contains all real individuals, whose body is made up of citizens but whose soul is sovereignty. We have to study power outside the model of Leviathan, outside the field delineated by juridical sovereignty and the institution of the State."[2]

Western democracies are, according to Foucault, still dependent upon this model because of their juridical structure. They are, then, secretly inhabited by the remnant figure of the sovereign; that is, of the king.

It thus seems that no form of sovereignty can exist independently of the figure of the sovereign. No sovereignty without the sovereign. No sovereignty without a king. This explains why the very notion of sovereignty has to be criticized or, as Derrida declares in his seminar *The Beast and the Sovereign*,[3] why it has to be deconstructed.

Is such a deconstruction on its way? Does it have any chance to attain its goal? To be accomplished? Have we, after Foucault, after Derrida—and I add, after Agamben—cut off the king's head? My answer, here, is no.

How can I justify such a position? In order to develop my argument, I first turn toward the concept of biopolitics, forged by Foucault and re-elaborated by Agamben and Derrida in two different ways. According to Foucault, sovereignty, as both a structure of power and a polity, has disappeared from the West with the emergence of modernity. A new form of organization, which has nothing to do with sovereignty, substitutes for it. At the turn of the seventeenth century, the pyramidal model of the Leviathan, described in political philosophy, appears as what it is in reality: the ideological mask that hides a disappearance or a void—precisely, the void of sovereignty. Foucault declares that from that time through the eighteenth century, a new form of power emerges that is "absolutely incompatible with relations of sovereignty"[4] and is occulted by the persistent ideological affirmation of sovereignty. This new form of power is constituted by the paradoxical dissemination of power, the existence of multiple networks, sites of control, the supremacy of the norm over the law, of discipline and technologies of conditioning over repression. "One must keep in view the fact that, along with all the fundamental technical inventions and discoveries of the seventeenth and eighteenth centuries, a new technology of the exercise of power also emerged which was probably even more important than the constitutional reforms and new forms of government established at the end of the eighteenth century."[5]

This new exercise of power is by no means reducible to the structure of sovereignty: "Power had to be able to gain access to the bodies of individuals, to their acts, attitudes and modes of everyday behaviour. . . . Hence there arise the problems of demography, public health, hygiene, housing conditions, longevity and fertility. And I believe that the political significance of the problem of sex is due to the fact that sex is located at the point of intersection of the discipline of the body and the control of the population."[6] The intersection of the discipline of the body and the control of population is constitutive of what Foucault calls, for the first time in 1974, "biopolitics."

Later, in *History of Sexuality*, volume 1, he writes: "For millennia, man remained what he was for Aristotle: a living animal with the additional capacity for a political existence; modern man is an animal whose politics places his existence as a living being in question."[7] Further, he wrote,

> Western man was gradually learning what it meant to be a living species in a living world, to have a body, conditions of existence, probabilities of life, an individual and collective welfare, forces that could be modified, and a space in which they could be distributed in an optimal manner. For the first time in history, no doubt, biological existence was reflected in political existence; the fact of living was no longer an inaccessible substrate that only emerged from time to time, amid the randomness of death and its fatality; part of it passed into knowledge's field of control and power's sphere of intervention.[8]

Biopolitics plays a double role. Because it inaugurates a new form of political authority made of micropowers that produce a "subjugation of bodies and control of populations,"[9] biopolitics is already, in itself, a deconstructive tool of sovereignty. It challenges its structure. At the same time, biopolitics covers its own deconstructive power to the extent that it hides itself behind the traditional ideological mask of sovereignty. If the emergence of biopower inaugurates the reign of the norm, it conceals the operation of normalization itself behind the old figure of the law. A normalizing society is the historical outcome of a technology of power centered on life. "We have entered a phase of juridical regression in comparison with the pre-seventeenth-century societies we are acquainted with; we should not be deceived by all the Constitutions framed throughout the world since the French Revolution, the Codes written and revised, a whole continual and clamorous legislative activity: these were the forms that made an essentially normalizing power acceptable."[10] The "right" to life becomes the biopolitical mask that dissimulates the normalization of life.

What, then, does the philosopher's task consist in? The philosopher has to deconstruct biopolitical deconstruction, that is, to unveil it and resist its ideological tendency. Such a task requires that we situate the point where biology and history, the living subject and the political subject, meet or touch.

The issue I am raising here appears precisely at that intersection. It concerns the philosophical discourse, more precisely, the structure of the philosophical critique of biopolitics. How do contemporary philosophers characterize the convergence of biology and history?

As Foucault affirms in several texts, the emergence of biopolitics is inseparable from the emergence of biology as a science. It is only at the turn of the seventeenth century, when biology is constituted as a science replacing natural history, that biopolitics becomes possible. The political subject becomes henceforth the living subject, the individual as it is determined by biology.

The problem is the following: for Foucault, as for Agamben or Derrida, even in different ways, biology is always presented as intimately linked with sovereignty in its traditional figure. Biology is always depicted as a science that transgresses its limits to repress, domesticate, instrumentalize life; that is, as a power of normalization, but a power that precisely occults its essential relationship to the norm and appears as what inscribes law within organisms. Function, program, teleology, organism: these are some examples of how biology conceptually and practically imprints the figure of law and of the sovereign at the heart of biopolitics, which is also at the heart of life. An organism always has the form of a micro–Leviathan. This explains why a thinker like Deleuze says that we have to think of bodies outside organisms. Biology plays the part of the sovereign, Derrida says, of the king.[11] This also explains why biology always appears, for philosophers, as an instrument of power, never as an emancipatory field or tool.

There can't be any *bio*logical resistance to *bio*power.

This means that biology—the biological determination of life—has to be transgressed. As if there were always two concepts of life in life. For the philosophers I am talking about here, there exists a nonbiological definition of life that transgresses or exceeds the scientific, objective one. This surplus of life is symbolic life. Symbolic life as opposed to biological life. This symbolic life appears as the resource or the potentiality of resistance.

This double-sided concept of life is easily noticeable in Foucault's discourse on the body, in Agamben's analyses of bare life, and in Derrida's elaboration of the notion of the animal.

In the *History of Sexuality*, Foucault declares: "Hence I do not envisage a 'history of mentalities' that would take account of bodies only through the matter in which they have been perceived and given meaning and value; but a 'history of bodies' and the manner in which the most material and most vital in them has been invested."[12] If biology invests what is the "most material" and the "most vital" in bodies, it means that there is a less material and less vital dimension. What can it be outside the symbolic body? The flesh?

In *Homo Sacer*, Agamben writes: "Bare life is no longer confined to a particular place or a definite category. It now dwells in the biological body of every living being."[13] It means that bare life is not reducible to the biological. It is the symbolic part of life that dwells within the biological body. A body within the body.

In the *Beast and the Sovereign*, Derrida characterizes the animal as a poem. The poem is irreducible to an organism. The poetic dimension of the animal is what forever escapes biopower and the instrumentalization of life. This poetic essence constitutes the sacred part of life. In a previous text, "Faith and Knowledge," Derrida had already declared that "life has absolute value only if it is worth more than life." More than the "natural" and the "bio-zoological." "Th[e] dignity of life can only subsist beyond the present living being." Life is "open to something and something more than itself."[14]

A border remains then, in these approaches, between two notions of life, between two lives. Deconstruction or critique of biopolitics maintains the old relationship between the biological and the symbolic, the discrepancy, the separation that exists between them. This is what prevents such a deconstruction or such a critique from superseding the traditional or metaphysical approaches to life. What do I mean by the "old relationship"? I refer here to Ernst Kantorowicz's famous book *The King's Two Bodies: A Study in Mediaeval Political Theology*.[15] The king has two bodies: a natural body and a nonmaterial one.

Let me recall the definition of the two bodies: "For the King has in him two bodies, *viz.*, a Body natural, and a Body politic. His Body natural is a Body mortal, subject to all Infirmities that come by Nature or Accident [. . .]. But his Body politic is a Body that cannot be seen or handled, consisting of Policy and Government [. . .]"[16] Eric Santner, in his beautiful book *The Royal Remains: The People's Two Bodies and the Endgames of Sovereignty*,[17] calls these two bodies the biological one and the symbolic one. It is then striking to notice that the critique or deconstruction of sovereignty is structured as the very entity it tends to critique or deconstruct. By distinguishing two lives and two bodies, contemporary philosophers reaffirm the theory of sovereignty, that is, the split between the symbolic and the biological.

Of course, for Foucault, Derrida, and Agamben "symbolic" does not mean immortal or infinite as opposed to biological (understood as finite and destructible). Yet the partition remains—and it is, in effect, a "royal remain"—between the empirical and the symbolic, between the natural and something that is irreducible to it, whatever its definition. In criticizing sovereignty, philosophy reveals its own sovereignty, that is, the two bodies of its discourse.

It has become urgent to deconstruct this deconstructive discourse, to put an end to the split between the two bodies. It has become of primary importance to stress the political force of resistance inscribed in most recent biological concepts. It is time to affirm that biology can play a part other than that of a royal remain. The time has come to free Continental philosophy from the rigid separation it has always maintained between the biological, hence the material, and the symbolic, that is, the nonmaterial or the transcendental.

Recent biological discoveries reveal the *plasticity of difference:* that is, the plasticity of the genome, of cells, of brain development—all elements that challenge the idea of a strict genetic determinism and allow us to go beyond the classical distinction between body and flesh, between a material, obscure, mechanically determined organism, on the one hand, and a spiritual body or incarnated spirit, on the other. What appeared, until recently, as irreversible or unchangeable—the genetic code, cellular differentiation, the phenotype, in general—is currently described as plastic, that is, mutable and reversible. Until recently, Continental philosophers have articulated the notion of difference. We now have to elaborate a theory of what changing difference may mean. The reversibility of difference, brought to light by current biology, opens a new perspective on the relationship between the symbolic and the biological. Their dialectical interplay is inscribed within the body, not outside of it, putting an end to the logic of the two bodies but consequently also challenging the structure of sovereignty inherent in this philosophical discourse. One of the most important of all current biological concepts, that of epigenetics, is a privileged factor in this total change of orientation.

What I develop here concerning philosophy is valid for any other discourse (political science, anthropology, law, etc.) where a fixed and rigid meaning of the symbolic that undermines the deconstruction of the Leviathan still prevails. The symbolic still colonizes all discourses in human sciences. It is as if we still need to affirm the existence of a beyond or an outside of the real to confer meaning to reality, as if a prior structure, necessarily nonmaterial, was requested to give sense to materiality itself. As if we need the two bodies to kill the king . . .

What does "symbolic" here mean? The contemporary signification of this term, as we know it, which is different from "symbolism," has been brought to light by Lévi-Strauss, mainly in his introduction to the work of Marcel Mauss. The symbolic designates the structural spacing of the different entities that compose a language, a political community, or the ethical values of a society.

According to Lévi-Strauss, such spacing has to do with the existence of what he calls the floating signifier, able "to represent an undetermined quantity of signification, in itself void of meaning and thus apt to receive any meaning." It is "a signifier with a vague, highly variable, unspecifiable or non-existent signified." As such, a "floating signifier" may "mean different things to different people: they may stand for many or even any signifieds; they may mean whatever their interpreters want them to mean." This floating signifier, which maintains the correspondence between signifiers and signifieds, is said to possess a "value zero," a *symbolic* value.[18]

Here, as we see, the symbolic means this empty space that gives language its mobility. It is because our language is full of these little nonsensical words, like "hau," "mana," and all the ones quoted from Lewis Carroll by Deleuze, that it can function. So the symbolic here designates the empty boxes or places or spaces, the value zero which determines the arrangement of any group of significant elements. What Derrida calls the supplement. An excess.

The symbolic, defined as the empty space, has, according to Lévi-Strauss, a double function: the empty space, the "mana," for example, is both the sacred and what is offered to sacrifice. The most preserved and the most exposed, both the sacred and the sacrificeable. Life, in modernity, appears precisely as both sacred and sacrificeable. This explains Agamben's famous book title *Homo Sacer*. "Sacer" designates something that is neither in nor out and both in and out at the same time. This is the status of "bare life": something that is nowhere, neither within nor outside the community. That is, both sacred and offered to murder. As we previously saw, bare life never coincides with biological life. Again: "Bare life inhabits the biological body of each living being." The space that separates bare life from the biological body can only be the space of the symbolic.

For Foucault, power mechanisms tend to obliterate, reduce, or restrict the emptiness of the symbolic, to fill it up with a content, to interrupt its mobility and transform it into an essence or a fixed entity. This is what sovereignty is: the result of a transformation of the floating signifier into a rigid figure, that of the king or of the law or of any central and centralized motif. Biology is thought of as what makes this transformation possible. Biological concepts are for Foucault immediately edible or assimilable by politics: hence, for example, blood and sex, which are constituted as organic-political values that appear as central and centralized entities obliterating the dissemination of both power and bodies.

Biology, again, is the ally of sovereignty. It never serves the cause of the symbolic but always tries to hide it. Of course, this eclipse is not a suppression. Politics itself, as well as sovereignty, is rooted, like every other reality, in the symbolic economy. Resisting sovereignty, then, amounts to reintroducing the excess, to unveiling it and making it ungraspable by power. Such a gesture necessarily implies a transgression of the biological. The resisting bodies, with their economy of pleasures (Foucault insists on the plural).

Deleuze, in "How Do We Recognize Structuralism?,"[19] shows that the symbolic, defined as a prior nonmaterial empty space, occupies a major role in Foucault's thought. Deleuze demonstrates that the empty or floating signifier for Foucault is the notion of subject, or subjectivity, which is not a substance or an essence but appears, on the contrary, as a pure void, a gap, that gets its content from its self-formative gesture. The self and the body that are thus formed and transformed are not the biological ones. Even if Foucault insists, particularly in his last seminars, on the importance of the biological body for philosophical discipline, as it appears in Cynicism, for example, it is clear that the formation and transformation of the self operates on the symbolic body in the first place. It is clear that we have two bodies in one. In all cases, biology is always dependent on the symbolic. Always derived from it. A secondary phenomenon. Biological life remains obscure, predetermined, genetically programmed, deprived of any meaning. Biology remains attached to control and sovereignty.

As I said at the start, the problem is that this critique of sovereignty is exactly structured as what it criticizes. The split between the biological and the symbolic is the scarlet letter printed by sovereignty on the philosophical body.

If we try to erase this mark, if we can affirm that plasticity inhabits the biological, that it opens, within organic life, a supplement of indeterminacy, a void, a floating entity, it is then possible to claim that material life is not dependent in its dynamic upon a transcendental symbolic economy; that on the contrary, biological life creates or produces its own symbolization.

Epigenetics is able to provide us with such a concept of biological supplement. I briefly explain what epigenetics means before I insist, in conclusion, on its political implications.

The term *epigenetics* (Greek: επί-, over, above) was coined by Conrad Waddington in 1942.[20] It designates the branch of biology that studies gene expression, that is, the molecular processes that allow the formation of an individual structure—the phenotype—out of the primary genome or DNA sequence. Gene expression concerns the translation or transcription from DNA into proteins via RNA. The passage from genome to phenotype involves the molecular mechanisms that constitute cell differentiation, extend genes' action, and give the organism its form and structure. This implies that certain genes are activated and some others inhibited. These operations of activation and inhibition depend on epigenetic factors, that is, factors of change that translate DNA without altering it. Epigenetics, in other words, studies nongenetic changes or modifications. These changes are of primary importance in the biological fashioning of individual identities.

What is extremely interesting is that such changes are both chemical and environmental. Environment, experience, and education appear to be epigenetic factors that play a major role in this fashioning. The brain's development, for example, depends for a great part upon epigenetic factors. The anatomy of the brain is genetically determined. But the innumerable synaptic connecting possibilities are not. Synapsis formation escapes genetic determinism and is indebted to contacts that the organism has established with its environment. The brain's connective development depends, throughout its long lifetime, upon experience and learning. It means that we are, for a great part, the authors of our own brains. As a contemporary neurobiologist affirms: "the brain is more than a reflection of our genes."[21]

Plasticity is in a way genetically programmed to develop and operate without program, plan, determinism, schedule, design, or preschematization. Neural plasticity allows the shaping, repairing, and remodeling of connections and in consequence a certain amount of self-transformation of the living being.

> The difference between genetics and epigenetics can probably be compared to the difference between writing and reading a book. Once a book is written, the text (the genes or DNA-stored information) will be the same in all the copies distributed to the interested audience. However, each individual reader of a given book may interpret the story slightly differently, with varying emotions and projections as they continue to unfold the chapters. In a very similar manner, epigenetics would allow different interpretations of a fixed template (the book or genetic code) and result in different read-outs, dependent upon the variable conditions under which this template is interrogated.[22]

In their important book *Evolution in Four Dimensions*, Eva Jablonka and Marion J. Lamb give a very similar definition: "Think about a piece of music that is represented by a system of notes written on paper, a score. The score is copied repeatedly as it is passed on from one generation to the next. [. . .] The relationship between the score and the music is analogous to the genotype/phenotype distinction."[23]

The becoming obsolete of the notion of program in biology opens new conditions of experience, new thresholds of rationality, as well as new philosophical and theoretical paradigms. If nature and culture are intimately linked in and through epigenetics, it means that nature and history meet within the biological, that there is a biological encounter between them. In that sense, biology ceases to be a pure deterministic field, with no symbolic autonomy, a simple raw material for political use. On the contrary, epigenetics is a biological notion that resists the political reduction of biology to a pure and simple vehicle of power. What epigenetics reveals is the originary intrication of the biological and the symbolic that never requires a transgression of the biological itself.

I have no intention here to negate the symbolic dimension of life or to affirm that life has only a biological sense. My contention is that if we admit that history and biology form a dialectical couple within biological life itself, we don't need to survey the biological from an overarching structural point of view, but on the contrary, we can discover the structural meaning of the empirical within the empirical, within "vibrant matter."[24]

If we keep the definition of the symbolic as an empty or vacant space, this empty space is currently becoming what I call the plastic space or the locus of plasticity, something that allows play within the structure, that loosens the frame's rigidity—the frame being biological determinism. The symbolic here appears as that which allows the interplay of determinisms and freedom within the frame or the structure. This symbolic biological dimension is the transformative tendency internal to materiality, the self-transformative tendency of life. It is life transforming itself without separating itself from itself. I would like to conceive of life as possessing its own modes of self-transformation, self-organization, and self-directedness.

What I specifically developed here about life may be extended to other contexts in which the symbolic, defined as a surplus or a supplement, an excess over the real, is conceived of as a critical political weapon. As we know, the structuralist definition of the symbolic was elaborated within the frame of the relationship with primitive societies, as a common feature to all human communities. To challenge the priority of the symbolic, thus defined, is then not only to touch on a particular point, for example, that of philosophy and biology, as I have done here, but to address the issue of the political legitimacy of such a priority in general. Do we still have to presuppose a gap between the structural and the material in order to render the material meaningful? Do we have to transcend the empirical organization of the real in order to produce a theory of the real? Or shouldn't we, on the contrary, consider such gestures as sovereign acts that reinscribe, just as kingship, the excess at the heart of meaning?

I wonder if the categories of excess, surplus, supplement are still accurate to approach any kind of organization. Bataille used to oppose the excess, the "accursed share," to the servility of Hegelian dialectics. As we know, for Hegel, energy never comes from outside the system but from the redoubling of the negative within it. What if he was right? What if the dialectical plasticity of difference was, more than the indifference of the symbolic, the most efficient way to materialize the deconstruction of sovereignty?

NOTES

1. Foucault, "Truth and Power," 121.
2. Foucault, *Society Must Be Defended*, 34.
3. Derrida, *Beast and the Sovereign*.
4. Foucault, *Society Must Be Defended*, 35.
5. Foucault, "Truth and Power," 124.

6. Foucault, "Truth and Power," 125.
7. Foucault, *History of Sexuality*, 143.
8. Foucault, *History of Sexuality*, 142.
9. Foucault, *History of Sexuality*, 140.
10. Foucault, *History of Sexuality*, 144.
11. See Derrida, *Beast and the Sovereign*.
12. Foucault, *History of Sexuality*, 152.
13. Agamben, *Homo Sacer*, 140.
14. Derrida, *Acts of Religion*, all quotations, 87.
15. Kantorowicz, *King's Two Bodies*.
16. Plowden (1816), quoted in Kantorowicz, *King's Two Bodies*, 7.
17. Santner, *Royal Remains*.
18. Translations from Lévi-Strauss, "Marcel Mauss," ix–lii.
19. Deleuze, "How Do We Recognize Structuralism?," 170–92.
20. Waddington, "Epigenotype," 18–20.
21. Schwartz and Begley, *Mind and the Brain*, 365.
22. Jenuwein (Max Planck Institute of Immunology, Vienna), quoted in "What Is Epigenetics?"
23. Jablonka and Lamb, *Evolution in Four Dimensions*, 109.
24. Bennett, *Vibrant Matter*.

CHAPTER 2

Whither Materialism? Althusser/Darwin

Catherine Malabou

■ Whither materialism? This title echoes another one, "Whither Marxism?," that of a conference held in 1993 in California where Derrida presented an oral version of *Specters of Marx*.[1] With regard to this ambiguous title, Derrida proposed that "one may hear beneath the question 'Where is Marxism going?' another question: 'Is Marxism dying?'"[2]

The same ambiguity will be at work throughout this chapter.[3] Where is materialism currently going? Is materialism currently dying? These two questions will of course allow me to address the problem of Marxism proper but from the point of view of what Marxism has repressed, that is, materialism itself. This strange approach to Marxism, according to which, in all Marx's work, an official materialism would be repressing a more secret one, is defended by the late Althusser in a fascinating text from 1982: "The Underground Current of the Materialism of the Encounter."[4]

In this text, Althusser brings to light "the existence of an almost completely unknown materialist tradition in the history of philosophy, . . . a materialism of the encounter, and therefore of the aleatory and of contingency. This materialism is opposed, as a wholly different mode of thought, to the various materialisms on record, including that widely ascribed to Marx, Engels, and Lenin, which, like every materialism in the rationalist tradition, is a materialism of necessity and teleology; that is to say, a transformed, disguised form of idealism."[5] Such a repressed materialism is the one I intend to interrogate here: a materialism which threatens necessity, order, causality, meaning, a "dangerous"[6] materialism, as Althusser characterizes it, a materialism—this is the central idea of the article—"which starts out from nothing."[7] I will constantly question this: what does starting out from nothing mean, and is it possible?

I quote Althusser again: "to free the materialism of the encounter from this repression; to discover, if possible, its implications for both philosophy and materialism; and to ascertain its hidden effects wherever they are silently at work—such is the task that I have set myself here."[8]

This task is clearly an answer to the first question: whither materialism? Where is it going? At the same time, the second question immediately appears. Is this materialism of the encounter still a materialism, Althusser asks. Is not the revelation of the repressed always the end of what is revealed? Will materialism whither in its contingent form, in the nothingness it presupposes? Will it open new paths, or will it die?

Again, I intend to show that these two questions are of particular philosophical and political relevance and urgency for our time.

Now, why Darwin? The list of authors Althusser considers representative of the new materialism includes Epicurus, Machiavelli, Spinoza, Hobbes, Rousseau, Nietzsche, Heidegger, Derrida, Deleuze, a certain Marx, and Darwin. Why Darwin? Is it an arbitrary choice? It is in a way. It has to be. Contingency alone can adequately respond to contingency. So why not Darwin. And it is not, of course. The encounter between Althusser and Darwin I am risking here helps to situate the specific problem raised by the notion of the encounter itself. Both share the same vision of this strange ontological point of departure: nothingness, nothing, the same critique of teleology, the same concept of selection—thus the same materialism.

Darwin? A materialist? Yes, indeed, according to Althusser, Darwin is a materialist of the encounter.

Let me propose some definitions before I start the demonstration. Materialism is a name for the nontranscendental status of form in general. Matter is what forms itself in producing the conditions of possibility of this formation itself. Any transcendental instance necessarily finds itself in a position of exteriority in relation to that which it organizes. By its nature, the condition of possibility is other than what it makes possible. Materialism affirms the opposite: the absence of any outside of the process of formation. Matter's self-formation and self-information is then systematically nontranscendental.

There are then two possibilities of explaining and understanding the origin of this immanent dynamic. Dialectical teleology is the first well-known one. The formation of forms—forms of life; forms of thought, forms of society—is governed by an internal tension toward a telos, which necessarily orients and determines every self-development. This teleological vision of materialism, which has long been predominant, is precisely the one Althusser rejects here. Such a materialism presupposes that "everything is accomplished in advance; the structure precedes its elements and reproduces them in order to reproduce the structure."[9] It amounts in reality to a transcendental analytics, which is why Althusser may identify it with idealism.

Materialism of the encounter, on the contrary, doesn't presuppose any telos, reason, or cause—such a materialism claims, against any transcendental structure, "the non-anteriority of Meaning."[10] From this second point of view, forms are encounters that have taken form. Althusser constantly insists on such a "form taking," or "crystallization": "The crystallization of the elements with one another (in the sense in which the ice crystallizes)."[11] Here, the formation of form has to be sought in what "gives form" to the effects of the encounter. The encounter has to "take form" and "take hold" in order to last and become necessary.

It is while explaining this very specific type of plasticity—the crystallization and taking of form out of nothing—that Althusser turns toward Darwin. "Instead of thinking contingency as a modality of necessity, [. . .] we must think necessity as the becoming-necessary of the encounter of contingencies. Thus we see that not only the world of life (the biologists, who should have known their Darwin, have recently become aware of this), but the world of history, too, gels at certain felicitous moments, with the taking hold of elements combined in an encounter that is apt to trace such-and-such a figure: such-and-such a species, individual, or people."[12] It is precisely the passage between a species, an individual, and a people that I will examine here. Are these forms equivalent? Can we transpose what happens at the level of nature to that of the political and of history?

I first ask to what extent social selection is assimilable to natural selection as Darwin elaborates it. I will then examine the difference between a natural encounter and a social and political one. Here I ask where in society is the void, the nothingness, the point zero from which a form can emerge? In conclusion, I attempt to situate Althusser's new critique of capitalism, its impact on our philosophical time, and the current emergence of new materialisms.

My use of the word "plasticity" a moment ago to describe the crystallization of form in the materialism of the encounter is not entirely my decision. An attentive reading of *The Origin of Species* reveals that plasticity constitutes one of the central motifs of Darwin's thought. Indeed, plasticity situates itself effectively at the heart of the theory of evolution. How does a "form" take form according to Darwin?

The concept of plasticity allows the articulation—as Darwin indicates at the beginning of his book—of a fundamental connection between the *variability* of individuals within the same species and the *natural selection* between these same individuals.

Variability first. There is no species without it. To refer to Althusser's terminology, variability is the "void" or "empty point" or "nothingness" from where forms can emerge. The most important characteristic of a species is its mutability; the great number of potential morphological transformations observable in the structure of the organism is a function of its aptitude to change forms. Contrary to a widespread misreading of Darwin, a species is never rigid or fixed. Filiation reveals the high degree of a species' plasticity. Considering descent, one has the impression that "the whole organization seems to have become plastic."[13] At the beginning of chapter 5, Darwin writes, "the reproductive system is eminently susceptible to changes in the conditions of life; and to this system being functionally disturbed in the parents, I chiefly attribute the varying or plastic condition of the offspring."[14] Characteristic of variability, plasticity designates the quasi-infinite possibility of changes of structure authorized by the living structure itself. This quasi infinity constitutes precisely the openness or the absence of predetermination which makes an encounter possible.

The form "takes" when variability encounters natural selection. Natural selection transforms the contingency of the former into a necessity. "I am convinced that the accumulative action of Selection . . . is by far the predominant Power [in the economy of mutability and variability]."[15]

One must therefore understand that selection guides variability and that it regulates the formation of forms. Selection allows the taking of *oriented* form, which obeys the natural exigency of the viability, consistency, and autonomy of individuals. The plastic condition—otherwise called the motor of evolution itself—therefore hinges on plasticity, understood as the fluidity of structures on the one hand and the selection of viable, durable forms likely to constitute a legacy or lineage on the other. The materialism of the encounter thus pertains to a natural process that assures the permanent selection and crystallization of variations.

The relation between variation and selection raises the fundamental philosophical question I would like to address here to Althusser. In nature, the relation between variation and selection is not, properly speaking, planned. Paradoxically, natural selection appears in Darwin as a mechanism deprived of all selective intention. The best is the fittest, but aptitude is here independent of all value judgments or all actual teleology.

Natural selection is ateleological, without intention. It is, again, an encounter. Insofar as it is not more than a mechanism—a term that, by definition, evokes a blind movement, the opposite or reverse of freedom—natural selection is paradoxically nonanticipatable, a promise of forms never chosen in advance, of differences to come.

However, this is again the central problem; it seems that this natural formation of forms cannot have, without disguise or misrepresentation, a social destiny. We know the errors of "social Darwinism," which is everything but a philosophy of plasticity to the degree that it reduces down to a simple theory the struggle of the strong against the weak. For many years, particularly in France, natural selection came to be understood as a simple process of eliminating the weakest and of life as a merciless struggle for power in all its forms. We may have also confused Darwinism and Malthusianism, despite precise precautions taken regarding this subject in *The Origin of Species*, taking natural selection as a simple quantitative dynamic governed by the ratio of the number of individuals in a population and the availability of resources.[16] This interpretation is absolutely not Darwinian and, again, is a misunderstanding.

If such a misunderstanding is possible, though, is it not because a materialism of the encounter seems to be socially and politically unsustainable because it can work only at the level of atoms or of forms of life, never when it comes to individuals or peoples? The automaticity and nonteleological character of natural selection seems definitively lost in social selection. Why—in the logic of exams, in competitions, or in professional selection in general, the discrimination of candidates regarding aptitude functions, of competencies, or of specific technical capacities—does selection seem to lack plasticity; that is, fluidity on the one hand and the absence of any predetermined selective intention on the other? Why, most of the time, does social selection give the feeling of being an expected or agreed-upon process, a simple logic of conformity and reproduction, whereas natural selection is incalculably open to possibility?

Is not the materialism of the encounter always doomed to be repressed by that of teleology, anteriority of meaning, presuppositions, predeterminations?

The plastic condition Darwin describes calls for a particular articulation of identity and difference. Identity, because individuals selected are able to reproduce and therefore to inscribe themselves into the stability of an identifiable type. Difference, because this identity is not rigid and is obtained precisely from variability. Specific identity is an identity produced by the differentiation of structures and types. However, in nature, there is an automatic and blind equilibrium between identity and difference, while it seems that, in the social order, there is always a predominance of identity over difference and that the natural grace of the balance is interrupted. The idea of choice, according to an apparent paradox, is again entirely absent from natural selection. In nature, selection is unconscious. As soon as selection becomes an intention of selection, which presupposes predefined criteria, certainly programmed this time, as soon as there is no more naturality or spontaneity in the promotion, the plastic condition is menaced or even inexistent. A materialism, again, is repressing another.

In nature, the fittest is never the one that accidentally fell upon a favorable environment for its survival. It is a matter of simply "adjust[ing] a response" to the environment, to restate it in François Jacob's terms.[17] Adaptation, the agreement between the environment and variation, can of course be unpredictable. There is no better "in itself." Certainly, Darwin described natural selection as a work of perfecting or as an "improvement," but these notions of "better" remain without intention. Darwin was very reticent to speak of "progress"; he himself never wanted to understand his theory as a theory of "evolution," a term that could risk suggesting a linear progress comparable to the Lamarckian law of complexification. The improvement of which Darwin speaks is not subordinated to a finalism. The form of survivors, its permanence over time, is in a certain way sculpted by the disappearance of the disadvantaged, by the return of eliminated living forms to the inorganic. In the words of Canguilhem, "death is a blind sculptor of living forms."[18]

The inanimate therefore becomes, negatively, the condition of sense or the project of the living.

Could we then consider that Darwinism stops itself at the threshold of society and culture and that all social destiny betrays it, which is to say, precisely, alters it? Selection would then be nothing other than a reproductive process of the identical.

Can we not envision, in spite of everything, a plasticity of social condition and recover the wealth of variations and deviations of structure at the heart of culture? Is it not possible to think a social and political equilibrium in the relation between variation and selection? Where are we today with Darwin on this point?

And where are we with Althusser? According to him, the same plasticity as the biological one should prevail in the social and political order. This is the profound meaning of his new materialism. Let's go back to individuals and peoples.

Althusser comes to the "taking form" of the individual when he talks about Machiavelli's *Prince*. Here is the political version of the materialism of the encounter at the level of the individual: "Machiavelli [. . .] moves on to the idea that unification will be achieved if there emerges some nameless man. . . . Thus the dice are tossed on the gaming table, which is itself empty."[19]

So we have here this void, this absence of meaning, telos, or predetermination. Form will emerge out of the encounter between fortune—that is, contingency—and the prince's virtue—that is, his ability to select the best possibilities fortune offers, yet a selection made with no intention to do so. As if there was a naturally plastic balance between the lion and the fox, fortune and *virtù*.

> Consequently, the Prince is governed, internally, by the variations of this other aleatory encounter, that of the fox on the one hand and the lion and man on the other. This encounter *may not take place*, but it may also take place. It has to last long enough for the figure of the Prince to "take hold" among the people—to "take hold," that is, *to take form*, so that, institutionally, he instils the fear of himself as good; and, if possible, so that he ultimately is good, but on the absolute condition that he never forget how to be evil if need be.[20]

But how can there exist, in the social, such a nameless man, able to begin from nothing, from such a nameless place, from such a nonteleological formation of forms?

The problem becomes all the more urgent when Althusser comes to the people or community via Rousseau. The specific political issue Rousseau raises is the following: to the extent that men have been "forced to have encounters"[21] when they were in the state of nature, forced into the social, is it possible to transform this imposed and illegitimate state of things into a legitimate one? That is, is it possible to re-create the conditions for a contingent and nonteleological form of encounter once the encounter has already taken place? To plasticize it retrospectively in some way? "To rectif[y] an illegitimate (the prevailing) form, transforming it into a legitimate form?"[22] Such is, according to Althusser, the leading question of *The Social Contract*. "The most profound thing in Rousseau is doubtless disclosed and covered back up [*decouvert et recouvert*] here, in this vision of any possible theory of history, which thinks the contingency of necessity as an effect of the necessity of contingency, an unsettling pair of concepts that must nevertheless be taken into account."[23] Again, where is the void, the empty square from where we can start undertaking such a shift? "It is in the political *void* that the encounter must come about,"[24] Althusser writes. But where is it and what can it be?

■ There seems to be no void in our societies. Let's have a look at the process of social selection—understood, for example, as the sorting and choosing of capacities or special aptitudes within the framework of examinations, contests, or recruitment interviews—which immediately appears as the antonym to the plastic condition that presides over the economy of natural selection and its nonsignifying sense.

The catalog of tasks, the outline of jobs, the protocol of exams always precede the real encounter with the variability and diversity of candidates, thus preventing differences from emerging by themselves. Such selection cannot, in fact, consist in the production of differences but, instead, only in the perpetuation of the criteria through which one chooses them. It is not the best that are selected or even those that exhibit an astonishing capacity for adaptation but those who are the most conformable. Agreement takes precedence over value. Ensuring the perpetuation and renewability of the identical, social selection therefore ensures the return of sociological heaviness, never the emergence of singularities out of nothing.

Marx, particularly in his *Critique of Hegel's Philosophy of Right*, was the first thinker to have denounced the conservative characteristic of the social selection of aptitudes. Taking the example of "functionaries," Marx shows that one expects of them no special competence beyond that which consists in perpetrating the established order.[25] Hegel writes in his *Elements of the Philosophy of Right* that these "individuals are not destined by birth of personal nature to hold a particular office, for there is no natural or immediate link between the two. The objective moment in their vocation is knowledge and proof of ability."[26] However, these capabilities, says Marx, are not capabilities; no "technique" is necessary to become a functionary, no specific expertise except for the talent of obedience, of respect for the state, and therefore of conformism.

Another critique of social selection would be conducted in the work of Pierre Bourdieu, notably in the famous text *The Inheritors*,[27] which he coauthored with Jean-Claude Passeron in 1964 and which concerns the class trajectory of students. Selection norms, always defined in advance, constitute a veritable program and coincide, again, with pure and simple values of conformity, those of the dominant class, that fix the criteria of "cultural legitimacy." The principal characteristic of this legitimacy is to be a dissimulated social authority. This is the function of social reproduction of cultural reproduction, founded upon "privilege"—by definition the most predetermined selective criterion ever.

Social selection has the goal of reproducing order, privilege, or the dominant ideology. One never selects the aptitude for action or political struggle, for example, but always aptitudes that respect order. Who among us has never been shocked by the injustice of this sorting, this triage, which retains only those individuals most compliant, never the most singular, and which, finally, elects so many mediocre, incompetent, and narrow minds? Who has never had the feeling that social selection was, in effect, a program and never a promise and that the morphological transformations of society were, deep down, only agents of conservation?

The question that arises then is whether the destiny of social selection is a fatality, or if selection could, in the political realm, join in any way the natural plastic condition. How can we ensure, within the realm of community and culture, the equilibrium between variation and selection, the future of difference, the promise of unexpected forms?

Althusser is in reality perfectly aware of these difficulties, of the discrepancy between the encounter in the ontological or natural order and the encounter in the political realm. There would have to be only one solution to this: to know that criteria do not preexist selection itself. In society, such would be the recovered plastic condition. The whole problem always concerns knowing how not to identify the difference in advance, since selection in the order is always an act that confers value and therefore creates hierarchies and norms. How must one think at once the evaluating character inevitable to all social selection and its possible indetermination or liberty?

The only philosopher to have clearly posed this question is Nietzsche, and that is why Althusser refers to him after dealing with Machiavelli and Rousseau. It is certainly not for him to condemn selection, for the latter is inevitable, and it has an ontological foundation: becoming is itself nothing other than selection. Do not forget the following saying by Heraclitus: "For even the best of them choose one thing above all others, immortal glory among mortals, while most of them are glutted like beasts."[28] Becoming is so rich in differences that it can occur only upon the mode of choice. The task of philosophy is essentially selective since it chooses the differences opened by the flux of life, sorts them, and interprets them. In *Ecce Homo*, Nietzsche asks, "What is it, fundamentally, that allows us to recognize *who has turned out well*?"[29] Which could be translated as "who has taken form"?

In *Difference and Repetition*,[30] Deleuze, to whom Althusser is also referring, shows that selection produces its own criteria *as* it operates. It therefore becomes sensitive to the validity and viability of differences. The difference will be selected, as it unfolds, demonstrating its aptitude for return, which is to say the possibility of engendering a heritage or tradition. Thereby "good" music, for example, engenders a tradition of interpretation, a great text engenders a lineage of readers. Selection should therefore happen *after* the emergence or springing of difference in the same manner that variability precedes natural selection.

Althusser perfectly knows that the "political void" in which the "encounter must come about,"[31] this political void which is also, as he says, "a philosophical void,"[32] may not exist; if we could be certain of its existence, if we were able to know in advance, the encounter would never take place, and we would fall back into teleology again. The determination of this void of nothingness, of this point of possibility that opens all promise of justice, equality, legitimacy cannot be presupposed and cannot be as blindly and automatically regulated as in nature either. It has to be made possible. This is the philosophical task that appears with the end of the repressed materialism.

Machiavelli's Prince is, Althusser says, "a man of nothing who has started out of nothing starting out from an unassignable place."[33] To find and give form to this unassignable place is what we have to do. "Unassignable" is the translation of the French *inassignable*, but I am not sure that the word has the same meaning in both languages. In French, it means indeterminate and infinite. In English, it means incapable of being repudiated or transferred to another: inalienable. But I also found unassigned: not allocated or set aside for a specific purpose. The English is then much more interesting because it opens a space within the idea of a proper, something that cannot be attributed to someone else, that cannot be denied without destroying the subject, that belongs to no one and has no destination. We can call this place, the unassignable place, the *properly anonymous*. Without qualities, without privilege, without legacies, without tradition. People of nothing, people of valor. From there and there only can new forms emerge—singular, unpredictable, unseen, regenerating—Althusser also says.

Before I ask a few questions about this "place," let me evoke the changes caused by this new materialism in Althusser's reading of Marx and consequently in his critique of capitalism. In the light of this new materialism, Althusser writes, Marx "was constrained to think within a horizon torn between the aleatory of the Encounter and the necessity of Revolution."[34] Hence, all his disavowals, debarments and philosophical betrayals. Very briefly: "In innumerable passages, Marx . . . explains that the capitalist mode of production arose from the 'encounter' between 'the owners of money' and the proletarian stripped of everything but his labour-power. It so happens that this encounter took place, and 'took hold,' which means that it . . . lasted, and became an accomplished fact, . . . inducing stable relationships and laws . . . : the laws of development of the capitalist mode of production . . ."[35] So initially, Marx analyzes the constitution of capitalism as an encounter starting from the plastic void, the nothingness of the proletariat—its fundamental dispossession. But instead of remaining faithful to this vision, to the vision of a mode of production as a form taking form out of nothing, aggregating different elements and becoming gradually necessary, Marx and Engels have inverted the process. They eventually affirmed that the different elements constitutive of the encounter "were from all eternity destined to enter into combination, harmonize with one another, and reciprocally produce each other as their own ends, conditions and or complements."[36] They substitute an analysis of the reproduction of the proletariat instead for its production.

> When Marx and Engels say that the proletariat is "the product of big industry," they utter a very great piece of nonsense, positioning themselves within *the logic of the accomplished fact of the reproduction of the proletariat on an extended scale*, not the aleatory logic of the "encounter" which produces (rather than reproduces), as the proletariat, this mass of impoverished, expropriated human beings as one of the elements making up the mode of production. In the process, Marx and Engels shift from the first conception of the mode of production, an historico-aleatory conception, to a second, which is essentialistic and philosophical.[37]

So again, the task is to free the repressed philosophical status of impoverishment, expropriation, dispossession, nothingness as the origin of any formative process. Poverty, dispossession, exploitation are the points of departure of philosophical thinking not because they would constitute objects or topics for philosophers but because practice and theory both owe their energy, the power of their dynamism, to their originary absence of determinate being. The same originary "virgin forest,"[38] Althusser says.

"The Underground Current of the Materialism of the Encounter" is no doubt a surprisingly anticipative text. The attempt at clearing a point of void, nothingness, and dispossession is at the heart of the most important current philosophical trends, which define themselves as materialisms. Speculative realism, for example, in its search for a noncorrelationist mode of thinking, elaborates a notion of an absolute which would be not "ours," which would remain indifferent to us.

Opening the unassignable place in a global world, where every place is assigned, has become the most urgent ethical and political task. The problem is to succeed in not constituting it as a transcendental structure. This is what I am struggling with myself, trying to disengage my plasticity from any symbolic grip and attempting to constantly empty it from its own sovereignty.

All this is extremely fragile; the waves are constantly, repeatedly, covering up the "open fields"[39] of singularity, surprise, nonanticipatable selection, recognition of aptitudes, the capacity to welcome new forms without expecting them. The waves of ownership, appropriation, reproduction are constantly and repeatedly covering up the originary deprivation of ontological wealth.

Whither materialism? The question won't ever lose its ambiguity. But as Darwin says, when considering the changing nature of species, one at times has the impression that the "whole organization seems to have become plastic."[40] Let's live for those times.

NOTES

1. Derrida, *Specters of Marx*.
2. Derrida, *Specters of Marx*, xiii.
3. This chapter was first given as a presentation under the auspices of the Centre for Research in Modern European Philosophy (CRMEP) and the London Graduate School of Kingston University London in May 2013.
4. Althusser, "Underground Current," 163–207.
5. Althusser, "Underground Current," 167, 168.
6. Althusser, "Underground Current," 168.
7. Althusser, "Underground Current," 189.
8. Althusser, "Underground Current," 168.
9. Althusser, "Underground Current," 200.
10. Althusser, "Underground Current," 169.
11. Althusser, "Underground Current," 170.
12. Althusser, "Underground Current," 194.
13. Darwin, *Origin of Species*, 12.
14. Darwin, *Origin of Species*, 131, 132.
15. Darwin, *Origin of Species*, 43.
16. On the relationship with Malthus, see the conclusion to Darwin, *Origin of Species*.
17. Jacob, *Logic of Life*, 8.
18. Canguilhem, *Vital Rationalist*, 212.
19. Althusser, "Underground Current," 172.
20. Althusser, "Underground Current," 173.
21. Althusser, "Underground Current," 185.
22. Althusser, "Underground Current," 187.
23. Althusser, "Underground Current," 187.
24. Althusser, "Underground Current," 173.
25. Marx, *Critique*, 21ff.
26. Hegel, *Elements*, 332.
27. Bourdieu and Passeron, *Inheritors*.
28. Fragment, 29.
29. Nietzsche, *Genealogy of Morals*, 224.

30. Deleuze, *Difference and Repetition*, 300.
31. Althusser, "Underground Current," 172.
32. Althusser, "Underground Current," 174.
33. Althusser, "Underground Current," 172.
34. Althusser, "Underground Current," 187.
35. Althusser, "Underground Current," 197.
36. Althusser, "Underground Current," 200.
37. Althusser, "Underground Current," 198.
38. Althusser, "Underground Current," 191.
39. Althusser, "Underground Current," 191.
40. Darwin, *Origin of Species*, 12.

CHAPTER **3**

From the Overman to
the Posthuman: How Many Ends?

Catherine Malabou

Forty-five years ago, in October 1968 in New York, Jacques Derrida gave the keynote address to an international conference called "Philosophy and Anthropology." The talk was published in *Margins of Philosophy* as "The Ends of Man."[1] In the first four pages, Derrida analyzes the meaning of the very gesture of giving a lecture in an international conference on the *anthropos*, that is, on the human. The problem, he said, pertains to the possibility for a speaker to open a space, in his or her address, between the differences of each national, ethnic, cultural, theoretical, and gendered identity and the massive immediate universality of the conference's theme. He writes: "At a given moment, in a given, political, and economic context, some national groups have judged it possible and necessary to organize an international encounter, to present themselves, or to be represented in such [an] encounter by their national identity (such, at least, as it is assumed by the organizers of the colloquium), and to determine in such encounters their proper difference, or to establish relations between their respective differences."[2] Is not a question as "the human" doomed to interiorize, assimilate, and in the end, erase these differences? Forty-five years later, we are facing the same problem. When talking about the human, will we, will I, let a certain diversity or minority come into language, or will we, will I, inevitably negate it?

In order to find his way through this question, Derrida chose to talk from his culture and identity as a French philosopher and asked: "Thus the transition will be made quite naturally between the preamble and the theme of this communication, as it was imposed upon me, rather than as I chose it. Where is France, as concerns man?"[3] Forty-five years later, I ask practically the same question. Not from the strict point of view of French philosophy perhaps—I doubt that such a thing still exists—but from that of Continental philosophy nevertheless. From somewhere where I am, trying to avoid universalizing my discourse and yet hoping to say something that all can hear. Paradoxical injunction.

If I present my discourse as a repetition of Derrida's, it is because, as I intend to demonstrate, the question of the human is that of a singular and unique destiny of repetition. It is not to say that repetition is specifically human. There are of course innumerable occurrences of animal repetitions; there are also many cases of nonliving repetitions, as in technology, all kinds of automatisms which again are not properly human. So it is not that the human would be the repetitive or repeating character per se. What I mean is that the human is sculpting a certain relationship to repetition and that, in return, this relationship is sculpting it.

Derrida himself observes that the human is what constantly repeats itself; but not only that, it is what repeats itself *beyond all deconstruction of its being*. The human is what repeats itself even when its essence is dissolved. I develop this point first,[4] then, returning to political issues, I ask what is repetition and what is the repetition of the human after deconstruction. Nietzsche will bridge these two moments.

Where is France, as concerns man? At the time when Derrida asked this question, French philosophy was undertaking a vast movement of deconstruction of the humanism which had reigned since Sartre's existentialism.[5] "Even if one does not wish to summarize Sartre's thought under the slogan 'existentialism is a humanism,' it must be recognized that in *Being and Nothingness*, *The Sketch of a Theory of the Emotions*, etc., the major concept, the theme of the last analysis, the irreducible horizon and origin is what was then called 'human-reality.' As is well known, this is a translation of Heideggerian Dasein."[6] It is true that in the fifties, the usual translation of *Dasein* was "human reality." Even if the "notion of 'human-reality' translated for Sartre and others the project of thinking the meaning of man, the humanity of man, on a new basis,"[7] non-Christian and nonmetaphysical, it revealed that philosophers were still believing in something like a unity of the concept of man, precisely in its universality.

Paradoxically, this Sartrean humanism was founded on philosophers—Heidegger but also Husserl and Hegel—who had, in their own way, pronounced the nonexistence of such a unified concept of the human and consequently also the nonexistence of "human reality" as such. Heidegger precisely decided to neutralize the term "man" by using *Dasein*, which implied an absence of any particular or specific qualities. *Dasein* is certainly not a "man." Nor is it a woman. It is a being there, regardless of any specific mark. As far as Husserl is concerned, we know that the "critique of anthropologism was one of the inaugural motifs of [his] transcendental philosophy [. . .] [For Husserl], one can imagine a consciousness without man."[8] As for Hegel, even if Kojève constantly identifies the consciousness of the *Phenomenology of Spirit* with human consciousness or subjectivity, it is clear that dialectical philosophy never refers to something as "human consciousness." The *Phenomenology of Spirit* is clearly not an anthropology.

So again, it is very striking to see that for a long time, all these philosophers have formed the basis for French existential humanism. At the time when Derrida wrote his text, as I said, the deconstruction of this humanism had nevertheless already begun. In the seventies, the nonhumanist ground of French contemporary humanism had started to get unearthed, and thinkers like Levinas, Ricoeur, and Hyppolite had undertaken new readings of Hegel, Husserl, or Heidegger, which cut them from the Sartrean influence. It is in the path opened by these new readings that Derrida first situated the initial impulse of deconstruction. A deconstruction which still had to free these nonhumanist readings from their still humanist remainder. Deconstruction then appeared right from the start as a second nonhumanist reading of these nonhumanist readings. As a critical repetition.

Such a repetition starts with the idea that the overcoming or sublation or *relève* of the human has not yet started. That the human always comes back, always returns, even in nonhumanist discourses. At that point, Derrida plays with the double meaning of his title "The Ends of Man." "End" meaning both disappearance and accomplishment. According to this double meaning, Man, or the Human, is what accomplishes itself in disappearing. What repeats itself out of its destruction.

What does this mean? Derrida explains in a fascinating analysis that the human's disappearance or the end—in the sense of coming to an end—of man is not something which happens from outside, like an accident or an historical state of things or event. It is in a way inscribed within the concept of the human or humanity itself. This is what Derrida calls later the apocalyptic nature of man: its destruction is its truth. Its end is its end, its telos. What Derrida means is that the human, as a supposedly rational being gifted with the *logos*, has to accomplish itself as nonhuman, that is as infinite, nonmortal, as a being able to spiritually, if not naturally, reach absolute knowledge. "*It is the end of finite man* ("*C'est la fin de l'homme fini*"). The end of the finitude of man, the unity of the finite and of the infinite, the finite as the surpassing of self."[9] Derrida then underscores the unity of the two ends of man, the unity of his death and of his completion, a unity which is immanent in the Greek concept of telos: the thinking of the end of man coincides with the thinking of the truth of man.

This contradictory unity is already present throughout the whole metaphysical tradition ("*the thinking of the end of man,*" Derrida says, "*is always already prescribed in metaphysics in the thinking of the truth of man*"),[10] but it is also present in nonmetaphysical discourse, that is, in these nonanthropological and nonhumanist discourses of Hegel, Husserl, and Heidegger. In deconstructing the human, they just accomplish or complete its concept to the extent, once again, that the human cannot remain what it is. It is a limit between two ends and end in itself.

I don't analyze in detail here the remnants of this motif of the human in the three mentioned nonhumanist philosophers Hegel, Husserl, and Heidegger. I just want to insist upon the main lines of Derrida's development. About Hegel, he writes that even if consciousness in the *Phenomenology* is not properly human, the "we" that Hegel sometimes uses is "the unity of absolute knowledge and anthropology, of God and man, of ontotheology and humanism."[11] We then understand why Kojève can interpret the figure of the lord in the master/slave dialectics in the *Phenomenology* as a consciousness which is ready to sacrifice its animality in order to reach its symbolic prestige, that is, "human" existence as such.

Same thing in Husserl. Derrida writes, "Despite the critique of anthropologism, 'humanity,' [for Husserl], is still the name of the being to which the transcendental *telos*—determined as [. . .] Reason—is announced. It is man as *animal rationale* who, in his most classical determination, designates the site of teleological reason's unfolding, that is, history. For Husserl as for Hegel, reason is history, and there is no history but of reason. The latter [quoting Husserl's *The Origin of Geometry*] 'functions in every man, the *animal rationale*, no matter how primitive he is . . . '"[12] As soon as we criticize or challenge the unity of the human, as soon as we thematize its end (disappearance or destruction), we accomplish the concept of the human which is just, *according to its concept*, a transition to a "more than human" being.

The double meaning of the "ends of man" is present even in Heidegger, who appears as the most radically nonhumanist of all philosophers. In *Letter on Humanism*, Heidegger precisely criticizes the notion of humanism, but he does so to demonstrate that "humanism" is a perversion of the essence of the human: "it is a threat to the essence of humanity [*Gefärdung des Wesens des Menschen*]."[13] Therefore Derrida can write that Heidegger's critique of humanism and the traditional concept of the human in fact amounts to "a kind of reevaluation or revalorization of . . . the essence of man, which here would have to be thought before and beyond its metaphysical determinations."[14] Again, every critique of the concept of the human seems to be oriented toward a better approach to the essence of humanity. The end is the end. The interruption is a completion.

Does this mean that all discourses on the human, albeit metaphysical or deconstructionist, political or juridical, anthropological or psychoanalytic, would share the same impossibility: that of overcoming the thinking of man as a moving limit—this old limit, which Aristotle described as the medium between God and the animal? This moving or flickering in-between point, always tending to its end?

And what about us today? Aren't we doomed to mime, to repeat infinitely this circle? When we claim that the human is now behind us, that we are entering the posthuman age, that we are opening the "interspecies dialogue," or that we cannot believe in cosmopolitanism for want of a universal concept of humanity, are we doing something other than trying to reconstitute, purify, re-elaborate a new essence of man?

Let me repeat Derrida one last time before I try to fail in my own way.

If we want deconstruction to break the loop of the ends of man, of this endless repetition of the two ends, we have to find the middle term between two apparently opposite strategies which in fact amount to the same:

> 1. To attempt an exit and a deconstruction without changing terrain, by repeating what is implicit in the founding concepts and the original problematic by using, that is, equally, in language.[15]

A *first possibility* would then be to admit that we can only repeat and have to stop creating new names for the human: *Dasein*, posthuman, whatever. We can only sculpt the human into itself, and if something new may occur from such a sculpting, it won't ever transgress the circle where it originates. This "continuous process of making explicit, moving toward an opening, risks sinking into the autism of the closure."[16]

A *second possibility*:

> 2. To decide to change terrain, in a discontinuous and irruptive fashion, by brutally placing oneself outside, and by affirming an absolute break and difference.[17]

This second possibility would imply a giving of new names, the elaboration of new theoretical perspectives, the invention of some "unheard of" concept of the other than man which would definitely break the looking glass. According to Derrida, this second possibility would perhaps get trapped in "inhabiting more naively and more strictly than ever the inside one declares one has deserted, the simple practice of language ceaselessly reinstates the new terrain on the oldest ground."[18] So again, how is it possible, then, to find an escape between these two aspects of the repetition, the same and the different, the different same or the same different? And the essence of the human, which is in fact the universal in both cases?

Derrida surprisingly does not provide an answer to these questions. On the last page of his text, he just sketches a way out by following Nietzsche's tracks. Of course, it may seem that Nietzsche himself is trapped in the circle he constantly describes: the eternal recurrence, here the eternal recurrence of the human. When he talks about the difference between the superior man and the overman, he seems to create a new name to describe an old reality and, in so doing, to announce the accomplishment of the essence of the human. Yet Derrida sees something else in Nietzsche, something different from other philosophical iterations. When man is on his way to the overman, because he is a "bridge" to the overman, man, at the same time, never turns back on himself. There is no reflective gesture in this end. Man "leaves, without turning back to what he leaves behind him. He burns his text and erases the traces of his steps."[19] This is what Nietzsche also calls "active forgetting" (*aktive Vergessenheit*).

Could it be possible, then, that the human actively forgets one of its ends? Actively forgets itself?

Derrida's text ends here, and here I come to modestly try to propose an "end" to it—and here starts the second moment of my development.

Let me follow the Nietzschean track in my turn and focus on repetition—on the necessity to repeat. What is there to say? Do we still have something to say about repetition and the human, about repeating the human? To what extent does this question orient the political and juridical context in which we currently raise it?

Let me refer to three extraordinary chapters of *Thus Spake Zarathustra*—"On the Vision and the Riddle," "The Tarantulas," and "The Great Longing"—and to their reading by Heidegger in volume 2 of his book *Nietzsche*.[20]

What is repetition for Nietzsche? Initially, primarily, repetition is another name for *revenge*. Heidegger writes, "Revenge, taking revenge, wreaking, *urgere*: these words mean to push, drive, herd, pursue and persecute."[21] If there is something like a specificity of the human, for Nietzsche, it is precisely *revenge*. The human is the only being that seeks revenge after an offense. This does not have to be confused with divine punishments, for example. Gods can punish men for their deeds, but they don't seek revenge proper. Revenge is a human, all too human characteristic. It does not have anything to do with struggle or fight either: animals can fight, can kill each other, but it is not out of vengeful instinct.

Revenge means the incapacity to forget. It is precisely the opposite of "active forgetting." The human is the kind of being who cannot forget the offense, who cannot erase the past and constantly repeats, ruminates, chews over. This incapacity to put an end to the past would be precisely the end of man, its essence.

Why? Where does this spirit of revenge and repetition come from? It comes from *time. It is time itself*. The human is the only being for whom time *is a spiritual injury*. There is in fact one single thing we are trying to get revenge from: the passage of time. Time is the utmost injury. The utmost offense. Nietzsche has Zarathustra say: "This, yes, this alone is *revenge* itself: the will's ill will toward time and its 'It was.'"[22]

Heidegger explains that revenge is not only revenge toward the past. It is toward time in general. Here, "past" means "passing away" in general. Heidegger writes:

> Revenge is the will's ill will toward time and that means toward passing away, transiency. Transiency is that against which the will can

take no further steps, that against which its willing constantly collides. Time [. . .] is the obstacle that the will cannot budge. Suffering in this way, the will itself becomes chronically ill over such passing away; the illness then wills its own passing, and in so doing wills that everything in the world be worthy of passing away. Ill will toward time degrades all that passes away.[23]

Let me quote a last passage on the same motif. Heidegger writes:

In converse with his soul, Zarathustra thinks his "most abysmal thought" [which is Eternal Recurrence . . .] Zarathustra begins the episode "On the Great Longing" with the words: "O my soul, I taught you to say 'Today,' 'One Day' and 'Formerly.'"[24]

This brief sentence contains something fundamental: that the proper of man is not language, that the proper of man is not to have soul or be able to talk to its soul; it is not perhaps time itself: it is the combination of language, time, and soul in a single structure which is repetition. "I taught you" refers to the past: my soul, I taught you about time, and I will again and again until the *end*.

Now, if only we try to cut this end from itself, if only we try to erase man's traces in order to attain a nonhuman mode of being which would definitely be cut out from the previous one. With no revengeful feeling.

This implies that we are able to free ourselves from the spirit of revenge. As Nietzsche writes, "For that mankind be redeemed from revenge: that to me is the bridge to the highest hope and a rainbow after long thunderstorms."[25]

The end of man would then be the end of revenge, but this end would not sound like an accomplishment or a telos (that is, like another end). It would on the contrary erase itself, give way to the overman who burst out in laughter, as he is, as Derrida writes, "directed toward a return which no longer will have the form of the metaphysical repetition of humanism."[26]

Shall we ever be liberated, freed from revenge?

Now, what is the link between all this development and the political and juridical question?

For Nietzsche, the link is obvious. Law is the political name for the spirit of revenge. It presents itself as a liberation from this spirit, as its end, but it is in fact its accomplishment, its end. The birth of written laws and codes appeared in Greece as the triumph of *logos*, or reason, over revenge and subterranean justice. Law is the rational reparation, as opposed to private ways of settling conflicts. It is true that *vendetta*, in Italy, in Corsica, as the mob's law, is seen everywhere as something behind the times, uncivilized. We think that law has won, at least in the West, over revenge.

Yet Nietzsche explains that law and the juridical concept of justice are just repetitions of revenge, a more subtle and refined spirit of revenge. This is the theme of the second treatise of the *Genealogy of Morals*. What is law? Law, Nietzsche writes, is the institution that tries "to sanctify revenge under the name of justice—as if justice were at bottom merely a further development of the feeling of being aggrieved—and to rehabilitate not only revenge but all reactive affects in general."[27]

The link between metaphysics and law is then clear: the hiding of ressentiment behind ideals. The hiding of repetition and haunting behind discourses and codes. Whatever the hiding, though, repetition repeats, the ghost of time comes back again and again. The human is still there. The question of the human is haunting us. We humans are seeking revenge from being human. From being humans.

Again, will we ever be able to be redeemed from the spirit of revenge and thus from our humanity?

Will we ever be able to invent a new relationship to time? To law? To justice? Will we ever be able to break the circle of the two ends?

"Redemption," Heidegger writes, "releases the ill will from its 'no' and frees it for a 'yes.'"[28]

Why is it important to utter this yes?

If I chose here to raise the question of repetition, it is not only because the human is what repeats itself, it is not only because I felt like repeating Derrida and praising in so doing his beautiful talk. It is because repetition has become the key notion to practically all theoretical and institutional domains. Repetition has become our topic. Repetition has become the raw material of our lives.

What do I mean?

In law, the major questions have now become that of *return* in general: return as restitution of indigenous lands in Canada or Australia, return understood as reparation and recognition in postcolonial law, as forgiveness in South Africa, and so on.

The issues of memory, ancestrality, genealogy seem to have a singular acuteness today, as if what comes back, what returns, what needs to be repaired, restituted was the most urgent of all problems. We know that Derrida thematized, in a recent text, this urge to forgive and repair and that the proliferation of scenes of regret and requests for forgiveness, of self-accusation, of repentance, of attendance, is a sign of the urgency of repetition. "The proliferation of these scenes of repentance and asking for forgiveness no doubt signifies, among other things, an *"il faut"* of anamnesis, an *il faut* without limit toward the past. Without limit, because the act of memory, which is also the subject of the auto-accusation, of the 'repentance,' of the (court) appearance [*comparution*], must be carried beyond both legal and national state authority."[29] Repetition, then, has become so important an issue and so strong an urge that it should transgress legal and national state authority . . .

Let me take another example of this phenomenon. As some of you know, I am interested in biology, molecular biology, in particular. If I had time, I would show that repetition plays a major role at all levels of contemporary molecular biology, particularly in genetics and epigenetics. I will just take an example: that of stem cells. These cells, which have been discovered quite recently, at the turn of the 1990's, have the capacity to transform themselves into any kind of specialized cells. They are able to *dedifferentiate* themselves. They also can self-renew to produce more stem cells. In mammals, there are two broad types of stem cells: embryonic and adult stem cells, which are found in various tissues. In a developing embryo, stem cells can differentiate into all the specialized cells (these are called pluripotent cells). In adult organisms, they act as a repair system for the body, replenishing adult tissues. They also maintain the normal turnover of regenerative organs, such as blood, skin, and intestinal tissues.

Regenerative medicine works on the possibility of using these cells to replace injured organs or tissues. Self-replacement has become the new paradigm: as if the possibility to duplicate and repeat oneself had substituted for other treatments, treatments like grafts or transplants, for example.

We can also think of biomimicry, that is, the use and imitation of natural processes in technology. As if nature repeated itself through techné. In her book *Biomimicry: Innovation Inspired by Nature*, Janine Benyus declares: "Biomimicry is a revolutionary science that analyzes nature's best ideas—spider silk and prairie grass, seashells and brain cells—and adapts them for human use."[30] Even computers today try to imitate brain functioning—which is all the more striking if we consider that it has long been the other way around: brains were frequently compared with computers!

This repetition of the "natural" is just another example of the fact that we are not only asking the question of repetition; repetition has become the question, what questions us.

All that I have tried to describe, thanks to the concept of plasticity, every act of shaping, reshaping, repairing, remodeling, might be developed here to illustrate the *return of repetition*.

You can now guess what the problem is: are we able to deal with this new urgency of repetition without seeking revenge toward it?

Are we able to repeat without seeking revenge? Without trying to crucify time and transiency, without trying to invent new forms of cruelty?

In the trembling opening of this question appears the possibility of sculpting the nonhuman, or the nonhumanist human.

What does giving a talk at an international conference mean? Did I erase my particularity as a French philosopher to sublimate it in a fake universalism or universality of repetition? Was it on the contrary too visible—French, all too French?

In looking for a definition of the human as the vengeful being, was I closer to Sartre than I imagined? After all, Sartre has written a good deal about revenge (cf. *The Flies* and all his other tragedies). Did I succeed in telling you something? Something able to concern you *all*? All *Dasein* present in this room?

I am absent anyway, celebrating the memory of the great human being Derrida used to be. Yes, I would like to conclude with these words: if we can one day get free from the spirit of revenge, we will become great human beings.

NOTES

1. Derrida, "Ends of Man," 109–36.
2. Derrida, "Ends of Man," 111, 112.
3. Derrida, "Ends of Man," 114.
4. This chapter was first delivered as the keynote address to the Association of Law, Culture and Humanities meeting in London, February 2013.
5. Cf. Sartre, *Existentialism Is a Humanism*.
6. Derrida, "Ends of Man," 115.

7. Derrida, "Ends of Man," 115.
8. Derrida, "Ends of Man," 117.
9. Derrida, "Ends of Man," 121.
10. Derrida, "Ends of Man," 121.
11. Derrida, "Ends of Man," 121.
12. Derrida, "Ends of Man," 122.
13. Heidegger, "Letter on Humanism," 198, quoted in Derrida, "Ends of Man," 128.
14. Derrida, "Ends of Man," 128.
15. Derrida, "Ends of Man," 135.
16. Derrida, "Ends of Man," 135.
17. Derrida, "Ends of Man," 135.
18. Derrida, "Ends of Man," 135.
19. Derrida, "Ends of Man," 136.
20. Heidegger, *Nietzsche*.
21. Heidegger, *Nietzsche*, 221.
22. Nietzsche, *Zarathustra*, 111.
23. Heidegger, *Nietzsche*, 224, 225.
24. Heidegger, *Nietzsche*, 218.
25. Nietzsche, *Zarathustra*, 77, "On the Tarantulas."
26. Derrida, "Ends of Man," 136.
27. Nietzsche, *Genealogy of Morals*, 73, 74 (II, §11).
28. Heidegger, *Nietzsche*, 226.
29. Derrida, *Negotiations*, 382.
30. Benyus, *Biomimicry*.

CHAPTER 4

Autoplasticity

Alain Pottage

▪ For Catherine Malabou, the science of "epigenetics" augurs "new conditions of experience, new thresholds of rationality, as well as new philosophical and theoretical paradigms."[1] "Plasticity"—her own philosophical work in progress—is enriched by the sense of epigenetics as the science of that which is "genetically programmed to develop and operate without program, plan, determinism, schedule, design or preschematization." The reception of epigenetics into critical thought might be construed as a peripheral effect of what popular science writers call "the epigenetics revolution."[2] And it may be more interesting to begin with a reflection on the underlying dynamics of this "revolution" rather than with the semantic potentialities of the notion of epigenetic agency itself. After all, the notion of epigenesis is old enough to have emerged as one of the archaeological[3] moments of modern philosophy. Kant's invocation of "the epigenesis of pure reason" in his explanation of how experience comes to be harmonious with "the conceptions of its objects" drew on a keen understanding of developments in the life sciences of the eighteenth century.[4] So what makes epigenetics so revolutionary and so generative for contemporary critical reflection?

One answer is suggested by the term itself, by the fact that we now talk about epigenetics rather than epigenesis. The "epigenetics revolution" was revolutionary because it came after the invention of genetics and after the twentieth-century paradigm of the genetic program, of which the ultimate flourish was the sequencing of the human genome and the consolidation of genomics as the primary conceptual and institutional framework for biomedical research. If genomics is the set of techniques and experimental settings associated with sequencing and mapping projects, then epigenetics reemerged[5] as a revolutionary science because of the need to explain, first, the density and complexity of the mechanisms involved in regulating gene expression and, second, the emergence of research findings that were incompatible with the paradigm of the genetic program.[6]

Arguably, the first experiments revealing epigenetic effects—crudely, durable changes in gene function that could not be explained by reference to changes in gene structure—can be retraced to the 1890s and the so-called Baldwin effect.[7] It has been plain for some time that the "reading" of gene sequences is conditioned by context, and these experimental findings remained in the background for reasons that are amply discussed in histories of molecular biology: the basic impulse of Mendelian genetics was to seek out traits that remained stable—or could be held steady—throughout ontogenetic development and across generations. It followed that the tools, techniques, and animal models of twentieth-century molecular biology were selected or designed to reveal phenomena that were stable across generations; after the discovery of the double helix, research focused on the structural and functional analysis of DNA as the "prime mover"[8] in the production and reproduction of life. So genetics and, then, the epigenetics revolution presuppose the set of infrastructural developments that social studies of science have made it their business to explore.[9] If one abstracts the semantic forms of epigenetics from the infrastructures that make (up) scientific knowledge, one loses sight of the fact that semantic potential is an effect of these sociotechnical *dispositifs*. We should recall the crude point that epigenetic process is not a dynamic inherent in life but a dynamic ascribed to life by these dispositifs.

We know that signifiers, such as "epigenetics," emerge and circulate as vehicles of the "promissory" logic of biomedical research programs[10] and that they function as attractors and intermediaries in the formation of nexuses of research funding, political imperatives, materialized standards, and experimental regimes. More specifically, we know that many of the trade journals in which these signifiers are retailed are the primary media for the articulation of this promissory logic[11]—material, textual, proof of the proposition that "fresh money and new information are the two central motives of modern social dynamics."[12] The speculative dynamic of biomedical research is one effect of the social-structural articulation of "information":

Information cannot be repeated; as soon as it becomes an event, it becomes non-information. A news item run twice might still have its meaning, but it loses its information value. If information is used as a code value, this means that the operations in the system are constantly and inevitably transforming information into non-information. The crossing of the boundary from value to opposing value occurs within the very autopoiesis of the system. The system is constantly feeding its own output, that is, knowledge of certain facts, back into the system on the negative side of the code, as non-information; and in doing so it forces itself constantly to provide new information.[13]

The effects of this compulsive dynamic are plain enough in the academic world, in the aesthetics of conference themes, in the coining of book and article titles, and in the imperative to come up with "new" ideas (to which one might add the use of personal websites and social media to "place" these novel productions). These phenomena are not merely incidental or supplemental effects. They are symptomatic of the role of the mass media in accelerating cognition by constituting and refreshing the baseline of "common" knowledge and in generating the techniques of schematization that are used in any specialized discourse.[14]

Luhmann's deceptively simple proposition is that "whatever we know about our society, or indeed about the world in which we live, we know through the mass media."[15] Here, the implication is that reflection on the question of how concepts such as epigenesis emerge and hold our attention opens into a reflection on the medial and social-structural processes in which philosophy and critical theory are enmeshed. My hypothesis is that these social-structural processes exemplify a mode of plasticity that illuminates and intensifies the sense of plasticity that Malabou elicits from the biological theory of epigenetics. For some, the question of what critical thought has to take into account in reflecting on its own conditions of possibility cannot rest with media in Luhmann's sense but should go into the technical "communication of communication."[16] But Luhmann's account offers a unique insight into the social-structural articulations in which critical philosophy or social theory is enmeshed.

There are strong resonances—and perhaps kinship bonds—between Luhmann's theory of autopoietic social systems and some of the theories of cellular self-organization that have been informed by or brought to bear on the observation of epigenetic effects. In the course of his discussion of how the mass media function to "increase society's capacity for irritation and thus also its ability to produce information,"[17] Luhmann refers to biological epistemology as one of the "empirical sciences" that corroborate the basic premise of radical constructivism—"no cognitive system, whether it operates as consciousness or as a system of communication, can reach its environment operationally."[18] So attention to the dynamics of the epigenetics revolution also yields a sense of the dynamic evoked by the notion of epigenetics—namely, a dynamic of "autoplasticity."

ENVIRONMENT

In the late 1990s, before the completion of the first map of the human genome was announced to the world in a carefully staged media event, epigenetics was already being cast as the "coming revolution" in biology.[19] The turn to epigenetics was informed by experimental observations that revealed variable "readings" of nucleotide sequences—more precisely, readings that were dependent on the state of cellular metabolism: "It is from the complex regulatory dynamics of the cell as a whole, and not from the gene itself, that the signal (or signals) determining the specific pattern in which the final transcript is to be formed actually comes."[20] The two basic mechanisms of epigenetic modification are DNA methylation and chromatin conformation. The expression of certain genes is affected by the presence of the chemical compound methyl on the promoter regions of the relevant gene. Because the bond between this methyl compound and the DNA sequence to which it is attached is produced by the action of an enzyme—methylase—the state of methylation is ultimately attributable to the functioning of the cellular program rather than chemical specificity or chemical action. And these programmed states persist throughout the life of an organism: "A given pattern of functional genomic activity is maintained in a state of nuclear and cytoplasmic enzymatic activities. This functional state is transmitted as such during cell division of differentiated cells although the DNA structures are always the same in undifferentiated and in all the differentiated cells of the various tissues of an organism."[21] On this basis one can speak of "epimutations"—so called because they affect the mechanisms which control the function of nucleotide sequences rather than the very structure of those sequences[22]—but it is less clear to what extent these mutations are transmissible through transgenerational inheritance rather than cellular division.

Some time before it was heralded as the cause of a revolution in molecular biology and as an exemplification of "plasticity" in Malabou's sense, epigenetics had already given rise to a biological-epistemological theory of plasticity in the shape of Maturana and Varela's theory of autopoiesis: "Living beings are autopoietic systems [in that] their being implies the ongoing participation of all their constitutive elements, such that no single one can be said to be solely responsible for its characteristics as such. That is why, stricto sensu, one cannot speak of genetic determinism or [say] that certain traits are genetically determined nor that a specific trait in an organism is determined by the DNA of its cells. More properly, every trait or character of the organism emerges from an epigenetic process that consists in an ontogenetic structural drift."[23] Here, "epigenetics" is given a particular meaning; the "genetic cause" of the organism is not its DNA but an ongoing process of self-production: "That living beings have an organisation, of course, is proper not only to them but also to everything we can analyse as a system. What is distinctive about them, however, is that their organisation is such that their only product is themselves, with no separation between producer and product. The being and doing of an autopoietic unity are inseparable, and this is their specific mode of organisation."[24]

Maturana and Varela's theory of autopoiesis is vital to any biologically informed reflection on plasticity because it makes an "autochthonous" linkage between plasticity and epigenetics within biological epistemology and because it gives us the essential sense of plasticity as a poietic rather than an ontic process. But to get at the complex nature of social autoplasticity we need to draw out a dimension that plays only a minimal role in Maturana and Varela's theory of self-production: namely, environment.[25] Although the biological theory of autopoiesis gives a particular meaning to "epigenesis," it has some affinities with Waddington's original program of epigenetics, which shifted the focus of evolutionary biology away from the emphasis on environment, in the Darwinian sense of a theater of competition between species, and toward the organization and agency of the organism itself: "It is by paying further attention to the nature of the evolving animal, rather than to that of the environment, that we seem likely to make the most rapid progress in our understanding of evolution."[26] From the perspective of evolutionary biology in the mid-twentieth century, this shift in focus

Autoplasticity 77

was an essential corrective, but, ironically, the effect may have been to foster neglect of the question of environment, and hence of an essential dimension of self-production.

Epigenetics in the contemporary sense necessarily raises the social-theoretical question of what we mean by "context" or "environment" but addresses it somewhat reductively. If the basic premise is that the agency of DNA sequences is conditioned by cellular metabolism, these metabolic processes already give us one sense of context or environment. But cells are themselves contextualized in organisms and in material and social environments, and these broader contexts are brought into view by environmental epigenetics (epigenetics has now become sufficiently well established to have its own subdomains). This branch of the science asks questions such as the following: "how do changes in the social and material environment have a physiological impact on individuals and on forms of sociality, and how may these be passed on to subsequent generations?"[27] This is associated with a certain way of modeling context or environment: "Spatial context includes 'genomic neighbourhoods,' for example, whether a DNA section is matrix-bound or not; the organism, for example, incorporating an organism's metabolic system into an experimental design by feeding methyl-donor enriched diets to mice rather than injecting them directly with methyl groups; and socio-material environments, for example, using data on child abuse in studies of receptor methylation or changing nesting and bedding material in animal studies to induce stress."[28] For this science, "reading up on twentieth-century social theory is not seen as the most useful way of advancing epigenetic research,"[29] so environmental epigeneticists work with a highly selective and formalistic set of ciphers that ultimately lead to the reductive "molecularization" of the environment.[30]

In his essay "Le vivant et son milieu," Georges Canguilhem briefly notices the phenomenon of epigenesis. In proposing his specifically biological conception of environment, Canguilhem takes the example of phenotypic variation in hybrids—"*les bâtards de deux espèces différentes*"—as evidence for the proposition that "the power of genes varies according to their cytoplasmic environment [*la puissance des gènes diffère en fonction du milieu cytoplasmique*]."[31] He makes no reference to the trajectory that (at that time) led from the directly contemporaneous[32] work of Waddington back to the work of Schmalhausen, Morgan, and Baldwin[33] and no reference to the genetics whose "beyond" is brought into view by epigenetics. It has been said of Canguilhem that he did not really think through the implications of the discovery of the double helix in 1962 or rethink his own theories in the light of that discovery,[34] but for present purposes the most interesting thing about this reference to epigenetics is the context in which it figures; namely, a discussion of "environment" as one of the most vital concepts of twentieth-century thought.[35]

In "Le vivant et son milieu," Canguilhem spends some time analyzing von Uexküll's sense of the environment [*Umwelt*] as a dimension relative to each species. Apparently, the biological sense of *Umwelt* was inspired by a sociological observation made by von Uexküll during a stay in his Italian villa. The coincidence of three entirely different descriptions of the Bay of Naples, one given in a guidebook, one by a local resident, and a third by "a bored American tourist," suggested to him that there was no such thing as an "objective" environment.[36] Ultimately, this insight informed the biosemiotic theory[37] that made the tick the celebrity parasite of philosophical literature:[38]

> The tick's life history provides support for the validity of the biological versus the heretofore customary physiological approach. To the physiologist, every living creature is an object that exists in his human world. He investigates the organs of living things and the way they work together, as a technician would examine a strange machine. The biologist, on the other hand, takes into account each individual as a subject, living in a world of its own, of which it is the center. It cannot, therefore, be compared to a machine, but only to the engineer who operates the machine.

The environment is not a universal plane or continuum but a horizon of signals that are apprehended and processed by the organism in accordance with its own vital preferences. As Canguilhem puts it, "the organism finds only what it seeks [*Si le vivant ne cherche pas, il ne reçoit rien*]."[39] Canguilhem derives from von Uexküll's notion of *Umwelt* the proposition that living beings are always normatively engaged with their environments; they exist through processes of discriminating, selecting, weighing, and deciding—"*Il n'y a pas d'indifférence biologique. Dès lors, on peut parler de normativité biologique.*"[40] These "preferences" call the organism's environment into being.

Although the most essential contribution of Canguilhem's essay might be its apprehension of "environment" as a basic figure of contemporary thought, it develops two particular notions that are vital to autoplasticity. First, there is the notion that environments are correlative to and constituted in a "debate" [*Auseinandersetzung*] with organisms: "To live is to radiate, to organise the environment from a reference point that cannot itself be referred to anything without losing its original meaning [*Vivre c'est rayonner, c'est organiser le milieu à partir d'un centre de référence qui ne peut lui-même être référé sans perdre sa signification originale*]."[41] And there is another sense in which environments are plural:

> From the perspective of biology, the relation between organism and environment is the same as that between parts and whole within the organism itself. The individuality of living beings does not end at its ectodermic borders, and nor does it begin with the cell. The biological relation between a being and its environment is a functional, and therefore mobile, relation, whose terms successively switch roles. The cell is an environment for infracellular elements, the cell itself inhabits an internal environment which is the dimensions of the organ or the organism, and this organism itself inhabits an environment which is to it what the organism is to its component elements.[42]

Taken together, these notions point toward the idea that we should focus not on "organism" or "environment," taken as existent terms, but on the difference between the terms or on the process that differentiates them. Canguilhem often makes the point that the environments imposed on organisms in experimental settings are not those that they make for themselves[43] and that environments are always constituted by an organism's vital schematizations; this is not yet the most essential idea in autoplasticity—the idea that both terms of the relation are effects of a process of self-differentiation.

This brings us to Niklas Luhmann's positioning of "environment" as a vital category of contemporary thought:

> The ontology of substance and essences has no concept of environment at all. The eighteenth century began to rethink this in reflections on the significance of "milieus" for the specification of genuinely indeterminate forms (e.g., human beings). This change can be seen in the concept of "milieu" (which originally meant "middle"). . . . The length of time required to learn this testifies to the difficulty of the idea. Ever since the sixteenth century, word compounds containing "self" and "Selbst" have proliferated in Europe. Yet a good two

hundred years were needed before anyone noticed that this presupposes an environment.⁴⁴

For Luhmann, the significance of the concept of environment is that it "leads to a radical de-ontologizing of objects as such" and hence "no unambiguous localization of any sort of 'items' within the world nor any unambiguous classifying relation between them."⁴⁵ Attention shifts from substantives such as "life," the "person," and "nature" to the differentiations that generate system-specific schematizations of the world. This mode of autoplastic "deontologizing" is also found in Foucault's reconstruction of classical "ethopoiesis."

ETHOPOIESIS

Foucault introduced the notion of ethopoiesis in his lectures *L'herméneutique du sujet*: "The Greeks had a word that we find in Plutarch, and also in Dionysius of Halicarnassus, a word that is very interesting. We find it in the form of a substantive, a verb, and an adjective. It is the expression, or the series of expressions, of the words *ēthopoiein*, *ēthopoiia*, *ēthopoios*. *Ēthopoiein* means to make *ēthos*, to produce *ēthos*, to modify or transform the *ēthos*, the manner of being or the mode of existence of an individual."⁴⁶ The difference between two kinds of knowledge, between those things it was useful to know and those it was not, lay not in the character of the things themselves but in the ethopoietic effects of knowing them. Useful knowledge was knowledge that was "capable of producing a change in the mode of being of the subject."⁴⁷ The techniques of ethopoiesis are summarized in Foucault's seminars on the "technologies of the self [*les techniques de soi*]," which explore how the classical techniques of self-knowing, self-scrutiny, askesis, and gymnastics were engaged in the fashioning of a self. What is in question is "a set of practices by means of which the individual can acquire and assimilate truth, and transform it into a permanent principle of action. *Aletheia* becomes *ethos*. It is a process of intensifying subjectivity."⁴⁸

The proposition that "*aletheia* becomes *ethos*" should be highlighted. It nicely expresses the idea of the self as a process that emerges from or as the differentiation of terms whose existence is referable only to the self that differentiates them. Foucault's characterization of the self as a trajectory—"the presence of self to self in the distance between self and self"⁴⁹—might be taken as a formula for this configuration, in which the self figures twice over in a recursive trajectory of self-observation. In this process of self-observation, the self comes into being in an "original" differentiating of itself from environment and then in managing or structuring that difference by means of mnemonic and expectational techniques that continually turn *aletheia* into *ethos*. The point of phrasing these terms as *aletheia* and *ethos* is that the constitution of the self unfolds the horizon against which the world is revealed, and in turn this process of revealing stimulates or informs the constitution of the self.[50] This is the celebrated Luhmannian notion of "openness on the basis of closure," where closure is not a matter of holding static, quasi-spatial, boundaries but of active self-differentiation. The exercises that Foucault characterizes as technologies of the self mobilize knowledge not for its epistemic benefits but for its effects in constituting the ethical or ethopoietic "equipment"[51] of the subject.

Techniques of meditation first evolved in the context of training for the rhetorical arts. Meditations were mnemonic exercises in which the student anticipated the strategies with which he might be confronted by an opponent. The point of anticipation was recollection. By imagining oneself challenged to mobilize an effective response, one could identify and commit to memory the discursive resources (*orationes* and *logoi*) that would form the premises of counterstrategy. This was not an exercise of stocking and cataloguing inert knowledge: the point was to incorporate precepts as equipment for improvisation. Training is a resource for spontaneous speech. When this form of technique is taken up by the Stoics, two themes come to the fore: imagination and memory.

In Stoic meditations imagination was exercised not to test out alternative objects of thought but to translate the subject into a situation in which it could experiment with itself. What was being actualized in imagination was not a set of variations of thought but a set of variations on or of the subject itself. So imagination became the medium of a kind of virtual gymnastics in which the subject tested its capacity to respond to specific events and measured its progress in developing these capacities. As with exercises in rhetoric, the point was to be prepared for an eventual challenge. . . . How would I react if? For the Stoics being prepared effectively meant equipping oneself with a schematization in which the event was already expected. The experience of an event prompts the formation of a correlative expectation, and that is true even if the experience is virtual or imagined. So what one was developing in this procedure was a set of forms or templates in which the potentialities of the event have already been selectively qualified or reduced by an expectational schema.

Ethical schematizations were formed and assimilated through re-memorization, and they were formed in the medium of precepts and doctrines. But the doctrines that were assimilated through meditation were not ethical rules or deontological algorithms. The object of meditation was not to learn new propositions or to locate oneself in a degree of relation to some body of ethical doctrine: precepts were not memorized as propositional forms one could consult from time to time. Rather, they were memorized as equipment for an ethical life, actualized in and by ethical activity. So how did ethical precepts become equipment?

We should begin with the quality of the precepts themselves. Marcus Aurelius suggested that maxims addressed to oneself as media of recollection should be brief and epigrammatic, the better to be recalled and the better to serve as equipment. They should "be memorable and capable of taking effect immediately in the aid and support of one's life." Maxims were framed as recommendations of how to address oneself to events, as aids to an ongoing practice rather than as prescriptions. Their epigrammatic quality meant that they were actualized in these practices, that it was only within the practice of a specific subject that they acquired their communicative value. Foucault emphasizes that the truth of such prescriptions was "assimilated,to the point of making it a part of oneself, a permanent internal principle that was continuously active with action [*toujours actif d'action*]."[52]

This is why writing was so significant as an "ethopoietic" function. More often than not, precepts were addressed to oneself. There was a kind of pedagogic or amicable economy in which maxims were recommended and exchanged between practitioners, but the central communication is that of the self with itself. And in some sense the message was the medium. What one might call the message of the maxim, its propositional content, was actually the medium of a particular kind of self-relation, a particular quality or focus of scrutiny, a particular mode of problematization. So the use of a precept as "an aid and support to one's life" actually meant folding it into an ongoing self-relation. In a sense the incorporation or actualization of precepts as media or occasions for self-relation is what is important to the notion of equipment. Again, whether imagined or actual, the encounter with an event forms a correlative expectation or schematization, and the ethical precept is simply the rubric within which this encounter is staged, the form that articulates *aletheia* and *ethos*. In a sense, the maxim is not an epistemic form but one that functions nonepistemically, as a device that enables the self to hold open and recursively regulate the difference between self and environment. The self is the set of accumulated competences that emerge from this recursive process of rememorization.

The exemplary ascetic technique was the exercise of *praemeditatio malorum*, premeditating or presuming the worst. For the Stoics, this was a basic meditation, which consisted in imagining that the worst that one could imagine had already happened. One had to imagine that one was already suffering an excruciatingly painful death or undergoing a particularly gruesome form of torture. Imagination transports the self to a future in which the worst is already happening, happening to its fullest intensity and with no prospect of remitting. Foucault suggests that this might be seen as an "eidetic reduction" of future misfortune or rather, perhaps, a process of double reduction: a reduction of the future itself and a reduction of suffering or misfortune as such.

To begin with, the exercise was premised on the Greek prejudice that an orientation towards the future was unethical or unphilosophical: to direct one's attention to the future was to neglect the past, over which one could exercise some mastery, in favor of a domain that was either inexistent or predetermined and, either way, unmasterable. Consistent with this prejudice, the exercise of *praemeditatio malorum* presumes the future in order to abolish it. In Foucault's terms it is not a simulation of the future as such but a simulation of the future—the whole expanse of the future—as present. So the exercise collapses duration or temporal succession into a kind of permanent present. This is the premise of what Foucault calls an eidetic reduction both of the future and of the misfortune that it holds. *Praemeditatio malorum* is an exercise in imagining the worst as "an actualization of the possible rather than a probabilistic calculation."[53] To be always already ready for something *whenever* it happens is in some sense to draw the sting of contingency from events and in the process to reduce the reality of the misfortune. All events have the same value, partly because if the distinguishing feature of before and after survives, it survives only as a formal abstraction, and partly because the event is almost completely saturated by the meaning ascribed to it by ethical training. This exercise might not allow one to stave off death or torture, but it does allow one to say what the Stoics said: either pain is so intense that one cannot bear it and one expires immediately, or it is bearable and therefore slight.

This is how truth becomes ethos. Truth is not propositional but performative, not epistemic but technical, and it is performed by being integrated as the medium of an ongoing self-relation. And the self with which Foucault is concerned is not ontic but poietic. The self consists in making, fabrication, *poiesis*. To return to the resonance between ethopoiesis and autopoiesis, Niklas Luhmann once recalled how the term *autopoiesis* was coined (not by him but by Humberto Maturana) by reference to a distinction between *praxis* and *poiesis*. Praxis is "an action that includes its purpose in itself as an action," an action that is virtuous or satisfying in itself, whereas *poiesis* implies action that produces something:

> *Poiesis* also implies action: one acts, however, not because the action itself is fun or virtuous, but because one wants to produce something.... Maturana then found the bridge between the two concepts and spoke of *autopoiesis*, of a *poiesis* as its product—and he intentionally emphasized the notion of a product. *Autopraxis*, on the other hand, would be a pointless expression, because it would only repeat what is already meant by *praxis*. No, what is meant here is a system that is its own product. The operation is the condition for the production of operations.[54]

Luhmann's autopoietic self or individual is more virtuosic precisely because it is not human, but there is a resonance here that goes directly to the question of plasticity.[55]

SOVEREIGNTY?

According to Malabou, Foucault's analytic of ethopoiesis falls short of true plasticity because it reintroduces the division between the symbolic and the biological: "Even if Foucault insists, particularly in his last seminars, on the importance of the biological body for philosophical discipline, as it appears in Cynicism for example, it is clear that the formation and transformation of the self operate on the symbolic body in the first place. It is clear that we have two bodies in one. In all cases, biology is always dependent on the symbolic. Always derived from it. A secondary phenomenon. Biological life remains obscure, predetermined, genetically programmed, deprived of any meaning. Biology remains attached to control and sovereignty."[56] So even in his lectures on technologies of the self, Foucault remains within a perspective from the "life" that detaches itself from (within); power can only be a "less material and less vital dimension," a "symbolic" counterpart to the "biological." The upshot is that sovereignty cannot be deconstructed because its foundational division persists: "The critique or deconstruction of sovereignty is structured as the very entity it tends to critique or deconstruct. By distinguishing two lives and two bodies, contemporary philosophers reaffirm the theory of sovereignty, that is, the split between the symbolic and the biological."[57]

It is true that the terms of Foucault's reconstruction of ethopoietic practices sometimes suggest that ethopoiesis fashions a quasi-biological body, a body in which biological substance becomes the medium of an essentially discursive or communicative process. For example, the technique of writing figures as a union of the spiritual arts of meditation and the physical practices of gymnastics. According to Seneca, writing gave things a body, "the very body of him who, in the course of transcribing his readings appropriates them to himself and makes their truth his own: writing transforms what is seen or heard into force and blood [*in vires, in sanguinem*]."[58] It is more interesting, however, to persist with the hypothesis that Foucault's technologies of the self point toward and resonate very closely with the general terms of Luhmann's autopoiesis. Again, ethopoiesis is a mode of autoplasticity in which the self differentiates itself from an environment that becomes the self-given "reality" of the self. Life, nature, or "biology" is "environmentalized." This has some crucial implications for the question of sovereignty and for the idea that the kernel of "sovereignty thought" is the division between the symbolic body and the biological body.

To begin with, the effect of "environmentalizing" biology is to dissolve the basic premise of the theory of biopower.[59] If life, nature, and biology are no longer ontic or universal realms but dimensions whose sense and configuration are dependent on the fashioning of the self that is correlative to the environment, then there is no such thing as "life itself." Nor is there such a thing as a symbolic order whose articulation is guaranteed by something like a *signifiant zéro*—the "empty space that gives language its mobility."[60] The environment does not function as a "supplement" or "excess" in the sense suggested by diagnoses of the hidden paradox of the symbolic order. The environment "exceeds" the self or system in the sense that its complexity cannot be matched by the processing capacities of the self, but whereas figures such as the "floating signifier" still start from a relation of reference, in processes of ethopoiesis or autopoiesis reference is eclipsed by self-reference. If the reality of a self or system is self-generated, then axes of reference are orthogonal to the basic process of self-production. Autoplastic processes are paradoxical, but they metabolize paradox rather than hide it; there is no longer any point to the old critical strategy of "reintroducing the excess, unveiling it and making it ungraspable by power."[61] Indeed, the effect of multiplying environments, centers, and worlds is simply and entirely to obviate the question of power and, hence, sovereignty.

NOTES

1. See chapter 1.
2. Carey, *Epigenetics Revolution*.
3. In the sense of Agamben, *Signature of All Things*, ch. 3.
4. Kant, *Critique of Pure Reason*, Deduction of the pure concepts of the understanding, §27. In the register of analogy, Kant distinguishes "the epigenesis of pure reason" from "a kind of preformation-system of pure reason." For an extensive commentary on this analogy, with reference to the historical-scientific context, see Brilman, "Georges Canguilhem," ch. 2.
5. Conrad Waddington first used the term "epigenotype" in *Introduction to Modern Genetics*.
6. Epigenetics can be folded back into the logic of sequencing and mapping. See, e.g., the blurb on the first page of the website of the NIH Roadmap Epigenomics Mapping Consortium: "[The] Consortium was launched with the goal of producing a public resource of human epigenomic data to catalyze basic biology and disease-oriented research. The Consortium leverages experimental pipelines built around next-generation sequencing technologies to map DNA methylation, histone modifications, chromatin accessibility and small RNA transcripts in stem cells and primary ex vivo tissues selected to represent the normal counterparts of tissues and organ systems frequently involved in human disease." www.roadmapepigenomics.org/.
7. After J. Mark Baldwin, particularly the findings discussed in Baldwin, "New Factor," 441–51.
8. For a discussion of Max Delbrück's Aristotelian formula, see Kay, *Who Wrote the Book?*, ch. 5.
9. See notably Kay, *Who Wrote the Book?*; Rheinberger, *Epistemic Things*; and Beurton, Falk, and Rheinberger, *Concept of the Gene*.
10. See notably Sunder Rajan, *Biocapital*.
11. See Mirowski, *Science–Mart*, xx.
12. Luhmann, *Mass Media*, 21.
13. Luhmann, *Mass Media*, 20.

14. "The mass media . . . are media to the extent that they make available background knowledge and carry on writing it as a starting point for communication" (Luhmann, *Mass Media*, 66).

15. Luhmann, *Mass Media*, 1.

16. "More than any other theorists, philosophers forgot to ask which media support their very practice" (Kittler, "Ontology of Media," 23). This observation does not apply only to philosophy before Heidegger; cf. Kittler's comments on Foucault, who, "as the last historian or first archaeologist, merely had to look things up . . . Even writing itself, before it ends up in libraries, is a communication medium, the technology of which the archaeologist simply forgot. It is for this reason that all his analyses end immediately before the point in time at which other media penetrated the library's stacks. Discourse analysis simply cannot be applied to sound archives or towers of film rolls" (Kittler, *Gramophone, Film, Typewriter*, 5). For the "communication of communication," see Winthrop-Young, "Silicon Sociology," 391–420.

17. Luhmann, *Mass Media*, 82.

18. Luhmann, *Mass Media*, 92. See also Luhmann, *Social Systems*, 179: "Scientific analysis . . . could hardly fulfil its task if it restricted itself to purely analytical distinctions and neglected the fact that within the systems it investigates, processes of self-observation are at work, making the difference between system and environment available within these systems themselves." For a discussion of what might be meant by "constructivism," see Luhmann, "Cognitive Program."

19. Strohman, "Epigenesis and Complexity," 194–200.

20. Keller, "The Century of the Gene," 63.

21. Atlan, "Biological Medicine," 271.

22. Holliday, "Epigenetic Defects," 168: "heritable changes based on DNA modification should be designated *epimutations* to distinguish them from classical mutations, which are changes in the DNA sequence (base substitution, insertion, deletion, or rearrangement)."

23. Maturana and Mpodozis, *De l'origine des espèces*, 25.

24. Maturana and Varela, *Tree of Knowledge*, 49.

25. See, e.g., Maturana and Varela, *Autopoiesis and Cognition*, 99: "to talk about a representation of the ambience, or the environment, in the organization of a living system may be metaphorically useful, but it is inadequate and misleading to reveal the organization of an autopoietic system."

26. Waddington, "Epigenetics and Evolution," 190.

27. Niewöhner, "Epigenetics," 284.

28. Niewöhner, "Epigenetics," 285.

29. Niewöhner, "Epigenetics," 286.

30. "The process that I refer to as the molecularisation of biography and milieu [consists in] the extraction of significant events from people's biographies,

from particular and situated socio-cultural histories and their embeddedness in particular milieu and everyday lives, and their conversion into standardised representations of particular forms of social change that can be correlated with the material body. The molecularisation of biography and milieu results in standard models of social change, which are able to travel between labs and into the wider public discourse" (Niewöhner, "Epigenetics," 291).

31. Canguilhem, "Le vivant et son milieu," 148.

32. Canguilhem, "Le vivant et son milieu" is the text of a lecture given at the Collège philosophique in 1946/47.

33. See Hall, "Organic Selection," 215–37.

34. See Lecourt, "Georges Canguilhem," 223: "In his own way, Canguilhem is saluting, by simply transferring his concepts, the latest developments in the theory of genetic codes. They seem to have realized, in ways that seemed to him impossible, the project he outlined in 1943! Hence the strangely disabused but triumphant tone in which he demonstrates that the 'concept' is inscribed within 'life' in the form of a code. . . . No doubt he attached too much importance to the formalist version of 'code' to which molecular biology almost surrendered in the mid-1960s." For analysis of this position, see Brilman, *Georges Canguilhem*, ch. 5.

35. Canguilhem observes that "the notion of environment is becoming a universal and essential way of grasping the experience and existence of living beings, and one might almost go so far as to say that it is being constituted as a category of contemporary thought [*La notion de milieu est en train de devenir un mode universel et obligatoire de saisie de l'expérience et de l'existence des êtres vivants et on pourrait presque parler de sa constitution comme catégorie de la pensée contemporaine*]" (Canguilhem, "Le vivant et son milieu," 165). See generally Brilman, *Georges Canguilhem*, ch. 3.

36. Uexküll, *Niegeschaute Welten*, cited in Brilman, *Georges Canguilhem*, 118.

37. Uexküll, xx. "The receptor signs of a group of receptor cells are combined outside the receptor organ, indeed outside the animal, into units that become the properties of external objects. This projection of sensory impressions is a self-evident fact. All our human sensations, which represent our specific receptor signs, unite into perceptual cues [*Merkmal*] which constitute the attributes of external objects and serve as the real basis of our actions. The sensation 'blue' becomes the 'blueness' of the sky; the sensation 'green,' the 'greenness' of the lawn. These are the cues by which we recognize the objects: blue, the sky; green, the lawn."

38. See notably Deleuze and Guattari, *Mille plateaux*, and Agamben, *The Open*.

39. Canguilhem, "Le vivant et son milieu," 144.

40. Canguilhem, "Le vivant et son milieu," 79.

41. Canguilhem, "Le vivant et son milieu," 147. Brilman cites Goldstein's critique of Uexküll, according to which "the environment is by no means something definite and static but is continuously forming commensurably with the

development of the organism and its activity," and speculates that the term that Goldstein uses for this continuous process—*Auseinandersetzung*—might follow Heidegger's use of the term in the 1930s in his lectures on Nietzsche: "In confrontation [*Auseinandersetzung*], the world comes to be" (Brilman, "Georges Canguilhem," 121).

42. Canguilhem, "Le vivant et son milieu," 144.
43. Canguilhem, "Le vivant et son milieu," 146.
44. Luhmann, *Social Systems*, 537–38.
45. Luhmann, *Social Systems*, 177.
46. Foucault, *L'herméneutique du sujet*, 227.
47. Foucault, *L'herméneutique du sujet*, 228.
48. Foucault, "Les techniques de soi," 800.
49. Foucault, *L'herméneutique du sujet*, 214.
50. In Luhmann's terms, *aletheia* is by way of "irritability": "Irritability is the most general structural characteristic of autopoietic systems, which in modern description occupies that place once accorded to nature and to the essence of things defined as nature. Irritability arises from the system having a memory that is actively involved in all operations and therefore able to experience and balance out inconsistencies—which means nothing other than being able to generate reality. This points to a recursive constitutive context of memory, irritability, information processing, reality construction and memory" (Luhmann, *Mass Media*, 98).
51. To borrow Paul Rabinow's felicitous translation.
52. Foucault, 'L'herméneutique du sujet' in *Dits et Ecrits*, vol. 4, 353–65, at 362.
53. Foucault, 'Les techniques de soi,' in *Dits et Ecrits*, vol. 4, at 801.
54. Moeller, *Luhmann Explained*, 12.
55. There is no point here in detailing the significant—and numerous—differences between Foucauldian and Luhmannian senses of poiesis.
56. Malabou, ch. 1, 42.
57. Malabou, ch. 1, 39.
58. Foucault, "L'écriture de soi," 422.
59. The insights of Foucault's writings on biopower might instead be framed in terms of a process of semantics. "The semantics of corporeality, with its undeniable influence on the experience and use of the body, correlates with the change of forms in sociocultural evolution, not because the human body is a mere substance (as a support for capabilities) or a mere instrument or social use, but because it is included in the interpenetration of human beings and the social system" (Luhmann, *Social Systems*, 251).
60. Malabou, ch. 1, 41.
61. Malabou, ch. 1, 42.

CHAPTER 5

Plasticity, Capital, and the Dialectic

Alberto Toscano

▪ What thinking of capital—in the objective and subjective genitive— is staged in plasticity? And what resources does the thinking of change animated by the concept of plasticity provide for envisaging the change in and out of capital? In an intellectual and political moment when linear conceptions of development have long lost any credence and enthusiastic celebrations of becoming ring increasingly hollow, Malabou's sustained inquiry into philosophical and scientific modalities of change is a welcome spur and inspiration for anyone wishing to rethink the dialectical character of contemporary social forms. In her attempt to endow plasticity with the character of an ethical and political conception of the world, in intimate dialogue with the sciences of the brain, Malabou has challenged the neoliberal formatting of change under the imperatives of flexibility, adaptability, and employability. The spiritual hegemony of such capitalist conceptions of change is evidently one of the extraphilosophical sources for the sense of urgency and intervention that marks her project. Malabou has also enjoined us to rediscover the Hegelian dialectic by recasting it in terms of the form-giving and form-receiving, reproductive and explosive features of plasticity. Yet in evident contradistinction to the rich and wide stream of interpretations of Hegel that present him as a thinker of social ontology first and foremost, Malabou's exploration of the dialectic has been almost exclusively philosophical in the specific sense of not treating the social as constitutive of the conceptual—a question to which I'll return below.

Yet the modern dialectic is synonymous with a thinking in and against the social forms of modernity, of bourgeois society in the wake of the French Revolution. It is also—and I would argue that this is the dimension of the dialectic most vital in our present—a thinking in and against capital (though we could also say, as Fredric Jameson has suggested, that it is also, paradoxically, a thinking which as a praxis could exist only on the other side of capital).[1] Definitions of the dialectic are rife, unsurprisingly contradictory, and arduous to totalize.[2] Here, I explore the notion that the dialectic is philosophy under condition of capital, a condition which implies the *expatriation* of philosophy, its not being at home in itself, its not being at home *tout court*. I'll try to specify this "expatriation" by outlining the manner in which, as an abstract thinking, philosophy may be outside itself, beside itself, beyond itself—in a sense that gives a social, political, and economic dimension to what Malabou calls "the *self-destructive* or *self-deconstructive tendency* of philosophy,"[3] but also allows us to explore "the ability of the dialectic to *negotiate with its destruction*."[4] This entails indicating the sense in which I distance myself from Malabou's lapidary declaration in *Plasticity at the Dusk of Writing* that the "new era" "is certainly no longer the era of the dialectic" (in effect, I would like to distance myself from the very idea of a "new era"). In fact, I want to suggest that the nondialectical sublation of the dialectic proposed by Malabou in *Plasticity* is troubled if we add to her polyvalent exploration of the W-W-V triad—*Wandel, Wandlung, Verwandlung* (change, transformation, metamorphosis)—the U of *Übergang*, or transition, the problem of the "other change" in Marx, the change against and beyond exchange. Or, to the extent that Malabou notes that her question is about transformation,[5] I want to think, in counterpoint to her work, what "transformation" may mean in and beyond capital or beyond the form of value as the principle of our social synthesis.

In a curious inversion, the problem of the social ontology of change is broached not in Malabou's writing on Hegel but in her more recent *Le change Heidegger*, a book that has the rare capacity of generating an "impious," profane illumination from Heidegger's work, of—to quote one of the few books, along with Malabou's, to recast Heidegger outside "Heideggerianism"—creating a "*topos* where the man Martin Heidegger undoubtedly would not so much have liked to see himself led."[6] And one of the topoi alien to "the man Martin Heidegger," but for some oblique and superficial remarks, is the question of the ontology of capital, understood as something other than the deployment of the essence of technology or an iteration of the epochal metaphysics of subjectivity. It is to this key question of dialectical thought that Malabou gestures in the conclusion of *Le change Heidegger*, where she writes: "There obviously exists a proximity between Heidegger and Marx, which rests no doubt on the thinking of a possible coincidence between the ontological and the economic in the definition of exchange, of exchangeability and mutability, of the metamorphosable and displaceable character of value and the impossibility of transgressing this plasticity."[7] But what if exchange, as an anoriginary, dispossessing origin of philosophy expropriated the self-sufficiency of philosophy, the consistency of ontology, and the sovereignty of the philosophical? To locate the crux of the dialectic in the real abstractions of money and exchange, in the seemingly autonomous logic of the categories of capital, as Marx and a number of his more speculatively oriented commentators have done, is to suggest the possibility that, to somewhat pastiche Heidegger, *the essence of philosophy is not philosophical*—in other words, that inasmuch as the unique ontology of capitalism sees abstractions having a social existence external to and in many ways indifferent to *mental* or *philosophical* abstraction, the problems of philosophy have a directly social character. This also means, as I will touch on below in terms of Malabou's critique of the neuronal ideology of neoliberalism, that philosophy can no longer propose its ethical or political mission as that of providing a conceptual synthesis for other disciplines or practices. If, as the likes of Adorno pointed out long ago, social life is already conceptual through and through, albeit in inverted and mystified ways, the notion that philosophy can propose concepts—such as plasticity—to reorient our practices is put into question.

Malabou's call to "put an end to the *dematerialization* and *demonetarization* of contemporary philosophy"[8] is a timely one. But I think for this not to remain simply a mutation in the reservoir of analogies, images, or metaphors of philosophy but a real challenge to philosophy's own ultimately sterile self-sufficiency, it involves exploring the ways in which the conceptual or speculative character of the existence of capital forces philosophy outside of itself, obliging it to reflect on how it is constituted by abstractions not of the mind. To put it paradoxically, philosophy can rematerialize only to the extent that it grasps the "spiritualized" character of capitalism. Inasmuch as capitalism is an *actually existing metaphysics*, philosophy is a crucial component of any transformative analytic of social life—as Marx amply demonstrated by mapping the inner dynamic of capital onto the logic of Hegelian categories; but philosophy is also revealed as increasingly obsolete in its image as a kind of ideological reservoir of worldviews that could be proposed *to* other practices and disciplines.

It is again with respect to Heidegger and not Hegel that Malabou poses the problem of the entanglement between metaphysics and capitalism. In Heidegger's philosophy, she writes, "*metaphysics* and *capitalism* coincide: hence too, 'other *thought*' and '*revolution*' coincide. The two logics at work in Western change are generalized equivalence (*Geltung*)—everything is equal to everything, any being can be exchanged for another according to the mercantile arrogance of calculus—and favor (*Gunst*)—the future exchange is exchange by *disappropriation*."[9] Homing in on the first of these logics, that of commensurability, indifference, or universal exchange, is crucial for any understanding of philosophy's relation to capital (and, a fortiori, for any elucidation of just what a nonphilosophical thinking and a revolutionary practice could mean in the present). But the coincidence or identity of metaphysics and capitalism is not a symmetrical one. In fact, it could be demonstrated that in Heidegger's work, as in most philosophical reflections on the constitution of capitalism, the latter is presented as the effect of a particular metaphysics that both precedes and underlies it. It is because being is metaphysically configured as indifferently exchangeable, as an ultimately abstract object at the disposal of arbitrary subjective will, that capitalism is possible. The perspective I would like to adopt instead, taking inspiration from Alfred Sohn-Rethel's pioneering reflections on "real abstraction"—that is, on the origin of philosophical thought and modern subjectivity in the nonmental practice of commodity exchange and the mediations of the money form—is that it is the extramental logic of commodity exchange which underlies "Western change" and that, consequently, to put it in somewhat exaggerated but I think pertinent terms, while *the essence of capitalism is not metaphysical, the essence of metaphysics is capitalist*. The consequences for thinking the "coincidence" of capitalism and metaphysics are considerable.

First of all, it requires, against any Eurocentric pieties about the singularity of philosophy's Greek origin, a radically profane expatriation: it is the contingent emergence of entirely mundane forms of social abstraction pivoting around monetary exchange that permitted the particular type of abstractions characteristic of ancient Greek philosophy to emerge, not any mysterious spiritual features of that civilization. Money is abstraction made tangible and visible, the representative, equivalent, and medium of a fundamentally impersonal exchange, a relationship without qualities. Ideal abstraction (philosophy) is derivative but also in a way identical to the real abstraction of exchange.

According to Sohn-Rethel's *Intellectual and Manual Labour*, the "act of exchange has to be described as abstract movement through abstract (homogeneous, continuous, and empty) space and time of abstract substances (materially real but bare of sense-qualities) which thereby suffer no material change and which allow for none but quantitative differentiation (differentiation in abstract, non-dimensional quantity)."[10] The same underlying schema accounts for the productive heuristic fiction of homogeneous spatiotemporal individuation and for the fact that "in the marketplace and in shop windows, things stand still,"[11] steeped as they are in the separation in time and space of the practices of use and the acts of exchange.

It is the spatiotemporal distinction between use and exchange which makes it possible to locate a "material" and historical basis for formal and ahistorical modes of thinking and practice. "The exchange-abstraction," Sohn-Rethel notes, "is the historical, spatio-temporal origin of atemporal, ahistorical thought."[12] The nature of exchange is such that the "abstract" activity of equivalence and commensuration is concrete, while use value becomes a matter of ideal representation and thus turns out to be abstract. This separation has to do with the "purely social postulate" that things can indeed be instantaneously frozen, a logical requirement for the exchange of commodities which is "then" projected onto the natural world. The "mental" reflection of commodity exchange takes place through money as an *abstract thing*. Coined money is the value form made visible and the token of a socially unconscious practice: "Abstraction is therefore the effect of the action of men, and not of their thought. In reality, it takes place 'behind their backs,' at the blind spot, so to speak, of human consciousness, that is there where the thinking and efforts of men are absorbed by their acts of exchange."[13] Unlike binding and embedded forms of precapitalist sociality, money as a social nexus is "formally unlimited."[14] This is a formal and logical echo of Marx's reflections about the manner in which money poses itself as the antithesis of any community other than itself. It is not only formally unlimited but tendentially exclusive.

In the second notebook of the *Grundrisse*, from November 1857, Marx noted the way in which money "directly and simultaneously becomes the *real community*, since it is the general substance of survival for all, and at the same time the social product of all. But as we have seen, in money the community is at the same time a mere abstraction, a mere external, accidental thing for the individual, and at the same time merely a means for his satisfaction as an isolated individual. The community of antiquity presupposes a quite different relation to, and on the part of, the individual. The development of money . . . therefore smashes this community."[15] Or, as the mention of "mere" abstraction suggests (which we could juxtapose to the *real* abstraction of money), it recodes the pre-monetized community as an auxiliary resource for the real community of money, deployed or retracted in keeping with the imperatives of accumulation.

But money is not just real community; it is also a *sensus communis*. Monetized exchange structures a whole socially transcendental aesthetic, which is not solely a matter of commensurability (and of its dialectical reliance on singularity or the appearance of uniqueness), but also that of a practical arrest of time and evacuation of space, which customary tools of psychology or, indeed, of philosophy itself are powerless to analyze. This monetized abstraction is an activity that is simultaneously relational and impersonal rather than in any sense primarily mental.

The crucial thing to grasp is that Sohn-Rethel's derivation does not move from the density of empirically observable and palpably material social relations to the supposedly distorting and transcendent illusions of philosophy; it takes its cue from Marx's conception of value as a social form to ground ideal abstractions in real abstraction. In this account philosophy can thus be seen to develop from the "socialized mind of man." As Sohn-Rethel declares in one of the most peremptory and provocative of his formulations, philosophy "is money without its material attachments, immaterial and no longer recognisable as money and, indeed, no longer being money but the 'pure intellect.'"[16]

The aim here is that of "putting Kant back on his feet," by analogy with Marx's notorious statement on Hegel; to show how the synthetic powers of the transcendental subject are really social powers. Or as Adorno noted in *Negative Dialectics*—partially acknowledging the considerable impact of Sohn-Rethel's thesis on the development of his own thought ever since their first contact in the late 1920s—the transcendental subject is "society unconscious of itself."[17] The elimination of society from abstract philosophical thought is a product of society itself; it is an abstraction that society makes from itself in intellectual labor and in the primacy of exchange as form of mediation. Capitalism is an abstract society where the social nexus is not generated primarily by custom, reciprocity, or tradition—though these are both the material and forms of appearance of capitalist society—but in the indifference of exchange. The profound theoretical originality of Marx is thus to be sought in the fact that he provides "the first explanation of the historical origin of a pure phenomenon of form."[18]

This perspective is very important, to my mind, if we are to approach the problem posed by Malabou, that of the seemingly intimate convertibility between philosophical exchangeability (or an ontological economy) and the exchange and accumulation of capital. In *Plasticity at the Dusk of Writing* she writes: "alterity can be thought without the aid of transcendence, if it is true that there is nothing outside, nothing beyond—outside the economy and outside the exchangeability or mutability of Being—then *there is no inconvertibility. Absolute convertibility, the migratory and metamorphic resource of alterity, is the rule. Absolute exchangeability is the structure.*"[19] But, if we are to accept Sohn-Rethel's interpretation of the singularity of Marx's relationship to philosophy and epistemology as lying in the capacity of the Marxian approach to establish the origination of the mental and philosophical forms of abstraction in the socioeconomic, practical form of exchange, then this structure is not to be thought of in terms of a general economy that would subsume the ontological economy and, so to speak, the economic economy, but as a determinate form of social synthesis which overdetermines the forms of ontology and metaphysics.

Malabou's challenge in her reflections on Heidegger—to think the bond between exchangeability as a capitalist and a metaphysical principle in the ambit of a radical thinking of change—is to be welcomed. But in treating exchangeability as the object above all of philosophical reflection, she risks, in the guise of an appeal for another thinking, reasserting philosophy's vocation to comprehend, in the sense of encompassing and exhausting, change itself—in a repetition of that primacy of philosophy over the domain of abstractions that the very notion of real abstraction so powerfully deconstructs. This is especially evident in her allegiance to the Heideggerian motif of the originary, itself convertible with the ontological. Malabou writes of an ontological mutability that "presupposes the originary economy of an exchange before exchange before economy. Before money, before price, before sex. Before commerce. Before history itself."[20] But the difference between a general, metaphysical thinking of abstraction and a thinking of the determinate, historical emergence of real abstractions is precisely that *there is no originary economy*, that economy, especially in its capacity to shape philosophical thinking "behind its back," is the dissipation of a thinking of the originary. Or, to put it another way, that the origin effect is a contingent but logically self-consistent effect of a social form. The essence of philosophy is not philosophical. If we wish to test philosophy's political valences, its potential to dislocate present impasses of thought and action, we will not do this by presenting philosophy's work on itself as the prelude to the creation (or reform) of concepts *for* other disciplines and practices. We would need to start instead from the moment of philosophy's expatriation, from a comprehension of philosophy being beside itself (in history, in science, in politics, in capital . . .); from the scandal that abstractions are in the social "before" they are in the mind. But this, unlike Heidegger's, is a totally profane "before," a strictly *meaningless* before—which can expatriate philosophy from its morbid pieties about its Greek or "Western" origins and truly terminate its dematerialization and demonetization.

This expatriation, as we encounter it in Sohn-Rethel and others who have located ontological convertibility in the social practices of ancient Greece, rather than in any misty realm of the spirit, is a matter of currency and coin. It is all the more interesting, in this respect, that Malabou brings our attention to some of the passages in Heidegger where the ontological scandal of money springs forth, closing *Le change Heidegger* on Heidegger's musings in the essay "Why Poets?" on Rilke and money. The encounter of poetry in a desolate time with the form of money takes the guise of a kind of threnody not so much for lost objects as for lost things, for originary relations not dissolved in the corrosive circuits of currency. Heidegger quotes the following verses from Rilke's "Book of Pilgrimage," the second book of the *Book of Hours*:

> The kings of the world are old,
> and they will have no heirs.
> The sons are dying as boys,
> and their pale daughters gave
> all the sickly crowns to force.
> The rabble grinds them into specie:
> the time-serving lord of the world
> distends them in the fire: makes them machines
> that grumble and serve his will;

but happiness is not among them.
The ore is homesick. Its desire
is to forsake the coins and the wheels
that teach it to live small.
And from the factories and from the tills
it will return into earthly veins:
the adits of the mountains
close behind it on its return.[21]

The plebeian sociality of labor timed and abstracted—*The rabble grinds them into specie*—is not the site of a possible emancipation, say, of a species-being finding in its daily "grind" the wherewithal to turn *the coins and the wheels* to better ends. As the juxtaposition between chthonic ore and worldly coin, or the natural-ontological and the social-ontic, suggests, the poetic gaze is here one of nostalgic distress. Two passages from Rilke's letters, quoted by Heidegger, reinforce this impression of poetic saying not traversing but simply resisting the onslaught of generalized exchangeability. The first is articulated in terms of European authenticity against the banal barbarism of the New World (a note echoed in Heidegger's own lectures): "Now, from America, empty indifferent things, sham things, *counterfeit life* are pushing their way across."[22] Capital's adoptive home simulates the ontology of the thing in the ubiquity of the commodity, whose dynamic is that of a devouring, unstoppable indifference. The second quotation is more ambiguous, finding in the "sensible-supersensible" nature of money a weird kind of spirituality: "The world withdraws into itself; and things, for their part, behave in the same way, by transferring their existence increasingly into the vibration of money and developing for themselves a kind of spirituality there that even now exceeds their tangible reality. In the period I am dealing with [Rilke means the fourteenth century]—money was still gold, still metal, a lovely object, the handiest, the most lucid thing of all."[23]

Yet in this contrast of the thing and the product, ore and money, as both allegory and reference point for Heidegger's confrontation with the question concerning capital, we encounter the absolute limits of his conception of change and the resources it may harbor for a contemporary thinking, such as the one proposed by Malabou, capable of thinking itself into and out of capital. What is most intriguing perhaps about the Heideggerian position, as viewed from the vantage of a theory of real abstraction, is its strangely "empirical" characterization of capitalism, understood not through its social forms (and above all not through the contradictory and self-positing form of value) but through the philosophical extrapolation of certain phenomenal contents. Thus, when Heidegger discourses about "the objectiveness of technical domination over the earth,"[24] we could note that he is confounding an effect with a cause. In the absence of an account of the social and economic forms—the value forms—that govern the expansion and intensification of capital, we are instead given a kind of ontological sublimation of economic terms: "What is human about humans and thingly about things is dissolved,[11] within the self-assertion of producing, to the calculations of the market value of a market that is not only a global market spanning the earth but that also, as the will to will, markets in the essence of being and so brings all beings into the business of calculation, which dominates most fiercely precisely where numbers are not needed."[25]

In Heidegger's sublimation and metaphorization of capital, the horizon of philosophy's expatriation—what should philosophers do once they take on the fact that capital *actually* "markets in essence of being" such that to speak of such an essence becomes otiose?—is rescinded by treating philosophy as a critical observer of the anthropology of capital in such a way that the sources and mechanisms of capital's real abstractions are ignored. This is evident in the way that Heidegger, rather than acknowledging the determinate character of the exchange abstraction under capitalism, treats exchange as a kind of exchange *in general*.[26] Thus, commenting on Rilke, he writes: "The self-willing man always calculates with things and people as he does with objects. That with which he has calculated turns into merchandise. Everything is constantly changed into new orderings. . . . Risked into defencelessness in this way, man moves in the medium of businesses and 'exchanges.' Self-asserting man lives by his will's stakes. He lives essentially in the hazard of his essence within the vibration of money and the validity of values. Man, as this constant exchanger and middleman, is 'the merchant.' He weighs and evaluates constantly and yet does not know the actual weight of things. Nor does he ever know what, in him, actually has weight and outweighs. . . . The usual life of today's man is the ordinariness of self-assertion in the defenseless market of exchanges."[27]

Now, though Malabou is rightly suspicious of Heidegger's tendency to treat the bad infinite of objective exchange as an inauthenticity that could be offset by recovering the horizon of true "things," the temptation in his work to "form an essence, to sculpt it, to coin it like one coins money," her deriving from Heidegger of the problematic of an economy "before" capitalism fails to confront the dialectical challenge of real abstraction, namely that such an originary dimension is a fallacious extrapolation—a one-sided abstraction, to put it in Hegelian terms— from the determinate abstraction of commodity exchange to general philosophical laws, as in the following formulation: "The economic law of being: every thing, beginning with being itself, constantly exchanges itself with itself, between presence and presence, value and favour, property and disappropriation."[28] Before returning to this problem of the ontology of exchange as it relates to the critical contrast between philosophical plasticity and capitalist flexibility, in Malabou's dialogue with the brain sciences, another brief poetic and monetary detour is in order.

> Gold? Yellow, glittering, precious gold?
> No, Gods, I am no idle votarist! . . .
> Thus much of this will make black white, foul fair,
> Wrong right, base noble, old young, coward valiant.
> . . . Why, this
> Will lug your priests and servants from your sides,
> Pluck stout men's pillows from below their heads:
> This yellow slave
> Will knit and break religions, bless the accursed;
> Make the hoar leprosy adored, place thieves
> And give them title, knee and approbation
> With senators on the bench: This is it
> That makes the wappen'd widow wed again;
> She, whom the spital-house and ulcerous sores
> Would cast the gorge at, this embalms and spices
> To the April day again. Come, damned earth,
> Thou common whore of mankind, that put'st odds
> Among the rout of nations.

This monologue from Shakespeare's *Timon of Athens*, quoted in the context of Marx's discussion of the fetish powers of money in the Paris Manuscripts of 1844, is intended to underscore the manner in which the quantitative indifference of money can unleash the most varied and uncontainable of metamorphoses, making a mockery of stable identities or hallowed oppositions—the very creative-destructive power borne by the buccaneering bourgeoisie of the *Manifesto*. Shakespeare's delirious vision and Marx's commentary also mime the way in which a world structured by the money form insistently tries to repel it, debasing it along with the threatening forms of otherness and mixture ("the yellow slave," "the common whore"). While not taking his distance from the gynophobic trope of prostitution as the dissolution of order, in his gloss on Shakespeare, Marx does note the intrinsic bivalence, or hypocrisy, of this monetized social ontology—which joins sovereignty and baseness, intercourse and separation, infinite dissemination and homogenizing unity:

> If money is the bond binding me to human life, binding society to me, connecting me with nature and man, is not money the bond of all bonds? Can it not dissolve and bind all ties? Is it not, therefore, also the universal agent of separation? It is the coin that really separates as well as the real binding agent—the chemical power of society.
>
> Shakespeare stresses especially two properties of money:
> 1. It is the visible divinity—the transformation of all human and natural properties into their contraries, the universal confounding and distorting of things: impossibilities are soldered together by it.
> 2. It is the common whore, the common procurer of people and nations.
>
> The distorting and confounding of all human and natural qualities, the fraternisation of impossibilities—the divine power of money—lies in its character as men's estranged, alienating and self-disposing species-nature. Money is the alienated ability of mankind.[29]

The affinity of capital's critique with capital is writ large. After all, what better name for communism than the fraternization of impossibilities? This affinity is perhaps best regarded as an ambivalence, a bivalent potentiality which haunts critical dialectical thinking's relation to its object. It is also a mark of immanence: the real critique of money is not an external critique—such as we may discern in Heidegger's Rilke—but one that roots itself in the possibilities opened up by this universal confusion of traditional categories, identities, and demarcations.

In this respect, Malabou's contention that a thinking of plasticity has to tarry with the languages and practices of capital's metamorphic indifference—above all with the mantra of "flexibility"—is testament to her dialectical intuition. A critical ontology of change must take seriously capital's "self-reflection" as an economy geared to transformation and novelty. Indeed, if we resist the tendency to call upon alterity and transcendence—as Malabou repeatedly does[30]—then in a sense we can think change only from within the forms that it takes within capital. In this respect, Malabou's proposal that we take political consciousness of the new image of the brain provided by plasticity while confronting head on its deep entanglement with the new languages of labor management and capital accumulation is in keeping with the Brechtian inspiration behind a number of recent Marxist interventions, from Jameson's musings on the utopian possibilities of Walmart to Virno's writings on the emancipatory potentials at the heart of subjective stances of cynicism: a critique of capital must not comfort itself with the good old things but tackle the bad new ones.

Though I remain sympathetic to this orientation, I think that Malabou's politicization of cerebral plasticity in light of shifts in contemporary capital is hostage to her reliance on a narrative about changes within capitalism which puts an undue emphasis on novelties in its "spirit," and on the "neural" character of such changes in particular. Resting her analysis on Luc Boltanski and Eve Chiapello's influential analysis—based on an ample corpus of French management writings—of the shift in the justificatory structures and practices, or "spirit," of the "new capitalism," Malabou wagers that a philosophical intervention into our understanding of the brain has a political charge precisely to the extent that contemporary capitalism thinks itself by analogy with the brain. It is certainly true that there has been a long and genealogically complex relation between conceptions of the brain (or more broadly, the mind) and visions of social organization and that, especially in the postwar period, the place of cybernetics (that "science of control") in the development of cognitive science, computing, social theory, and social policy laid the groundwork for a particularly dense resonance between the mental and the political. Sensitive to how neurobiological developments can be enlisted in the legitimation of insidious forms of exploitation and a naturalization of capital overall, Malabou calls for a critique of the kind of neuronal ideology that would picture us as flexible individuals putting our flexible brains to work in a flexible labor market. Yet this stress on ideology critique is unsteadied by two broad ontological claims: the first is that there is a real mirroring between the brain and capitalist globalization; the second is that the plastic brain can be recast as a site of resistance, the basis for a biological alter-globalization.

For critique to be both immanent and dialectical, it requires, to a certain extent, that one begin with the assumption that the object of said critique is not mere falsity or manipulation. A critique of classical political economy, accordingly, is not a refutation of Smith or Ricardo but an inquiry into the constitutive limitations, the blind spots, in systems of thought which nevertheless contain a considerable adequacy with regard to their object—the emergent capitalist economy—but are incapable to fully account for their own categories and thus come to be sublated in an account which is more capacious and starts from a radically different perspective (that of the agency of the proletariat, in the case of Marx's critique). That said, there are of course authors and discourses (the majority, in fact) that don't require this kind of critique. Mere *apologists* for capital, such as Malthus was for Marx, for instance, are more aptly treated by means of refutation, sarcasm, and invective.

How do we stand then towards the contemporary "neuronal" ideology or spirit of capitalism? This is what Malabou writes in the preface to the new French edition of *Que faire de notre cerveau?*

> the structural relationship between the biological subject and the political subject matter is always already determined by the functioning of capitalism at a given moment in its history. One could say in Marxist terms, quite simply, that brain plasticity is now the superstructural or ideological expression of global capitalism or post-Fordism that replaces industrial capitalism. Organization in networks, absence of hierarchy, decentralized control, emotional lability, mobility—the new management is the objective version of the structure of the nervous system revealed by contemporary neurobiology. Brain plasticity can be considered as the preferred form of naturalization of capitalism.[31]

Somewhat facetiously, I would say that this statement is both too Marxist and not Marxist enough. It is too Marxist (in the sense of a rather orthodox Marxism) because the functioning of capital is not ideologically univocal and capitalism need neither require a single regime of organizing labor (e.g., post-Fordism) nor a single ideological superstructure. Arguably, the mirroring between capital and the brain has had much more effect on the sciences of the mind than on the organization of capital: as Bo Dahlbom has shown in an acute essay on the work of Daniel Dennett, models of cerebral functioning often unconsciously replicate prevalent modes for organizing work or, rather, discourses about the organization of work (the machinic brain and the Fordist factory; the connectionist brain and the distributed production network).[32] Though, as Boltanski and Chiapello detail, the network has had ample discursive and material effects since its emergence across the social, biological, and digital sciences, there is little evidence—outside of the world of popularized science, whose impact on the organization of capital is very debatable—about the importance of "brain plasticity" as an organizing principle for the control of work, exploitation, and profit.

The reasons why Malabou's account may be too Marxist in its fit between capitalist base and biological/ideological superstructure are also the ones why it is not Marxist enough (in the sense of following through Marx's own dialectical intuitions). To think that the social is *like* the brain is no more enlightening today than to think that the economy was like a large organism in the nineteenth century or like a hydraulic machine in the twentieth. Dialectics—precisely because of that attention to the modeling and deflagration of form, that attempt to combine relational continuity and destructive interruption, which Malabou so elegantly explores—should be wary of the trap of analogical thinking. Marx's reflection on the dialectic of the abstract and the concrete was aimed, among other things, at having done with the "picture thinking" that plagued economic and political thought. In this respect, I would suggest that to do justice to the philosophically empowering dimensions of the thematization of plasticity in the neurobiological sciences requires rejecting *any* mirroring between our thinking of society and our thinking of the brain and stressing their discontinuity.

Since Malabou mentions Althusser as a possible reference for a renewed materialism in her preface, I think that our engagement with the interferences between the brain sciences and political economy would benefit from his penchant for *demarcation*. In his sympathetic critique of Jacques Monod, collected in *Philosophy and the Spontaneous Philosophy of the Scientists*, Althusser tries, with characteristic schematism, to distinguish in the French biologist's discourse the statements of science (i.e., the discovery of DNA and its reflection in novel concepts of biological theory like "teleonomy" and "emergence"), the spontaneous philosophy of the scientist (which in Monod combines a dialectical and materialist elaboration of how there can be living systems but there is no living matter, on the one hand, and an idealism about the "noosphere," on the other), philosophy (Monod's "atheist idealism"), and worldview (a practical ideology drawn from but discontinuous with his scientific work) from one another. The danger of not heeding these demarcations is to draw an illegitimate continuity between scientific theory and a practical ideology—a political inference that relies on overextending the reach of a concept across these four domains, something which Althusser (prescient here in terms of its later use) ascribes to the idea of emergence.[33]

When Malabou assumes the ontological and social reality of this "mirroring" between brain and capital she risks, in order to bolster her argument about the political meaning of plasticity, to give excessive credence to one among the many apologetic discourses of capitalism. Managerial discourses on delocalization and (especially) the abolition of hierarchy are in the main thin veneers over practices of labor exploitation which have in many ways grown fiercer since the days of "Fordism." The idea that it is no longer possible to struggle against a boss or a father[34] treats the notion of a horizontal capitalism as a social truth, while—notwithstanding momentous transformations in logistical systems, ownership structures, and commodity chains—changes in contemporary capitalism have little if anything to do with a decentralization of command, which could either "reflect" a new understanding of the brain or legitimate the notion that power has become particularly diffuse (the gargantuan growth in military and policing apparatuses, the increase of monopolistic tendencies, and the astronomical rises in inequality put paid to that notion quite quickly).

Though attention to different historical and political regimes of labor and subjectivity is of paramount significance, the premium on flexibility is not an invention of "post-Fordism," nor is it constitutively linked—despite the incessant temptation to naturalize capitalism that permeates management apologias—to our shifting understanding of the brain. It is a primordial, axiomatic imperative of capitalism, reflected in the metamorphic capacities of money, in the "bad infinite" of capital accumulation and in the transformation of all workers, as Marx notes in the *Grundrisse*, into "virtual paupers" whose "organic presence" is a matter of "indifference" to the system of production and exchange.[35] Does this mean that plasticity cannot be, as Malabou proposes, a site of resistance? Not necessarily. In spite of Malabou's welcome reversal of Continental philosophy's abiding neglect of the neurosciences, I remain unpersuaded that the brain is the "sensitive and critical biological site of our time, through which pass, in one way or another, the political and cultural evolutions and revolutions which began in the 1980s and continue into the early 21st century"[36] and that becoming conscious of cerebral plasticity harbors political consequences. I think that her conception of plasticity as a kind of form taking and form leaving that is *not* infinitely malleable, reversible, renewable can help us resist certain tendencies within contemporary philosophy whose celebration of novelty and change puts them into unwitting resonance with capitalist fantasies of novelty.[37] In other words, rather than heralding a new "worldview" to rival that of the scientific apologists of capitalist flexibility, plasticity could serve as one of the components of a resistance, *within the field of philosophy*, against two ways of thinking change which impede a sober and transformative reflection on the challenges for a thinking opposed to capital: the first, a thinking of finitude anchored to a notion of the subject which neglects neurobiology and finds succor in quasi-religious forms of transcendence or messianism; the second, a thinking of becoming which disavows the fact that form (be it neural, biological, economic, or political) is affected by irreversible transformations and is not the object of unlimited powers of metamorphosis. In setting plasticity apart from elasticity,[38] flexibility, becoming, and other names for indefinite, reversible change, Malabou is making a significant contribution to the renewal of a dialectical thinking that is capable, at one and the same time, of an immanent critique of capital's real abstractions and a prospective inquiry into what ideas of form can aid us in thinking what substantive change would mean when it is not a change dictated by a system which is in the last instance indifferent to our organic presence, be that of our bodies or of our brains.

NOTES

1. Jameson, *Valences of the Dialectic*.
2. Jameson, "The Three Names of the Dialectic," in *Valences of the Dialectic*.
3. Malabou, *Plasticity at the Dusk*, 20.
4. Malabou, *Plasticity at the Dusk*, 27.
5. Malabou, *Plasticity at the Dusk*, 27.
6. Schürmann, *Heidegger*, 293.
7. *Le change Heidegger*, 352. Needless to say, the coherence of the political horizon of Marx's work depends on the prospect of the "transgressing" of the plasticity of capitalist value or, better, on its abolition.

8. Malabou, *Plasticity at the Dusk*, 45.
9. Malabou, *Plasticity at the Dusk*, 45.
10. Sohn-Rethel, *Intellectual and Manual Labor*, 53.
11. Sohn-Rethel, *Intellectual and Manual Labor*, 25.
12. Sohn-Rethel, *Intellectual and Manual Labor*, 96
13. Sohn-Rethel, *Intellectual and Manual Labor*, 65
14. Sohn-Rethel, *Intellectual and Manual Labor*, 67
15. Marx, *Grundrisse*, 225-26
16. Sohn-Rethel, *Intellectual and Manual Labor*, 130
17. Adorno, *Negative Dialectics*, 10.
18. Sohn-Rethel, *Intellectual and Manual Labor*, 45
19. Malabou, *Plasticity at the Dusk*, 47. Parenthetically, though the brevity of her remark makes it difficult to engage with it critically, it is somewhat perplexing that in the same book Malabou presents the question of fetishism as one of the appearance of an externality to exchange: "The assertion of inconvertibility lies, for Marx, at the heart of fetishism. On the face of it, the fetish always occurs outside the operation of exchange, outside the market. From then on, when otherness is fetishized by its resistance to plasticity, when hospitality continues to be thought as the 'counter' to plasticity or, in other words, against form, it is no longer possible to distinguish cosmopolitanism rigorously from hypercapitalism" (Malabou, *Plasticity at the Dusk*, 77). Commodity fetishism is not distinguished by inconvertibility but rather by the "objective illusion" that exchange enacts a "social relation between things," that human beings are mere vehicles for the infinite convertibility of the goods they produce. Rather than pose an otherness to convertibility, the fetishes of capital, money, and value occlude (not in a mental but in an operative and social sense) the alterity of laboring bodies.
20. Malabou, *Le change Heidegger*, 361.
21. Heidegger, "Why Poets?," 219.
22. Heidegger, "Why Poets?," 218.
23. Heidegger, "Why Poets?," 218.
24. Heidegger, "Why Poets?," 219.
25. The echoes of the *Manifesto* are evident enough, except it is no longer the bourgeoisie but an impersonal "mastery" that "has drowned the most heavenly ecstasies of religious fervour, of chivalrous enthusiasm, of philistine sentimentalism, in the icy water of egotistical calculation."
26. Heidegger, "Why Poets?," 219.
27. In this perspective, it would be useful to consider the manner in which Marx's distinction between the abstract and the general (viz., between abstract labor and labor in general) in his remarks on method could serve to undo the underdetermined, epochal hypostases that drive Heidegger's monotonous panorama of the history of Western metaphysics.

28. Heidegger, "Why Poets?," 236; Malabou, *Le change Heidegger*, 354.

29. Marx, *Early Writings*, 377.

30. See, e.g., her declaration that "The philosophy to come must explore the space of this collapse of messianic structures." Malabou, *Ontology of the Accident*, 88.

31. Malabou, *Que faire 2ème édition*, 11-12.

32. Dahlbom, "Mind Is Artificial."

33. "Emergence proliferates: a true *deus ex machina*. Each time something new happens—a new idea, a new event—Monod utters the magic word 'emergence.' As a general rule, it might be said that when a concept is used to think everything, it is in danger of not thinking anything at all. This is the failing Hegel once denounced in Schelling, who applied his theory of poles everywhere: formalism." Althusser, "Appendix: On Jacques Monod," 152.

34. Malabou, *Que faire*, 158.

35. Marx, *Grundrisse*, 604.

36. Malabou, *Que faire*, 109.

37. On this question, see the introduction to Noys, *Persistence of the Negative*, in particular, his critique of the contemporary philosophical tendency he dubs "accelerationism."

38. See the critique of Deleuze in Malabou, *Ontology of the Accident*, 36.

CHAPTER 6

Plasticity and the Cerebral Unconscious:
New Wounds, New Violences, New Politics

Catherine Kellogg

The recent anthology New Materialisms: Ontology, Agency, and Politics, charts a path through what its editors identify as a renewed materialism in the humanities and social sciences. Acknowledging that the great materialist thinkers of the nineteenth century—Marx, Nietzsche and Freud—were all inspired by developments in the natural sciences, this new materialism reworks understandings of matter, agency, and capitalism on the basis of the dizzying advances in physics, medicine, genetics, and biology over the last fifty years. The editors suggest that engaged social and political analyses are confronted with a world ineradicably changed by technological advances predicated on those very researches—climate change, new forms of war and terror, bio- and nano-technology—and that new understandings of the composition of matter and life, as well as the changed world we inhabit, has brought forth a renewed commitment to materialist approaches to politics and ethics.[1]

Catherine Malabou's recent work on plasticity—what she calls the triple movement of receiving, giving, and destroying form—is clearly an important contribution to this endeavor.[2] Emphasizing the many semantic extensions of plasticity, including synthetics, explosives, and so on, she has worked this term from an initial book on Hegel and futurity toward feminist theories of the body, questions of affect, and most recently, the sciences of the brain.[3] In this most recent work she points out that what is called *neuroplasticity*, the insight that our brains are capable of forming themselves in variable ways and are also very sensitive to the world they encounter, is a well-established point of departure in neuroscience. Her signature term is thus already widely used in the neurosciences, and it suggests an opening that is being explored between the natural sciences and philosophy, particularly in the relatively new field of psychoneurology. Opening up the relationship between what we think of as materiality (the brain, neural pathways, etc.), on the one hand, and ideality (the psyche or soul and so on) on the other, this field is a natural new research area for her, coming from her book *What Should We Do with Our Brain?* There she asked, "what should we do so that consciousness of the brain does not purely and simply coincide with the spirit of capitalism?"[4] Recalling Marx's point that our physical organs are always also social organs, Malabou advances the deceptively elegant argument that our brains—like the eye or ear as Marx describes them—are social organisms with a history and with the capacity to both be transformed by us and to transform us.[5] If it is true that an ear must develop the capacity to hear certain kinds of music as beautiful and that "the forming of the five senses is a labour of the entire history of the world down to the present,"[6] so, too, is our research into those senses and our conception of the brain itself. We think that our brains make us ("we are our brain chemistry," or "we are nothing but our synapses") and forget that we, too, make our brains. This is true at the level of the production of neural pathways (an obvious way that we make our brains) but also at the level of the differential and transdifferential nature of brain cells; the plasticity of the brain refers to the fact that neurons must die in order to generate a self and experiences must be forgotten in order that an identity might be formed. Distinguishing plasticity from the term so often associated with capitalism—elasticity—she makes the powerful call that we not replicate the world through how we reproduce our brains, that we refuse to be the "flexible individuals who combine a permanent control of the self with a capacity to self-modify at the whim of fluxes, transfers and exchanges for fear of explosion."[7]

In her 2007 book *Les nouveaux blessés*, Malabou turns the question of the brain's plasticity towards the psychoanalytic understanding of trauma.[8] She identifies a constituency she names the "new wounded," those whose brains are ineradicably changed as a result of brain damage (Alzheimer's disease) or severe trauma. These wounds can neither be explained nor offered help by way of psychoanalysis as it presently understands itself. This is so because the psychoanalytic rendering of trauma deals with a phenomenon that is understood in connection to memory and a kind of psychic economy she calls the "regime of sexuality," wherein all trauma owes its properly traumatic character to a resonance with an earlier trauma that was sexually charged. But what marks the wounds Malabou identifies as *new* is the fact that there is effectively no *before* for the new wounded; those who are fundamentally altered in the ways she describes are not "traumatized" or pierced by the repetition of an old wound. Rather, because they attain an essentially new identity, any prior trauma is effectively wiped out by the new injury; these new wounded *are no longer who they once were*. Specifically, like sociopaths or those who are severely autistic, the new wounded have lost their capacity to care and display a distinct emotional coolness, a profound indifference to the world and those around them.[9] Because they are "beyond love and hate," they can no longer meaningfully be understood as *parle-êtres*, or subjects who can "work through" by way of transferential relationships. In this sense, they mark the limits of psychoanalysis as therapeutic technique.

Perhaps more radically still, Malabou argues that the discovery of "the emotional brain," which regulates the brain's life through affect, has invalidated the Freudian hypothesis of the libido as the source of psychic energy. In fact, she says that whereas the psyche cannot feel itself, such thinkers as Antonio Damasio, Mark Solms, and others have shown that certain kinds of affect or emotions produce "an elementary form of attachment of the self to itself and to its own life."[10] This emotional auto-affection is not self-conscious; there is no direct experience of it. However, "cerebral self-affection is the unconscious of subjectivity." She argues that the "cerebral unconscious," directly linked as it is to the processes of the brain, "is the only truly material unconscious."[11]

The challenge she issues to psychoanalysis, then, is a radical and profound one. And the bridge she proposes between neurobiology and psychoanalysis is without peer. Elegantly and meticulously argued, she reads the psychoanalytic text deeply and with attention both to its systematicity as well as to the ways it unfolded in a heterogenous manner first in Freud's clinic and then in subsequent other clinics over the last hundred years. Her concern is specifically with psychopathology because, as she points out, this field is no longer dominated by the neurotics who populated Freud's nineteenth-century Viennese clinic but rather with those whose brains have been injured by way of an event that no longer fits comfortably with the map of "eventuality" that made sense in Freud's day. As she says: "Beyond the controversies and discussions about the efficacy or scientificity of psychoanalysis that currently divide the field of psychopathology, we should, instead, devote our attention to the *change in the concepts of event, wound and trauma*. This gesture does not entail taking sides against Freud. On the contrary, I will undertake a reading of Freud that will turn upon the elaboration of the notion of the psychic event."[12] There is such a host of questions that can be posed vis-à-vis her work—for she is surely tapping a deep mine—that I deliberately pose questions that simply try to follow her own: how exactly *does* Freud's theory of trauma articulate itself with the event, with memory (and time generally) and with "the matter of the body"? Is it possible to consider a theory of trauma in terms of a sexual psyche that could still account for the loss of personhood and affect Malabou describes? While it may be that there is something to be gained by introducing a regime of cerebrality to psychoanalysis, replacing the regime of sexuality with one that is open to understanding the kinds of processes that give rise to these new wounded, I wonder what also might be lost? To get at this loss, I ask how Freud's notion of the "death instinct" as the desire to return to inorganic life, coordinates with Lacan's elaboration of the death drive, most powerfully and fully elaborated in his notion of surplus pleasure, or plus-de-jouissance? If surplus pleasure (or jouissance) can be understood as coextensive with Freud's notion of the death drive (as Lacan insists), how do we understand its relationship with a more general understanding of trauma and specifically with a theory of libido which is, at root, a sexual libido? In proposing a theory of subjectivity that has the "matter" of the brain and its relationship to the psyche at its root, does her new materialist approach to psychic events threaten to alter a theory of psychic life that was materialist all along? In short, is it possible that Malabou risks throwing out the psychoanalytic baby along with its immaterial bathwater? In what follows, I bring into a kind of preliminary focus, the relationship (or, alternatively, the point of non-passage) between those whom Malabou describes as "speechless," those for whom trauma is meaningless because of the extent of the trauma and who therefore have, in fact, lost themselves, on the one hand, and Lacan's notion of the subject as one who has already survived its own death, on the other.

NEW WOUNDS, NEW VIOLENCES

Malabou ended her first book on Hegel by saying that in the current moment we live under the shadow of "saturation and vacancy," in which there is no event that is not a world event (saturation), and yet we are left with the sense that it seems there is "nothing left to do" (vacancy).[13]

She indicates that this closure of the world and the crisis of its meaning are the contemporary modes of subjective anticipation, our way of experiencing the future, so to speak. She goes on to say that it does give rise to a "new opening," but beyond naming it as plasticity itself, she does not say much about what that opening would consist of. What she does say is that from the perspective of this opening, life must be thought of in terms of a circulating automatism that may be at once "self-engendering and self-destructive."[14]

In her new book, she comes back to saturation and vacancy on the very terrain of this automatic self-destruction. Specifically, as I said, she identifies a new constituency, the "new wounded" who have been indelibly changed by the trauma of war, earthquakes, tsunamis, violent attacks, or rape, on the one hand, and those who have had their personhood destroyed by brain traumas, such as Alzheimer's or Parkinson's disease, on the other.[15] Those in this new constituency are robbed precisely of the capacity *to make sense* of their wounds such that they can no longer be considered who they once were. Indeed, she claims that for these new wounded, "no interpretation of it is possible."[16] The saturation of the world, then, consists of the illegibility of the line between the brain accident, on the one hand, and crime, war, and natural catastrophe, on the other. And its vacancy consists in the fact that there is no sense to be recouped for those who are severely traumatized, or gravely and permanently changed, by events we name in this way. The saturation of the world and the vacancy of its meaning are such that she says we have entered a new age of violence. Indeed, Malabou says that the peculiar lack of sense or meaning in the violence that gives rise to the "new wounded" is such that in this new age, "social conflict [is] without dialectic, as anonymous as a natural catastrophe."[17] From the vantage point of those so injured, no distinction can be made between social and neuronal disasters. In this sense, not only is this a new age of violence; this violence can not be given *meaning*.

Malabou's invocation of a new age of violence and a new kind of wound, along with the idea of a self-destructive automaton that functions in every life is a direct reference to Freud's "death instincts." And in fact, the death drive's position as a central operator in the psychoanalytic theory of trauma, along with its conceptual coordinates, repetition compulsion, libido, and so on, is central to Malabou's dispute with Freud. Malabou takes specific issue with Freud's idea that all trauma owes its properly *traumatic* character to its resonance with prior traumas. Because, as she explains, for Freud, sexuality is the regime that decides the meaning of all psychic events; on his account, all trauma is linked in some way to early or infantile experiences of oedipality, to the fear of castration, and so on.[18] Malabou's rejoinder is that there are certain kinds of relentless destructivenesses that make the "post" inherent in this kind of trauma impossible simply because they destroy any *prior* to that event. As Slavoj Žižek puts it, "for those in a war torn country like Sudan or Congo, trauma is the permanent state of things, a way of life. They have nowhere to retreat to and cannot even claim to be haunted by the specter of an earlier trauma."[19] On the terms of the regime of the sexual psyche, all trauma is given its meaning as traumatic by virtue of its relationship to neurosis, infantile sexuality, and the so-called beyond of the pleasure principle. The knowledge regime of the sexual psyche, then, stands in the way of a psychoanalysis robust enough to account for these "new wounds." This is the claim that stands at the center of the present chapter. On the basis of research undertaken in the neurosciences, Malabou proposes to replace Freud's regime of sexuality with a regime of cerebrality, one that is not marked by the death drive but rather one that displays a *destructive plasticity*. This destructive plasticity is not the so-called positive capacities associated with plasticity of holding or giving a form but rather the capacity to become someone completely other than who one has been, the constant possibility of the destruction of the *form of subjectivity* itself. This, then, is the view from the new perspective of saturation and vacancy; the automatism at work in every life is a neuronal automatism, and it operates in such a way that "at every instant, we are all susceptible to becoming new wounded."[20] This susceptibility, this vulnerability to the erasure of the distinction between political and other forms of violence, on the one hand, and the destructive plasticity of the brain, on the other, is in fact, as she calls it, a "new form of life."[21] Taking specific aim at Freud's libido theory as governed by the instincts of life and the instincts of destruction, she asks if, instead of a "death drive," there might be something even more soberly destructive at work in the brain itself that psychoanalysis has avoided confronting. As she says: "Might there be a type of plasticity that, under the effects of a wound *creates a certain form of being by effacing a previously existing identity*? Might there be, in the brain, a destructive plasticity—the dark double of the positive and constructive plasticity that moulds neuronal connections? Might such plasticity make form through the annihilation of form?"[22]

DESTRUCTIVE PLASTICITY VS. DEATH DRIVE

As I said, in her book *What Should We Do with Our Brain?* Malabou first turned her attention to the plasticity of the brain. There she said, "Talking about the plasticity of the brain thus amounts to thinking of the brain as something modifiable, "formable," and formative at the same time. Brain plasticity operates, as we shall see, on three levels: (1) the modeling of neuronal connections (developmental plasticity in the embryo and the child); (2) the modification of neuronal connections (the plasticity of synaptic modulation throughout life); and (3) the capacity for repair (post-lesional plasticity)."[23]

It is this third kind of plasticity that Malabou discusses in *Les nouveaux blessés*, but it is not understood as a restorative plasticity. Instead, among the most important insights she has gained from her engagement with neuroscience is that the brain damage that occurs as a result of severe trauma or as a result of brain lesion means that the person in whose brain these changes occur becomes unrecognizable as who he or she once was; the person has, in effect, a new identity. This way of being changed is a kind of post-traumatic plasticity that "is not the plasticity of reconstruction but the default formulation of a new identity with loss as its premise."[24] The loss that this way of being represents is a total loss of the self that had been before. Thus, Malabou warns, plasticity in this case also designates the capacity to annihilate the form that it receives or creates. The victims of severe geopolitical violence—victims and perpetrators of rape, terrorism, torture, and so on—as well as those whose brains have been injured by a lesion are all radically changed; *they are not who they were* before they underwent their wounding.

On this view, the kinds of destructive changes she sees in the "new wounded" cannot be understood as a result of damage against the *sexual* functioning of the organism, however widely we can construe the meaning of sexuality. As she says, "*The complexity of the concept of a cerebral unconscious inheres within the relationship of the cerebral psyche to its own destruction.*"[25] The fact that the brain is susceptible to lesions and/or shocks that radically change personality means that the study of psychopathology requires entirely new understandings of what constitutes a "psychic event" and "new etiological principles."[26]

Reformulating the guiding principles of philosophy and science that regulate our dealings with trauma in terms of "cerebrality" and the destructive plasticity of the brain, as opposed to Freudian "sexuality," changes the terms of what decides the meaning of an event in psychic life. This is also to say that it changes the terms of the meaning of "the border between the outside and the inside of the psyche."[27] If psychic events are understood in terms of the "brain" and a regime of "cerebrality," if it becomes possible to talk about the injuries to these new wounded in terms of what it has done to their brains, it might be possible to both incorporate the new range of cerebral damages (and their accompanying suffering) and, at the same time, reconsider the relationship between psychoanalysis, neurology, and philosophy.[28] "Cerebrality" here, in an ingenious twist, is constructed the same way as "sexuality" in Freud: in terms of its capacity to "determine the course of psychic life."[29] The concept of "cerebrality" then, functions as a kind of umbrella under which a new discourse can unify various discourses about the brain, especially when it comes to dealing with various types of injury.[30]

On this view, the brain appears as the privileged site of affect, and this cerebral organization presides over a new libidinal economy. As she says, for most neurobiologists today, cerebral and psychic life are indistinguishable. And as Malabou says, "insidiously, but unmistakably, cerebrality has usurped the place of sexuality in psychopathological discourse and practice."[31] This substitution, she says, is the main cause of the conflict between neurobiology and psychoanalysis. In order to enact a meaningful encounter between neurobiology and psychoanalysis, then, Malabou produces a bridge between them, one that allows for the possibility to think the brain's capacity for a kind of autoaffection, as well as the possibility of a "clinic to come" that would "integrate the conjoined results of Freudianism and neurology."[32]

Indeed, unlike the psychoanalytic version of the unconscious mind, cerebral autoaffection, what she calls "cerebral unconscious," is not a story that the subject tells itself about itself. It is not symbolic, nor is it symbolizable. As she says, "no one can speak of 'his' brain. Between 'my' brain and myself, there is a sort of opaque wall, an absence of mirror, even as it is the most intimate part of myself, the 'me' who thinks and feels within 'me.'"[33] The matter of the brain, if you will, "solicits itself *without seeing itself*" in the sense that it regulates its own changes without any representation of itself to itself. The brain "in no way anticipates the possibility of its own damage."[34]

Notwithstanding the fact that contemporary neuroscientists are convinced about this capacity for the brain to regulate itself without any part of that regulation being accessible to consciousness, the cerebral plasticity acknowledged by contemporary brain scientists all too quickly moves away from its destructive dimensions. As Malabou says, "it must . . . be recognized that the explicit elaboration of this negative plasticity is *my intervention* . . . neurology always stresses that *illness is a compensatory creation* that functions to repair the world. No sooner is negative plasticity invoked than it is conjured away."[35] The destructive significance of plasticity is kept "in shadows." If we are all at every moment susceptible to becoming "new wounded," unrecognizable to ourselves and those around us, victims of an accident we could not see coming, how do we think the new form of life that emerges from the destruction of subjectivity that is destructive plasticity? Unlike the neuroscientists upon whom she relies, she is determined to think "a plasticity without remedy."[36]

EVENT, TRAUMA, AND THE TIME OF THE MATTER

How does this "plasticity without remedy" compare with the psychoanalytic account of psychic piercing? On Freud's account, psychic events can be understood as exogenous (from without, such as extreme trauma) or endogenous (from within). But what makes psychic events *traumatic* is their unexpected quality; there is something shocking about them for which the subject was not prepared, and thus they cannot be recuperated or integrated by subjects who experience them. As Malabou points out, for Freud, trauma reactivates an earlier trauma that has become meaningful through what she calls a "regime of sexuality." That is to say, that all psychic events—exogenous or endogenous—come to have the quality of "eventness" by virtue of their capacity to resonate with the fear of castration that marks the subject's entry into subjectivity, as well as oedipality, and its attendant psychoanalytic cognates. And traumatic events produce the kinds of psychopathologies Freud puzzled over throughout his career by virtue of the ways that they resonate with the earliest traumas that mark human life. The question at issue here is the relationship between the term "castration" and its fear (what Freud called neurotic anxiety) and the regime of sexuality Malabou says governs the psychoanalytic field. What is this regime of sexuality that decides the meaning of a psychic event such as trauma? Understood as much more than a set of practices, she points out that in the Freudian scheme, sexuality is a term that governs a regime of meaning. It is a "law" in the sense that it is *"a specific form of causality."*[37] To unpack this idea, I turn first to Freud's writings on anxiety as a *specific* kind of neurotic affect—one that implicates psychoanalytic debates about the place of memory, loss, repetition, and the body, as well as the meaning of a psychic event—before discussing his more general theory of trauma.

In his famous study on anxiety, *Inhibitions, Symptoms and Anxiety*, Freud first suggested that anxiety is a signal of some kind that is different from fear.[38] Because anxiety is an unpleasant affect, we develop various symptoms and inhibitions in order to cope with it. Inhibitions, for example, try to prevent us from finding ourselves in situations that provoke anxiety, and symptoms try to replace anxiety's effects, and so on. What *really* interested Freud, however, was distinguishing *Realangst* (realistic fear) from neurotic anxiety. *Realangst*, he said, is fear in the face of a real danger, an *external* situation that threatens our safety. Neurotic anxiety, by way of contrast, is a pathological response to an *endogenous*, or inner, "event." But it is not the organism that is threatened (as it would be in the event of an attack from a wild animal) but rather the ego. Indeed, Freud says that "the ego is the actual seat of anxiety," and in *The Ego and the Id* Freud says that "what it is that the ego fears . . . cannot be specified; we know that the fear is of being overwhelmed or annihilated; but it cannot be grasped analytically."[39] The dread associated with the affect of anxiety has *no object* because the danger to which the organism responds is to the *ego*.

It seems, first, important to note that there is something about the *status* of the ego that is at work in differentiating "natural" fear from "human" anxiety. And second, for my purposes, it is also important to note that when distinguishing between neurotic anxiety and fear, Freud linked neurotic anxiety to the *future*, noting that whereas fear has an object (in the present, one might say), anxiety has no object but is rather a mode of waiting or distressed anticipation as though the threat was impending from the future. A double structure is thus opened by the problem of anxiety. On the one hand, we see a temporal structure insofar as anxiety involves memory (both repetition and anticipation) that shapes the time of anxiety in particular ways. On the other hand, we see a peculiar relation to the object, since anxiety is distinguished from fear in having no object and being a relation to "the nothing." Anxiety is not only a temporal structure then, but also a relation to the void or the absence that philosophers—from Kierkegaard to Heidegger to Sartre—have addressed. Freud referred to this relation to "the nothing" as the threat of castration. As he says "I am . . . inclined to adhere to the view that the fear of death should be regarded as analogous to the fear of castration and that the situation to which the ego is reacting is one of being abandoned by the protecting superego—the powers of destiny—so that it no longer has any safeguard against all the dangers that surround it."[40]

Peculiar to the human and unlike an "adaptation" to our environment, then, anxiety is linked to the destructive processes Freud came to name as "beyond the pleasure principle"; the self-destructive thoughts, impulses, and repetitions that lie beyond the simple animal-like response to danger and safety.

It was precisely these destructive instincts that sustained his attention once he began looking at the soldiers returning from the First World War. He discovered that they had a curious tendency to repeat in their dreams the traumatic events they had lived through in combat.[41] Committed as he was to the central insight of *The Interpretation of Dreams*, which was that dreams were a form of wish fulfillment, he tried to understand why these men lay awake in the middle of the night, troubled by traumatic dreams that did not fulfill any wish, breaking the principle of pleasure. His answer connected these dreams to the repetition evident in a game he witnessed his grandson playing with a spool. After experiencing his mother's coming and going, Freud observed the child sending the spool away, saying "Fort" and reeling it back, saying "Da." This activity, like the dreams of the war neurotics, staged a repetition of an unpleasurable event. Asking "how the repetition of this distressing experience as a game fit in with the pleasure principle," Freud thought that the child was able to gain a sense of mastery of the loss of a desired object through repeatedly enacting it on the child's own terms.[42] The game turned the tables on the object by making the child the agent of the loss rather than the passive victim.

Thus, Freud speculated that while each of us is looking to maintain a consistency of tensions (*eros*), we are also compelled to go *beyond* this limit in a quest for mastery, which, by going beyond the pleasure principle, would take us in the direction of death (*thanatos*). Freud also speculated that with every repetition of the "distressing experience," there is also a reduction of stress or excitation. A tension that initially overwhelmed the organism is slowly dissipated through repetition, which is itself a kind of slow death. As the repetition of traumatic dreams and masochistic games of mastery indicate, "life only ever returns there via paths that are always the same, ones it has previously traced."[43]

DEATH DRIVE, PLUS-DE-JOUISSANCE

Freud's theories about the relationship between pain and pleasure, about fear, anxiety—in particular, that castration is the subject's greatest fear—instigated an extensive debate among his disciples over what kind of loss the subject is most anxious about. From Melanie Klein to Joan Riviere to Ernest Jones, the question of what loss is at issue in anxiety has been a debate that has structured the terms of psychoanalytic engagement throughout the twentieth century. Perhaps the most significant advance psychoanalysis has made over the question of anxiety and its relationship to castration was made by Jacques Lacan in his infamous "return to Freud." Specifically, Lacan, as we will see, organizes Freud's discussion of the ego with reference to the "imaginary" with the consequence that the danger to which anxiety responds is neither a "real" internal threat nor an internal conflict (in unconscious thought) but rather the threat of *imaginary fragmentation and disintegration*. If anxiety is a response to a threat, what is threatened is not life but the imaginary structure of the ego, and this ego is not the center of consciousness.

Freud himself insisted that the ego is not equivalent to "consciousness" and should not be construed in terms of what he had previously called the "perception-consciousness system." Rather, the ego is the imaginary border between the outside and the inside; it is always, as Freud says, "a bodily ego; it is not merely a surface entity, but is itself the projection of a surface."[44] The meaning of "castration anxiety" can be clarified this way, since in the course of the child's maturation, the organ that Freud says is privileged in the child's negation of sexual difference is not a *real* organ but rather an imaginary one. The threat of "castration" then, as Lacan details in his early discussion of the mirror phase, is a *threat to the imaginary integrity of the body*.

Thus, while many have dismissed Freud's notion of a castration and its fear, of a beyond to the pleasure principle that is coextensive with a destructive or "death drive" as nonsensical, Lacan develops it in a variety of places. Taking his cue from Freud's insight that there is something "beyond" the pleasure principle that works against it and also serves as the cause of the strange, painful repetition that Freud discovered in his grandson, in neurotics, and in war veterans, Lacan begins from what Freud only speculated: the idea that death itself is a final kind of pleasure. Lacan connected this final kind of pleasure to what he called an "ancestral knowledge" that causes life to dawdle on its road to death. In other words, if death is a final kind of pleasure, the repetitions and returns we take proceed from the fact that "the organism wishes only to die in its own fashion."[45] Indeed, these repetitions and returns, this "ancestral knowledge," is actually what Lacan calls jouissance.[46]

As Žižek points out, what Lacan means by jouissance, particularly the ways that it is different from either pleasure or pain, is precisely what Malabou fails to take into account as she otherwise painstakingly reads the psychoanalytic account of trauma, pain, or even cruelty.[47] For while it is true that, as Malabou says, Freud ultimately concludes that there is no "beyond" to the principle of pleasure as "a fundamental law of psychic regulation," her reading of Freud takes his own ambivalence about the ways that the repetitions of unpleasurable experiences point towards a kind of "dying in our own way" too literally.[48]

On Malabou's account, Freud is clear about the possibility of a "beyond" to the pleasure principle. As she says, "Is there or is there not a beyond of the pleasure principle? To this question, Freud ultimately responds in the negative. Nothing, in the end, seems to shake the mastery and authority of the pleasure principle as a fundamental law of psychic regulation. As painful and unpleasurable as it might be, experience of the repetition of trauma or the accident in fact serves to bind [*binden*] an energy that would otherwise purely and simply annihilate the psyche."[49] To put this in different terms, as Adrian Johnston says, citing Jonathan Lear, for Freud "what lies behind the pleasure principle isn't another principle, but a lack of principle . . . There is just the dysfunctional pleasure principle and nothing more."[50] While the principle of pleasure tries to tame experiences of overwhelming pain and make them tolerable by way of repetition, this tactic doesn't work, which is the entire psychopathological problem to begin with. Freud made use of a dual-drive system that borrowed from ancient cosmological cosmic clashes between the forces of life and death, but Malabou says that in looking for a *representative* for the death drive, Freud cast about. He looked at sadism, the drive of mastery, or even primary masochism. But as she says, these figures "are all derived from the love-hate dyad, from love inverted into hate—that is, once again, from *the intrigue of pleasure*."[51] Importantly, Malabou claims that this failure to admit the existence of a beyond of the pleasure principle is psychoanalysis's limit.[52] Claiming that "the most vulnerable" problem in her work is thinking "the plastics of death" situated between the "Freudian hypothesis of the death drive . . . and contemporary neurological hypothesis of a *death of the drive,*" her argument is that the "new wounded" are "figures of the death drive" itself.⁵³

However, there is a way to read the equivocal nature of Freud's speculations concerning the death drive that accounts for the "death of the drive" as well as shows us "figures of the death drive." Rather than ask if Freud ever found a "beyond" to the pleasure principle, if one looks at the distinction Freud drew between pleasure and *enjoyment*, it becomes possible to notice that the psychoanalytic account of the "new wounded" need not replace a sexual etiology with a neuronal one at all. In fact, Malabou's invocation of the "new wounded" as striking figurations not for the death drive but for the *death of the drive* is extraordinarily close to Lacan's own account of living "between two deaths." Indeed, with the Lacanian notion of "surplus jouissance," it becomes possible to find a psychoanalysis and a reading of the destructive instincts that accounts for the kinds of events Malabou says can be accounted for only as neuronal.

JOUISSANCE, OR BEYOND THE PLEASURE PRINCIPLE

In Lacan's early work the term "jouissance" was essentially the French translation of the German word *Genuss*, which Freud used to refer to an intense satisfaction at the level of the ego, in contrast to *Befriedigung*, which is a word Freud reserved for the satiation of needs or instincts.⁵⁴ But in his later work, he thought of "jouissance" in terms of the distinction between pleasure and enjoyment that Freud drew in his lectures on sexuality. Freud noted that sexual excitation is not uniformly pleasurable even if it is always *enjoyable*. This is so because sexual excitement also has the character of an unpleasant tension that compels one to take action to release it, to "alter the psychic situation."⁵⁵

> The character of the tension of sexual excitation is connected with a problem the solution of which is as difficult as it would be important for the conception of the sexual process. Despite all divergence of opinion regarding it in psychology, I must firmly maintain that a feeling of tension must carry with it the character of displeasure. For me it is conclusive that such a feeling carries with it the impulse to alter the psychic situation, and acts incitingly, which is quite contrary to the nature of perceived pleasure. But if we ascribe the tension of the sexual excitation to the feelings of displeasure we encounter the fact

that it is undoubtedly pleasurably perceived. The tension produced by sexual excitation is everywhere accompanied by pleasure; even in the preparatory changes of the genitals there is a distinct feeling of satisfaction. What relation is there between this unpleasant tension and this feeling of pleasure?[56]

Thus, sexual enjoyment involves both an unpleasurable tension and the pleasurable release of tension. Freud's explanation for the pleasure involved was that the human organism seeks to maintain a constant minimum level of excitation needed to sustain life. The pleasure principle, Freud writes, "is a tendency operating in the service of a function whose business it is to free the mental apparatus entirely from excitation or to keep the amount of excitation in it constant, or to keep it as low as possible."[57] Sexual pleasure, Freud suggested, comes not from what excites but from the diminution of excitation back to the minimum threshold. What was peculiar about sexual enjoyment for Freud, therefore, was not that the diminution of tension was pleasurable but rather that something drives us to increase the tension in the first place and to do so repeatedly only to come back to the starting point. It is a pleasure *beyond* pleasure (or a kind of surplus).

The key aspect of this formulation for understanding what Lacan means by jouissance is the idea of going beyond the pleasure principle exemplified by sexual excitement. The repetition of transgressing the tendency to persist at a constant level of excitation suggests there is an enjoyment that exceeds the pleasure principle and compels us to move in its direction. "Jouissance" is a term that captures this factor of enjoyment *beyond pleasure*. Thus, even if Freud does seem to conclude that there is no beyond to the pleasure principle, Lacan's reading shows that Freud concluded that there *was* a beyond, even if he didn't think so. Jouissance as a kind of painful pleasure expresses the paradoxical satisfaction the subject derives from the symptom.[58]

The term jouissance does refer to a bodily experience, but as the satisfaction from the symptom might suggest, this painful pleasure is an experience that is possible only with and through language and knowledge or what Lacan refers to as "the signifier." Indeed, on the one hand, language is precisely what produces the *break* between the child and its parents because with the advent of language, the child lives forever in exile from an imagined wholeness or oneness with them. In this sense, the signifier is the cause of the *loss* of oneness; it is the cause of the division between the "subject" and its body as a pure organism, as well as the cause of the division between the subject and the Other. The signifier is thus the cause of the impossibility of reaching full ecstatic oneness. At the same time, the signifier (or meaningful speech) is the only available path back to the (impossible) attainment of that lost oneness (impossible, because this oneness *never was*). The signifier thus relates to jouissance not only as surplus pleasure—pleasure *beyond* pleasure—but also in the sense of *no more pleasure*. The French phrase plus-de-jouissance renders this equivocality in a way that no English phrase could. The surplus here, as Žižek puts it "is the part of *jouissance* which resists being contained by the homeostasis, by the pleasure principle."[59]

This also marks a decisive moment of departure between Freud and Lacan. According to Freud, what is beyond the pleasure principle is death. And this is why, on Malabou's account, for Freud, what is "beyond" the pleasure principle is simply a "certain time," which is the *death that comes before life*. Freud's reading of the "death drive," in other words, relies on postulating a beyond of life even if it is posed in the terms of a *before* to life to which we long to return. The negativity Freud describes with his "nirvana principle" displays no plasticity, and thus, "Freud ruins the possibility of thinking precisely what he wishes to think, the plastic coincidence between creation and destruction of form." Put in slightly different terms, if the time of materiality is that *between* life and death, this time would be "prior to the time of pleasure."[60]

However, Lacan associated this "beyond" of pleasure not with a death before life but rather a death *drive* and, more specifically, with jouissance, which is bound to the signifier. I hope it is becoming clear that here jouissance, originally just a way of describing intense satisfaction, moves decisively away from Freud's conception of *Genuss*, whereby the subject has such complete access to objects of desire that he/she can (imaginarily) cancel out the possibility of their loss—to a notion of loss *as such*, one that is much closer to a notion of *waste*.

Linking jouissance to the signifier and repetition is what leads Lacan to reference the thermodynamic concept of entropy, of repetition compulsion. As Freud suggested, repetition introduces entropy, a loss of energy in the drive's move towards satisfaction. And the aim of repetition is both enjoyment itself and a blocking or *slowing down* of the drive's satisfaction. Each repetition will be less than what it tries to repeat, and with that loss, there is also a loss of enjoyment. As Lacan says, "Freud insisted on this loss—in repetition there is a reduction in *jouissance*."[61]

But this loss of enjoyment is not *lack*, or something missing. It is *waste*, a useless surplus, very much here as something to be added to signification and to be reckoned with as such.

The relationship Lacan describes between the subject and loss, whereby the subject is the subject of loss, sounds remarkably like the "formation of identity with loss as its premise" that Malabou says is unique to the new wounded. To put this in other terms, when Lacan insists that anxiety is not a response to the loss of an object but is rather what arises when *lack fails to appear*, what he is suggesting is that it is not the loss of the mother or an object that is the source of neurotic anxiety nor is anxiety the index of a lack that must be somehow ameliorated.[62] Rather, Lacan presents us with a lack or a loss that is the condition of the subject's emergence. The lack of lack—the absence of the distance between the "real" and its symbolization—is what gives rise to neurotic anxiety. For Lacan, anxiety is not a response to the loss of the object but is rather the affect that emerges when the Other is too close and the order of symbolization (displacement and substitution) is at risk of disappearing.

For Lacan, then, the problem of anxiety is not an isolated problem or merely a local detail of his theory but, as I have shown, leads to a reflection on the status of the ego, on the beyond of the pleasure principle, and the strange painful pleasure we seek as we look to die, slowly, in our own way. For Lacan, anxiety is not a "thought-like" process (whether this is linked to the "perception-consciousness system," as in the case of "realistic anxiety," or to the activation of an unconscious conflict, as in the case of neurotic anxiety); he rather regards it as an overflow of internal excitations that cannot be contained by the imaginary integrity of the body. If desire animates the body and structures its possibilities, this overflow of jouissance has a very different function. The conflict in anxiety is not a matter of conscious or unconscious thought but rather a matter of the *discontinuity between the real of the organism and the imaginary unity of the body*.

And here I find myself agreeing with Žižek, who argues that what Malabou points towards with her idea of posttraumatic subjectivity, is precisely what, on the Lacanian reading, is the subject. As Žižek says, "the subject is, as such, the survivor of its own death, a shell that remains after it is deprived of its substance . . . for Lacan, subject as such is a 'second subject,' the formal survivor of the loss of its substance."[63] Thus, while Malabou's magisterial description of the "subject of loss," the subject who has lost himself through trauma or brain injury, from terror to rape to brain lesion, is a radical and new one, it is perhaps not the case that the entire psychoanalytic frame, the regime of sexuality that determines the meaning or sense of psychic events, must be replaced with a neuronal one.

Indeed, the "formation of death in life, the production of individual figures that exist only within the detachment of existence" and that are the "representatives of the death drive" Malabou insists cannot be explained in the frame of psychoanalysis as it understands itself turns out to be a frame provided by Lacan all along.[64] When she argues with Antonio Damasio that "Spinoza was right" insofar as he claimed that "a man can die before being dead" she has recalled the point that Lacan makes so well in his Ethics seminar, that the Antigone demonstrates that between the dead and the alive are those who are "undead," neither alive nor dead. This is the domain Lacan describes as "between two deaths."[65] What makes Antigone "unnatural" is the way that she coolly walks out of her social life, out of any legal or symbolic life, and towards death itself. In so doing, she is literally acting "beyond the pleasure principle."

CONCLUSIONS

I began this paper with the claim that Catherine Malabou's contribution to the debate between psychoanalysis and neuroscience is a decisive one for many reasons but that I would focus on the way that it raises the question of the "materiality" of the psyche and the possibility of thinking the destruction of subjectivity that she witnesses in the "new wounded" in terms other than psychoanalytic ones. As I hope I have shown, while the materiality of the psyche has always been in question for readers of psychoanalysis, replacing the "sexual etiology" of trauma with a neuronal one does not finish the question. As Malabou is well aware, to separate out the "bad" Freud who cannot think the materiality of the brain from the "good" Freud who is able to think the destruction of the drive, even as he can find no representative of it, is to already play into the problem of the "two bodies" always at play in psychoanalytic accounts of trauma. Some commentators have suggested that Lacan's great accomplishment in his "return to Freud" was the killing off of the first body, the "natural" or material body, to replace it with the signifier-shaped body image. However, if Malabou has asked the question of whether psychoanalysis is able to think the destruction of the form of subjectivity itself (and found it wanting), as I hope I have shown, there is another psychoanalytic tradition wherein the question of the destruction of subjectivity does not require a turn to neuroscience.

At the same time, her description of new violences that wipe out the distinction between geopolitical and biological "accidents" or events and her description of contemporary forms of subjective anticipation—or contemporary forms of anxiety, if you will—in terms of saturation and vacancy in which it seems there is nothing left to do are utterly compelling. The term I have said is decisive for separating out the psychoanalytic tradition upon which she draws from the one that she eschews—plus-de-jouissance—is deliberately borrowed from Marx's notion of surplus value. It is a jouissance that is produced as a useless remainder to the subject. The logic whereby a surplus like this is appropriated and "put to work"—in the service of meaning and in the service of profit—is precisely the logic of enjoyment that Lacan suggests is endemic to the capitalism that produces us as beings with brains unable to be anything other than elastic.

NOTES

1. Coole and Frost, New Materialisms.

2. As she says, "I continue to defend the thesis that the only valid philosophical path today lies in the elaboration of a new materialism that would precisely refuse to envisage the least separation, not only between brain and thought but also between the brain and the unconscious. It is thus such a materialism, as the basis for a *new philosophy of spirit*, that determined my definition of cerebrality as an axiological principle entirely articulated in terms of the formation and deformation of neuronal connections." Malabou, *New Wounded*, 211–12; Malabou, *Les nouveaux blessés*, 342.

3. See, e.g., Malabou, *Future of Hegel, You Be My Body, What Should We Do, Plasticity and the Dusk, Changing Difference*.

4. Malabou, *What Should We Do*, 12.

5. As Marx says, "The senses and enjoyments of other men have become my own appropriation. Besides these direct organs, therefore, social organs develop in the form of society; thus, for instance, activity in direct association with others, etc. has become an organ for expressing my own life, and a mode of appropriating human life. It is obvious that the human eye gratifies itself in a way different from the crude, non-human eye; the human ear different from the crude ear, etc."; Marx, "Manuscripts of 1844," 74.

6. Marx, "Manuscripts of 1844," 75.

7. Malabou, *What Should We Do*, 78.

8. Malabou, *Les nouveaux blessés*; Malabou, *New Wounded*. In some instances I provide page numbers for both the French and the English citation, particularly where it seems to me that there is a slight transformation in the meaning from the French to the English.

9. Malabou, *New Wounded*, 214/346. "That the victim of trauma is totally incapable of symbolically reappropriating in one way or another, the destructive event; that the executioners are not implicated in what they do (one thinks of the coolness of serial killers) and thus are not responsible."

10. Malabou, "Subjectivity," 114. She says, "No one can feel his or her own brain; nor can he or she speak of it, hear it speak, nor hear himself or herself speak within it . . . Within my inner self, my brain never appears. The brain absents itself at the very site of its presence to itself." Malabou, *New Wounded*, 42–43; *Les nouveaux blessés*, 85.

11. *Les nouveaux blessés*, 235; cited in Žižek, *End Times*, 301.

12. Malabou, *New Wounded*, 11–12.

13. Malabou, *Future of Hegel*, 192.

14. Malabou, *Future of Hegel*, 293.

15. Malabou, *New Wounded*, 10–11: "The behavior of subjects who are victims of trauma linked to mistreatment, war, terrorist attacks, captivity, or sexual abuse display striking resemblances with subjects who have suffered brain damage. It is possible to name these traumas "sociopolitical traumas." Under this generic term, one should group all damage caused by extreme relational violence. Today, however, the border that separates organic trauma and sociopolitical trauma is increasingly porous." It is perhaps important to note that Malabou suggested that the English title for her work might better be the "new injuries" or the "new wounds" rather than the "new wounded." See her interview in Vahanian, "Conversation."

16. Malabou, *New Wounded*, 5. This is slightly more emphatic in the French, where she says "*toute herméneutique en est impossible*"; Malabou, *Les nouveaux blessés*, 29.

17. Malabou, *New Wounded*, 160; emphasis in original.

18. As Freud says: "The patient cannot remember the whole of what is repressed in him, and what he cannot remember may be precisely the essential part of it. . . . He is obliged to *repeat* the repressed material as a contemporary experience instead of . . . *remembering* it as something belonging to the past. These reproductions, which emerge with such unwished-for exactitude, always have as their subject, some portion of infantile sexual life—of the Oedipal complex, that is, and its derivatives." Freud, "Pleasure Principle," 18.

19. Žižek, *End Times*, 293.

20. Malabou, *New Wounded*, 213/344.

21. Malabou, *New Wounded*, 66.

22. Malabou, *New Wounded*, xv; Malabou, *Les nouveaux blessés*, 15.
23. Malabou, *What Should We Do*, 2008, 5.
24. Malabou, *New Wounded*, 48/94.
25. Malabou, *New Wounded*, 63.
26. Malabou, *New Wounded*, 63.
27. Malabou, "Psychic Event," 2010.
28. Malabou, *New Wounded*, 2/24: "*sexuality* appears as the concept that determines *the sense of the event within psychic life*"; emphasis in original.
29. Malabou, *New Wounded*, 2.
30. Malabou begins the book by saying, "I will allow myself to invent one word and only one: *cerebrality*. My hope is that such a barbarism will come to be accepted as the mark of a concept"; 1.
31. Malabou, "Psychic Event."
32. Malabou, *New Wounded*, 214.
33. Malabou, *New Wounded*, 140.
34. Malabou, *New Wounded*, 140–141.
35. Malabou, *New Wounded*, 180.
36. Malabou, *New Wounded*, 188.
37. Malabou, *New Wounded*, 1.
38. Freud, "Inhibitions," 77–175.
39. Freud, "Inhibitions," 57.
40. Freud, "Inhibitions," 130.
41. Freud, "Pleasure Principle."
42. Freud, "Pleasure Principle," 15–17.
43. Lacan, *Other Side*, 18.
44. Freud, *Ego and the Id*, 26.
45. Freud, "Pleasure Principle," 188.
46. "This pathway . . . this ancestral knowledge . . . this path towards death is nothing other than what is called *jouissance*." Lacan, *Other Side*, 18.
47. Žižek, *End Times*, 304.
48. Malabou, *New Wounded*, 169.
49. Malabou, *New Wounded*, 169.
50. Johnston, "Weakness of Nature," 160.
51. Malabou, *New Wounded*, 191.
52. Malabou, *New Wounded*, 189.
53. Malabou, *New Wounded*, 20, 214; emphasis mine.
54. What Freud referred to with the word *Genuss* was an intense satisfaction of the ego. It occurred when the subject experienced its relation to a desired object as so complete that the ego essentially disappeared and became one with the object. Thus, the subject's lack of the object is overcome to such an extent that the ego itself disappears. In his early seminars, Lacan worked with this paradox through his tripartite division of the imaginary, symbolic,

and real, suggesting that the subject could reach this kind of enjoyment only at the imaginary and symbolic levels. The subject could cancel out all lack only by either (imaginarily) misrecognizing it or by (symbolically) repressing it, but the lack—which is constitutive of subjectivity itself—continued at the level of the real. As I show, the shift in the meaning of "jouissance," especially as it is articulated in the seventeenth seminar, hinges on the nature of the way that the subject, in a sense, destroys itself through the experience of jouissance and, in particular, what this means for the status of the real.

55. Freud, *Three Contributions*.
56. Freud, *Three Contributions*.
57. Freud, "Pleasure Principle," 62.
58. Evans, *Lacanian Psychoanalysis*, 95.
59. Žižek, *End Times*, 304.
60. Malabou, "Plasticity and Elasticity," 78.
61. Malabou, "Plasticity and Elasticity," 78.
62. Weber, *Return to Freud*, 159.
63. Žižek, *End Times*, 304.
64. Malabou, *New Wounded*, 199.
65. Lacan, *Ethics of Psychoanalysis*, 270–85.

CHAPTER 7

"Go Wonder": Plasticity, Dissemination, and (the Mirage of) Revolution

Silvana Carotenuto

I do not know any more . . . these words belong to an idiom, which I am not sure any more of being able to understand . . . in order to let one understand, in this idiom, my own incomprehension, a certain increasing and stubborn non-intelligence, on this stubbornness precisely, of an idiom, of more than one idiom, perhaps, at the crossroads of the Greek and of its other, go wonder . . .
—Jacques Derrida

In the following pages I "wonder"[1] at two of the most significant traits of contemporary thought: an emphasis on or a return to Hegelian philosophy and the resistance of deconstruction to dialectical thought.[2] After the "queering" of Hegel by Judith Butler, it is the French philosopher Catherine Malabou who today interprets the revaluation of the Hegelian speculative system.[3] I read the origin of Malabou's "return" in *The Future of Hegel*, originally her doctoral thesis, then published with a preface by Jacques Derrida, "A Time for Farewells."

The relationship between Catherine Malabou and Jacques Derrida started with his supervision of her research for this work, then continues in *Counterpath*, and returns in various essays where Malabou critically interacts with deconstruction, particularly concentrating on Derrida's insistence on "writing."[4] Malabou maintains that today deconstruction is experiencing a definitive decline; writing inscribes itself in its unavoidable "dusk," "twilight," or "death"; the grapheme does not characterize our epoch any longer. We must go back to the thought—according to Malabou, a real and proper "philosophy"—of dialectics in its "plasticized" form: "plasticity" is the future of philosophy, the future "in" Hegel and "of" Hegel and the future tout court. Derrida, in his turn, has left the philosophical scene well aware of the necessity of thinking and practicing deconstruction in the future-to-come. At the end of his career, he insistently asked, does "postdeconstruction" exist? Will our epochal transition require the recuperation of ontology? Is it necessary to insist on the demise of dialectics as inscribed in the histories of culture, politics, and institutions and as advocated by the Hegelian system in its dedication to Absolute Knowledge?[5] In deconstruction's future-to-come, is it not the system of the philosophical question—"What is it?"—and the right to question—"Who interrogates whom?" or "Who interrogates for what?"—to be deconstructed and, in so doing, opened up to the call of the other, who arrives—if and when she arrives—to break with any sovereignty of expectation, appropriation, and interpretation, freed from all absolutistic pretenses of (the system of) philosophical thinking and from the order of history in its controlling "succession" and its "force of law"?

The writing here presented shares these deconstructive perplexities. If it is true that writing is the trait overcome by our epoch, it still remains relevant in a system—the graphosphere—that lasts and will last for a period that remains to be defined, inscribing its "dissemination" or the "survival" of its philosophical and political reflection on the present and on its à-venir. The "return" of dialectics and its radical "dissemination": these are the two traits that I want to countersign with my intervention in the debate. They represent two interpretations of subjectivity, two conceptions of the critical energy that supports them, two positions in the face of philosophical systematicity. They are the assumptions that involve, in the reflection carried out by Malabou, an attention on the "work of the negative" and, differently, in the work by Derrida, the infinite affirmation of life (*Learning to Live Finally* was his last intervention before his death in 2004).[6] From these two assumptions follow an emphasis on a "plastic mourning" on one side and on "laughter" on the other side, a "laughter" that does not avoid death but knows how to illuminate its coming with a different "intimacy."[7] In one case, at the core of the philosophical circle, the translation of dialectics into plasticity appears; in the other case, dissemination is precisely interested in the critique of dialectic. In one case, *kenosis* assumes the destinies of plasticity; in the other, there is an emphasis on the uncontrollable inscription of the trace.

"The trace will never pierce the figure": the confrontation between plasticity's "return" to Hegel and the resistance of deconstruction are here framed in a "project" and a "program." Catherine Malabou develops her "invention" of plasticity in Hegel by making its concept traverse Continental philosophy and Western sciences, with a determination to "trans-form" the system of philosophy itself. The "ject" of her speculative energy is directed, it takes place, it explicates itself in favor—a "protension" (121)—of plasticity, in its established meaning of "giving and receiving" form, "reforming," "exploding" (the plastic) and "transforming" that same system.[8] Her critical interventions seem to again expose philosophy to its own "death"; in this mortal face-to-face, "plastic mourning" offers philosophy a fluidized and mobile self-defining process—one that is able to absorb, appropriate, incorporate, and at the same time unify both tradition and change. This process implies the act of kenosis ("without" is a key word in Malabou, who asserts that we must philosophize "without identity" and "without difference")[9] and of the Eucharistic, which together celebrate philosophy's final *relève*.[10] Malabou would say that this implies *voir venir* the speculative automatism, the "selfless" of the Hegelian—desired, announced and realized—"plastic reading." For Derrida, though, what appears at the center of the practice of deconstruction is not the "trans-formation" of the philosophical system but its "deferment"—dis-location, dis-adherence, post-ponement—capable of bringing "elsewhere"/*ailleurs* all instances of vital affirmation and their surviving ghosts. Without intending any "before" or "after" the political engagement of deconstruction, the legacy left by Derrida becomes a "pro-gram" produced while practicing the survival of writing, along the axis of its resistance, in the historical shadow of its *survie*.

I here try to read "plastically" the interview "Paper or Me" that Derrida gave *Les Cahiers de Médiologie* (1997) by untying some of its nuclei of attention in their impossible relevance to Malabou's plasticity.[11] For Derrida, time is now and the future cannot be anticipated because calculation would negate its promise and, consequently, its "advent" or "event."[12] "Now," beyond any plastic progress of the *substance-subject*, what we are witnessing is a "seismic earthquake" of the very system of "subjectedness" carried out by writing itself. In its advanced technological outcome, the "force of law" of writing continues to provoke, in its contemporary "withdrawal," some important effects and affects (Derrida speaks of "symptoms"). For example—and "exemplarity" is here the question—the authoritarian incorporation of the "paper principle" is causing global discrimination toward people who do not comply with its parameters of identification, the ones who do not possess the "base" of any certification on "paper": the *sans-papiers*." Today this displaced community emerges on the "scene" (here the word is not metaphorical but implies the real—"theatrical"—scene of necessary encounters and dialogues)[13] of the political agenda, necessarily claiming "true" forms of hospitality, actions of collective engagement, and common denotations of words—in other terms, "a program of the baseless."

"The pro-ject of plasticity" / "The pro-gram of the baseless": I conclude my "wonder" inside the philosophies and practices of present-day critical thought with a reference to the contemporary work taking place within the "plastic" art par excellence: the "sculptures" of the transnational performer Zoulikha Bouabdellah. I let myself wonder at this work because her brief but intense productions seem to indicate a "return" to plasticity, countersigned by an insistence on some deconstructive assumptions. Beyond any "trans-formation" or "dis-semination" of the system, Z.B. is determined to "deviate"; in particular, her artistic attention is focused on the cultural motif of "eros." Her experimentation is not inscribed with any dialectics of negativity and/or affirmation, death and/or life; it is vindicated as a wholly other "birth," experienced in geographic and identity displacement and tainted by childish, infantile, and "soft" transgressions of both plasticity and deconstruction. Z.B.'s art "softens" the performative screen and, by operating an infinite "jet" of ironic inscriptions, manages to pierce the surface of her figures. It is the contradictory rendering of plastic philosophy marking the birth of "chance": from the "holes" practiced on her *subjectile*, the twinkling of an eye might induce belief that we are "seeing coming" a new epoch, another history. In truth, the simulacrum of the traversed surface merely produces "mirages"—for example, the *Mirage*, the title and content of one of Z.B.'s last performances: of the ongoing Arab revolutions. Here the Hegelian sentence "God is dead," Malabou's conviction that "writing is dead," and the Derridean resistance of their cinders recall another death: "Marx is dead." Z.B.'s art keeps questioning the veracity of "Marx is dead"; her reply is that only the future-to-come will respond to the "dis-order" of history, without expectation or calculation, affirming life in the next collective actions and resting open to the promises of alterity, "incalculable" and "ungraspable" beyond any plastic "project" or deconstructive "program" . . .

"GOD IS DEAD": THE "PROJECT" OF PLASTICITY

... if God is dead, is it an accident? Is he dead by accident? If by accident, would he have seen it, and seen it coming—or not? Would or could he have seen it come in this sense (foresight) or in this other sense (unexpectedness) of the plasticity inherent to the expression "to see (what is) coming"? If this accident becomes essential, the expression "to see (what is) coming" would be the future anterior of some sort of providence or theodicy . . . : no more explosive surprise, no more letting come, farewell to the future! For the future to have a future—and becoming God himself remains still to come—should not his death, if it has ever taken place, be *purely* accidental? Absolutely unpredictable and never reappropriable, never re-essentializable, not even by some endless work of mourning, not even, above all, by God himself? A god who would have, without ever seeing it come, let an infinite bomb explode in his hands, a god dead by some hopeless accident, hopeless of any salvation or redemption, without essentializing *sublation*, without any work of mourning and without any possible return or refund, would that be the condition of a future, if there must be such a thing called the future? The very condition for something to come, even another God, an absolute other God?[14]

Catherine Malabou appears in the milieu of contemporary philosophy with a "project" to realize: the rethinking, the thinking anew, or the thinking *otherwise* of the Hegelian system. The emphasis, the energy, the "jet" of her determination is itself systematic and precise, strategic and schematic: Malabou vindicates the marginal element of "plasticity" in Hegelian philosophy, translating it as the comprehensive element of the whole, able to produce a different comprehension of—the necessary return to—Hegel in the present and for the projection of his system into the future. Plasticity is actually cited by Hegel as that character of Greek sculpture that emerges in the "forward march of spirit" when Man gives himself a face, supported by the work of "habit" liberating him from the structural pathology of his "inside," his self-feeling and (his)torical self-determination. For Malabou, "plasticity" becomes the fluidification of dialectics, a necessary force that establishes the dynamism by which Man interacts with the negativity that is himself, in his constitutive encounter with the "alterity" that is in the world and that reflects itself in Man's self-feeling, the structure that "anticipates" heterogeneity and that knows how to trans-form itself—dialectically, plastically—into a force of advancement, the progress of history, the "jet" toward the new conditions of existence. For Hegel, this dialectical achievement marks the final acquisition of the speculative; for Malabou, it means *voir venir* plasticity as the future in/of Hegel and for the future in general.[15]

"Negativity programmes substance."[16] At the center of Hegelian thought and, conversely, in the philosophy of Malabou, there is a specific interest: the passage, the elevation of the *substance*-subject to the substance-*subject*, the coming out from vital organicity in its progressive movement toward philosophical speculation, passing through teleological modernity, and concentrating on the "negativity" in the human (and the vegetal and animal) kingdom.[17] Initially, negativity constitutes the incapability of Man to erect himself as the example of the species, due to an internal "alienation" that can verge on idiotic pathology (the concentration on one's own incapability) or on madness, the mental illness or the heterogeneous presence assumed as an incurable "split" in subjectivity. In the historical origin of this process, the Greek moment, the remedy to such alienation, is provided by "habit," the appropriation of one's self, that adapts, exercises, practices continuity and change, producing the adaptability, the reproducibility, and the connivance of Man with his own species. Man feels negativity, alienation, and heterogeneity "within" him and, by fluidizing, plastifying, acquiring the habit to the new conditions of existence, knows how to project himself in his historical progress, in the overcoming or *relève* of his own structure of temporalization. Subjectivity anticipates alterity, and by "possessing" and "appropriating" it—if the etymological meaning of "habit" lies in *habere*—it sends itself in advance of time, in "excess" over time, towards the future: "the same project: how to characterize the subject as a structure of anticipation, and, by the same token, a structure of temporalization" (130).

The strength of the "negative," however, is not arrested here. Malabou advances her project by noticing that "Habit murders man . . . it is also a force of death which, once the aim is achieved, puts the individual to death" (76). The plastic thrust of Man towards the new era, his project after his death: it is the second and central "step" by which we move from the Greek moment to modernity. "God is dead" here marks the scandal of reason in establishing the advancement, the evolution, and the progress of the "project" of subjectivity. God divides himself in the triad of the Father, the Son, and the Spirit; God "incarnates" in Christ, accepting the negativity inside him; he then sacrifices himself on the cross, to finally resurrect in the Spirit. This passage is the apotheosis of plasticity: God assumes to himself the pain and suffering of the human, plastifying himself in Man; from Man he receives the form, giving it to Christ, who in his turn incarnates human destiny in a "representation" that puts "at a distance" the assumption of negativity, death, and sacrifice. The evil that determines God's sacrificial death turns into the motif of his resurrection. If God represents himself in Christ, Christ is then produced by kenosis (the emptying out of God's divine attributes, his absolute spoliation, his assumption of the "without" of divine traits, which will plastically resolve into his resurrection) and, even more strategically, in the "Incorporation," the "Eucharistic," as the final assimilation of God by the believers (who then become God himself) and by the community of cult, which knows how to appropriate God's death and, in so doing, projects itself towards the advent of a new history.

It is now time for the third "step" of the "forward march of the spirit," the one it accomplishes in traversing, fluidifying, and appropriating its limits and its own negativity. If initially the accidental becomes essential and if in a second moment the essential becomes accidental, now, on the stage of human progress, the *substance-subject* opens to the Speculative. By constituting the definitive *relève* of the past and the present, the systemic automatism, which can do "without" identity, difference, and heterogeneity, announces its sheer and pure future: the transcendental imagination, Absolute Knowledge, the end of history, and the coming of the new epoch. By taking place as the synthesis of the Greek moment and the modern moment, it establishes the new era of plasticity. In its absolute form, the form of the system, the completion of the subject's self-determination now becomes the self-thinking idea, the absolute freedom of thinking-for-itself: "I think" gets established in the *eidos*, freed from all attachment or alienation, finally capable of self-feeling, self-determining, self-causing, self-distributing, self-regulating. In this last passage, the project of plasticity reaches its "resting place" (of the Spirit): the event of the abandonment of the "I" of all its internal fracturations in order to place itself in the speculative automatism. The Hegelian scheme is in place (and time); for Malabou, it functions as the "outline" of her own project in favor of plasticity: the production of the discursive conditions for the advent of Absolute Knowledge and the emergence of the Philosopher, who can finally form his own idiom, the formal expression of the Spirit, the discipline of "plastic" reading that gives and receives form by deforming, exploding, reforming, and transforming philosophical thinking along the line of its absolute continuity and change.

Malabou's discourse is not abstract or metaphorical. The energy she assumes from the thought of Hegel, *from* the future in/of Hegel and *for* the future in general; the "outline" or "overarching structure" of his system turns, precisely, historically, plastically, into Malabou's project of her plastic writing.[18] After *The Future of Hegel*, the author starts the mirroring of what she has discovered (in fact, it was already there, like a "purloined letter") in the German philosopher into a series of passages, "steps," or "trials"—leading to a closure, a circular composition, the final *relève*—that are foundational of her philosophical elaboration.[19] The following text, *Le change Heidegger. Du fantastique en philosophie* (2004), plasticizes the Heideggerian thought of imagination into plastic "metamorphosis." In *Plasticity at the Dusk of Writing: Dialectic, Destruction, Deconstruction* (2010), she vindicates the "end" or "death" of the grapheme as the end of an epoch which "sees coming" the emergence of plasticity as the historical future of thought. In *Que faire de notre cerveau?* (2004), in an important move toward neurosciences, Malabou acquires the "representability" of the cerebral synapsis in order to *voir venir* the plastic liberation of the brain itself. In *Les nouveaux blessés: De Freud à la neurologie, penser les traumatismes contemporains* (2007), the kenosis of Hegelian inspiration finds its exemplary form in the Alzheimer patient, in total emptiness, the absolute loss of memory, the traumatic, painful, and "human too human" indifference to the world. In "The Eternal Return and the Phantom of Difference" (2010), Malabou plastically reads the intervention of Gilles Deleuze and Jacques Derrida on the "eternal return" in Nietzsche against any principle of difference, *seeing coming* the philosophical future in the task of thinking "without" identity and "without" difference.

But what would a reading of Nietzsche give that would refuse to turn difference into its guiding thread? With this question I end this text, leaving open the possibility of a new understanding of the eternal return—that is to say also, of life—that would substitute synthesis for difference and the equally unsettling figure of the *clone* for that of the phantom. I thus state very simply, in the form of an announcement, the possibility of reading the doctrine of *the eternal return as a thought of ontological cloning*. And what if, in the end, everything were to redouble, if all the ontological knots were to reduplicate, without being different but without returning to the same either? What if the philosophical challenge of our epoch, prefigured by Nietzsche, was precisely to come to think without identity and without difference?[20]

It is, however, in *Sois mon corps* (2010), the dialogue with Judith Butler on Hegel's "Domination and Servitude," that Malabou finally turns to the absolute, pure, and simple vindication of the philosophical system, claiming the Hegelian "absolute detachment": "Plasticity acquires its definitive meaning . . . The form of 'self' explodes . . . This explosive detachment is presented by Hegel as an '*Aufheben*,' an 'abandon.' This '*Aufheben*' is not exactly a *relève* but a free abandon."[21]

"WRITING IS DEAD": THE "PROJECT OF THE BASELESS"

I have learned words,
They have taught me things.
In my turn I teach them a new way to act
—Antonin Artaud

The Hegelian scheme—its *betwixt* and *between*—"anticipates" and "advances" plastic thought; Malabou's project vindicates it in the emergence of its sheer automatism by drawing the "outline" of a new philosophy corresponding to a new epoch, which is in fact the same epoch but rethought, to be thought *otherwise*. Still, the "wonder" would question precisely what happens if the (Hegelian) system—the *substance-subject*, the order of history that produces it, the negativity that inhabits it, the plastic mourning that incorporates it, and the *relève* that resolves it—comes to be exposed to a series of "seismic shake-ups" that no plastic structure might ever contain, absorb, or return to itself? Here, the "outline" of a reply can be provided by the "interview" "Paper or Me" that Jacques Derrida gave *Les Cahiers de la Médiologie* (1997), in an issue devoted to *pouvoirs du papier*, where he offers a radical "other" perspective in the face of plasticity.[22] Positioning his reasoning neither in the subject's "anticipation" nor in the "excess" of time over time, Derrida concentrates on "a period of history of a technology and in the history of humanity" where critical attention is on today's specific condition of the *substance-subject* par excellence: the contemporary destinies of "paper," the support, the *being-beneath*, "the submission or subjectedness of subjectivity in general" (42–43).

This too has a history: "a technological or material history," "a symbolic history of projections and interpretations, a history tangled up with the invention of the human body and of hominization." This history, however, is not tainted with negativity, death, or dusk; the energy of a constant "affirmation" supports it, affirming not the actual decline or *demise* of paper but its resisting *resistance*. Today, by being exposed to a series of "telluric earthquakes," paper is not dying in order to transform itself into something else, even in its "plastic" otherness, but it survives in its "getting small," "shrinking," "reduction," or "withdrawal"—if we are witnessing the announcement of its "loss" or "end," the *substance-subject* of paper continues to hold us, now and for a stretch of incalculable time, through every sense and every fantasy, "with the interest, investment and economy it will continue to mobilize for a long time to come" (42): "Paper is the support not only for marks but for a complex 'operation'—spatial and temporal; visible, tangible, and often sonorous; active but also passive (something other than an 'operation' then, the becoming-opus or the archive of operative work) . . ." (42). The survival operation of paper constitutes the radical deconstruction of all the dialectical efforts that still labor in trying to control paper's dynamism, producing the dominant conventions that still want to appropriate the historical economy of the backing of the paper's surface. Always and already exposed to its unstable hierarchy ("fine paper" can easily be delivered to abasement; its immaculate virginity, together with its sacred, safe, and indemnified value, can always verge on discredit; its valorization turns into depreciation), paper is what allows the disseminating trace to appear on the "stage" of the deconstruction of dialectics and plastic mourning. On this stage paper, beneath its surface, holds a volume in reserve, a series of folds, the enigmatic drawings of infinite labyrinths. Its reserve is provided by the body that experiences its inscription on the *subjectile*: the hands, the eyes, the voice, the ears, the traces inscribed in the paper's withdrawal. They are the ones that carry out the breaking of all typographical habits (simultaneity, synopsis, and synchrony) and the disturbance of the idea of a flat, transparent, and reflective surface by failing it, occupying it, reinventing its formatting devices, its "unilinear" continuum and "monorhythmical" line. Instead of habit, appropriation, and possession, these bodily traces affirm their work of "disadherence," the opening up of "hollows," "gaps," and "holes" on the withering support of paper, through which the task of ethical responsibility is to insist on reading the incalculability, dissemination, *restance*, and *retrait* of its "order":

> Thus the order of the page, even as a bare survival, will prolong the afterlife of paper—far beyond its disappearance or its withdrawal.
>
> I always prefer to say its withdrawal (*retrait*) since this word can mark the limit of a structural or even structuring, modelling hegemony, without that implying a death of paper, only a *reduction*. (46)

The "reduction" of paper—without end or death, "an endless murmur, the underlying existence, the bottomless depth"[23]—signifies a specific double bind: if paper remains a constraint, it will continue to provoke the permanent desire of transgressing it; at the same time, the technological mutation or reduction experienced by paper does not liberate the strategy of a plastic reading but, instead, provokes a retrospective interpretation, the anterior future of the past resources of paper itself. In this case, there will be no kenosis, the emptying out or the "without" of paper's graphospheric traits, but rather the interrogation of the superimpositions, overimprintings, overwritings, and overinterpretations of the remains of paper; the concepts and fantasies, the projections, cathexes, and desires inscribed on its *beneath*; the inhibitions, the symptoms and the anxiety, the abandon and the arrest, sedimented on its material surface.[24] What is important to note is that this incalculable and infinite interrogation is necessarily governed by a deconstructive anamnesis, which will never produce any *relève*, *dénouement*, or untying of a new posthistorical era but will keep insisting on the "remains" of the present time:

> Another epoch, then: but isn't an *epoch* always the suspension of prohibition, an organization of withdrawal or retention? This new epoch, this other reduction, would also correspond to an original displacement, already, of the body in displacement—to what some might perhaps be quick to call another body, even another unconscious . . . the eroticization of fingers, feet, hands, and legs. While it is tied to the "paper" system (just a few centuries, a second in regard to the history of humanity), this furtive eroticization also belongs to the very long time of some process of hominization. Do tele-sex or internet sex alter anything in this? A program with no base. A program of the baseless. (54–55)

The "program of the baseless" is, for Derrida, not only a hint towards a future-to-come; it is a task urged by the present state of things. By turning the metaphoric progress of the *substance-subject* into its materiality, the philosopher again constructs the difference of his philosophy from the Hegelian scheme in a very specific way. If in Hegel, as read by Malabou, "God is dead" in order to be sublated in the arrival of the Speculative, which marks its assimilation, digestion, and incorporation by his community of cult, then in "Paper or Me" Derrida focuses on "Incorporation" as a real "force of law" of the subject of the paper-substance. If paper is withdrawing—at a scandalous speed—then the modes of its appropriation are not disappearing; on the contrary, they are becoming "spectral," virtualizing, fantasizing, undergoing a process of abstraction that make them more operative because they've become "incorporated schemata," ghost members, supplements of a structuring prosthesis. If paper once protected subjectivity, providing the "resting place" of the self's appropriation, the certification of the construction and institution of its identity by means of the autograph, the signature, the identity document, then the shrinking of paper, its substitution by electronic supports, cards, and numeral codes, provokes a series of anxieties due to which "a certain legitimating authority of paper still remains intact" (57). This authority does not represent the responsibility of the Philosopher in view of the advent of the "Speculative"; it presents the urgent move to "the essence of politics and its link with the culture of paper" (61). It is what moves public attention, for example, to the question of the *sans-papiers*, the community of "baseless people" or undocumented immigrants who struggle to get identity papers throughout the worlds of their exiles or migrations. In truth, this "well-determined category of people subjected to an un-admissible discrimination" announces a "program" to the public space: the urgency of a "new legal imminent age," a "new economy," a "new international and national law," and a "new politics." It is, indeed, a "common" program, because the incorporation of paper, turned into its force of law," affects the *sans-papiers* and, at the same time, humanity in its whole, producing the awareness that "we are all baseless people": "there are processes of technological transition at work: the recording of marks of identification and signature is computerized. Computerized but, as we were saying, via the inherited norms of paper that continue to haunt electronic media. It is computerized for citizens and their citizen status (consider what happens at passport controls), but it can also be computerized for the physical-genetic identification of any individual in general (digital photography and genetic imprints). In this, we are all, already, paperless people" (61).[25]

"MARX IS DEAD": THE "JET" OF ART

> One of the most striking sculptors involved is Giuseppe Pennone, whose work is devoted to forming the trace, as if the trace were the raw material of an *ultrametaphysical development of the concept of form* and hence an *ultrametaphysical development of the understanding of sculpture*: "a trace formed by the images I have on hand."
> —Catherine Malabou

> Do you know Richard Long's sculptures? He lays down the archive, so to speak, of certain trajectories, often with stones or even with dried mud that draws a circle in a landscape literally sculptured by the artist's memory—and what rests of the *oeuvre*-in-progress is then exposed, the journey makes *oeuvre*.
> —Jacques Derrida, referring to Long's "A Walk of Ten Days in High Sierra California 1995," "Asia Circle Stones," "Gobi Desert Circle," and "White Mud Circle"

"God is dead" and paper is dying: what will take place in the future?[26] Derrida closes the "outline" of his interview with an interrogation and a chance of reply:

> Writing, literature, even philosophy . . . would they survive beyond paper? Survive beyond a world dominated by paper? Survive the time of paper? These inexhaustible questions . . . would stay that way, impossible to deal with, as theoretical questions, on a horizon of knowledge—on a horizon, quite simply.
>
> The response will come from what future decisions and events, from what the writing of a future that cannot be anticipated, will make of it, from what it will do for literature and for philosophy, from what it will do to them. (64)

Let me finish the "outline" of my own (plastic?) reading with some of the "decisions," "events," and "actions" that belong to contemporary plasticity par excellence: the sculptures animating the performance art of Zoulikha Bouabdellah, the artist who, in her brief but intense career, has worked to translate the philosophical reading of plastic "subjectivity" and the political dissemination of the "subjectedness" of paper into the investigation of the "subject" of plasticity in art, its communicative potentiality when inscribed on the screen of her performances. In her artistic position, Z.B. is not aiming at "trans-forming" the Hegelian system nor at "de-constructing" the "force of law" of the graphosphere; she wants to "de-viate" a specific motif of today's cultural system, that is, the rigid codification of eros, especially for women in the Muslim world. She wants to "plastify" this cultural motif by transgressing it in a "soft" fashion: "Deviation for deviation, I proceed by transgressing things in a noninvasive or judgmental way. I push limits in accordance with a positive rhythm by going from one element to another, from one structure to another, from one shape or from one concept to another. . . . Despite the paradox, my transgression actually aims to reconnect links. A transgressive dynamics that reflects the world's biological and historical mutations or a connection between beliefs and values, subjects, symbols, stereotypes, genres and sexes."[27]

Soft Transgression is the title of the text that "outlines" the force of Z.B.'s experiments. "Soft transgression" is also what allows the artist to "see coming" the interaction of the philosophy of plasticity with the incisive strength of deconstruction: her work seems to directly face Malabou's assumption that "the grapheme will never pierce the figure," giving her own interpretation of the philosopher's conviction. By refusing to position herself either in death and "negativity" or in the "survival" mode of existence, Z.B. "receives and gives" form to her art in the instance of a new birth, her own "birth" diasporically displaced in Russia: "I imagine: she would scream her state of woman in pain in French? In Arab? Would the midwife give her advice in Russian? I have been unconsciously marked by the cultural boilings that filled the room . . . there must have surely been Ukrainian, Georgian, Lithuanian nurses."[28] This birth assigns the story to her mother while designating the task of "imagination" to the artist herself. The form taken by Z.B.'s imagination is the "deviation"— *l'écart* allied to women since Scheherazade[29]—of the limits of representation. In her imaginative practice, formal transversality is what realizes the link *betwixt/between* elements, structures, concepts, beliefs, values, symbols, genders, and sexes: ". . . the plasticity of form involved in its process of formation."[30]

How can Z.B. establish such a "schema"? What "tactic" will she adopt? According to a plastic strategy, after her "different" birth, Z.B. wants to imagine a wholly other birth of art, an *otherwise* imagination of artistic birth, according to an obstetrics performed by a "forceps" that, beyond all dialectics of life and death, nature and culture, anticipation and excess, will practice a new act and a new "sense" (*forcenner* also means *hors sens*, to be gifted with "another" sense).[31] Since 2002, in her residencies in South Africa, in America, in Palestine, in Syria, the "jet" of her creations has been un/measuring itself against/with all possible matters, genders, and genres. Her projects include installations, anecdotes in the shape of brief videos and photographs, sheets of paper (in *Chéri*, 365 drawings are accompanied by written sentences in red lacquer), ink and acrylic, wood, transparent Plexiglas, gelled polyester, loudspeakers, nets (*Carre blanc sur fond noir*, 2006), even modified *couscoussières* that the artist entitles *Moresque, Marranos* (2006).[32] In her performances, installations, and single pieces, she uses clay and gold leaf (*Autoportrait ou la pucelle*, 2008); lacquer iron, lacquer wood, resin, dust, neon lights, paillettes, lamps, mannequin busts, veils, bras, embroideries on velvet. Her works ex-scribe in triptychs or dioramas; they choose the color red, the blue monochrome, the white; they involve poetry, music, and cinema. These materials constitute the "outline" of Z.B.'s "subject" and "subjected" surface, the artistic matrix where to inscribe the *forcenned* "jet" of her writing (made, literally, of letters and words), softly transgressing.

To reconnect figurative representation and nonrepresentative representation raises the question of figuration and its opposite, the status of images, such as videographic images, and their intrinsic connection to light. It also raises the question of an "image's opposite—and therefore light's opposite—black."[33]

In her first *Écran* (the "screen" defined by Malabou as the "representation-stereotype or philosophical resistance to neuroscience and vice versa"),[34] Z.B.'s "deviation" takes place with/in a written gesture established on the threshold of light and darkness.[35] A woman, illuminated by the light that comes from a television showing the face of a man, covers the screen from high to low, her hand using a plastic substance. While the television light gets darker, the light allowing the shooting extinguishes; the scene stops existing when the whole screen is covered up. White and black, light and darkness, constitute the full and the emptied *écran*: the image, in order to reveal itself, needs light (solar, electric, internal, external), indissociable from it; its dialectical pair is darkness, marking the absence of images in the void. Darkness is what constitutes the bottom from where the image is born. It is within the richness of this black that the image-to-come exists, if only virtually. For Z.B. the "moving image" is the link between the opposites of light and darkness, where the act of transgression is realized by the woman's hand performing a "caress" that recalls the ancient gesture of *Amadou*, the "softening" of the screen's surface: "this substance whose Provençal name designates the amorous behaviour of the *amador*, is used to rub and caress. Rubbing and caressing in order to enflame is done with the help of a colored substance known for its facility to set fire. To soften with *amadou*: to appease, domesticate, flatten, tame the other, seduce or win over the enemy by caressing, but also to burn, inflame, set fire to him . . . leave holes of fire in the page. Those were *working*.[36] The workings of plasticity and Z.B.'s own "soft" transgression are producing their creative actions.

In her next work, *Silence*, the artist stages another deviation—one that "propagates"[37]—of the cultural motif of eros by presenting a praying carpet (in fact, many carpets!) with burnt "holes" inside which golden high-heeled shoes inscribe the female "hosts," the parasites, incubi and succubi of a religion that expels women's desire. If the matter of the screen's surface has been fluidized, softened, and plasticized, it now needs to be "traversed":

To probe: the probing element works by penetrating . . . perforating the surface and passing through to the other side—"I could probe" . . . means that: I could make the most intimate of moves, by transgressing a limit . . . a *mine* . . . I could probe to find out, to discover the truth under the subjectile, behind the veil or the screen . . . try to learn, to decipher the sign or the symptom of a truth . . . by refusing or exposing the inertia of a sick body is to prepare oneself to treat them for their good, starting with their own truth.

To cut: . . . with scalpels, scissors, shears, knives, needle tips, or feathers: cut, notch, diminution, castration. But to cut is also to regenerate, to strengthen by loping off everything restraining the growth, to prune, thin, cut back; rejuvenate . . . in short, to save, physically or symbolically . . .

To scrape: . . . I could irritate the surface . . . In scraping I risk wounding . . . But in scraping I purify, I appease, I efface what is written to write again . . . accede to the other surface as it is hidden, asphyxiated, interred under the deposit.

To file: "I could . . . file," *break into* the figure . . . according to the obliqueness of the metal teeth, molar against millstones . . . but the aggression . . . is destined to polish, make delicate, adjust, inform, beautify . . .

To sew: I could . . . sew . . . make holes in the skin of the figure, but I can sew, and even suture and scar, in order to close the wound that I open in sewing . . .

To unsew: "I could . . . unsew," unmake, do the preceding operation in reverse, and it was already the reverse of itself. The link itself, like the link between these two operations that consists precisely in a certain treatment of linking and unlinking, the obligation of this ligature is a *double bind*, a double conjuncture. . . .

To shred: . . . cut into pieces, into tatters or shreds, slash, hack, wound, mutilate the body with a cutting instrument . . . *Shredded* linen also names the old cloth (textile is always along with paper, the best paradigm of the subjectile) from which threads are taken to make bandages, generally in wars. The act of war would be perhaps purely aggressive and devoid of any repairing counterpath without this virtual allusion to the act of bandaging . . .

To stitch: . . . never to cease *covering with scars* . . . the body . . . covered with traces, the scars of blows and wounds. But to cover with scars may mean at the same time to multiply the bows and wounds and the gestures of reparation, sutures, and bandages, which belong to the moment of scarring. Surgery does both, successively or simultaneously.[38]

Z.B.'s plastic and/or deconstructive action "pierces" the surface by "probing, cutting, scraping, filing, sewing and unsewing, shredding and stitching" the textile of the carpet; in the emptied hole of its surface, she inscribes the material fetish of female jouissance, the written marks of women's play, desire, and resistance. Is this the instance when, "inside-outside" sense, as a "soft" transgression, Z.B.'s perforating "jet" might allow one to perceive the other side of another epoch—"to see oneself on the other side of the target, already on the other side, and from the other side of the wall that I also am. I traverse the membrane, and my own skin?"[39] In truth, in envisioning the "traversal" of time, identity, and body, what matters is that the creative journey, its thrust and "jet," is always and already offering a "chance" to "chance": "But I do not traverse, or in doing so, I keep a trace of a traversal, even if the trace is in its turn subjected or promised to the trajectory that it recalls, which in truth it calls. . . . . This *arrest* of the journey makes a work. I understand the arrest as the

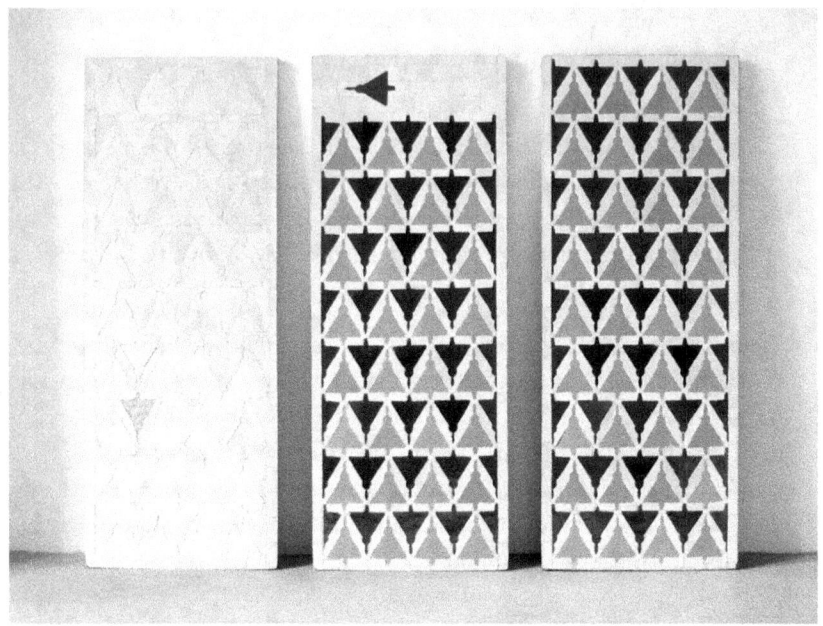

Figure 7.1. Zoulikha Bouabdellah, *Is your love darling just a mirage?*, 2011. Zellige ceramics, 100 × 120 cm. Ed. 2/3. Courtesy Sabrina Amrani Gallery and the artist.

sentence that makes the law, and as the interruption of thrust, the tonic immobilization of a would-be-lancer. Both giving birth to chance."[40]

Zoulikha's jet "arrests" on her last work, *Mirage*, an installation that shows her artistic perspective on the events taking place in North Africa, the Arab "revolutions": "In a few months, history has changed its side. It is now being written in the south, across the Mediterranean, where after Tunisian and Egyptian revolutions, civil war in Libya and the rising of Syrian people, the spreading revolution has arrived to Bahrain and Yemen. And while Morocco launches unprecedented political reforms, Algeria is committed to strengthening the democratic process. How will all this end up? No one can say with certainty. . . ."[41] To celebrate the structural "uncertainty" of the "revolution," Zoulikha produces the picture of the Mirage aircraft of Gadhafi's air force, shot down in flight by the rebel forces, with its beak pointing toward the Lebanese soil (see Figure 7.1).

The image resounds with Z.B.'s question: "Will the image inspire the continuation of the story or, agitated as a broken promise, will it remain in the state of mirage?"[42] *Mirage* takes the form of a geometric composition, inspired by a specific idiomatic repertoire: like the concepts underlining the tradition of Arabic tiles, the "unattainable" is inscribed inside a visual experience that exceeds contemplation in order to provoke interpretation, offering its "future" to *l'à-venir* of history. For Zoulikha, the forms of *Mirage*, by combining rhythmic movements that the eye cannot see accurately, are the "shapes that attract the brain with their lack of certainty that characterizes each revolutionary episode . . ."[43] Is it still necessary to "comprehend" the (mirage of) revolution on the edge of its "plastic reading" and/or the "disseminative break" of its surface? In truth, art will have already produced her "inedited" events calling for another responsibility that, without certainty on the forms of their "resolutions," in the very caesura or derangement of the order of time, will promise the coming of the other. If the "revolution" breaks with subjectivity, history, and knowledge, art will have always already plasticized and deconstructed its "representation," offering its absolute hospitality—without "identity" and in "radical difference"—to *l'à-venir*, where the "unknown" can only be "wondered" at. "The inedited waits for us, there, we repeat, where we don't know any longer what waits for us . . ."[44]

NOTES

1. Derrida, "Time for Farewells," xl. This preface, first published as Derrida, "Le temps des adieux," appeared in Italian as a single text entitled *Il tempo degli addii*. In "go wonder . . . ," the translation proposed by Joseph D. Cohen for the Derridean "*allez savoir*," there is an echo of the expression "*voir venir*" that Malabou invents for "the coming of plasticity." In my reading, "go wonder" associates with Derrida, "Quelqu'un s'avance et dit" (in Derrida, Guillaume, and Vincent, *Marx en jeu*, dedicated to the play *Karl Marx*, in *Théâtre inédit*, by Jeanne-Pierre Vincent), on the "scene" of politics and to his "faire arriver quelque chose" ("Marx, c'est quelqu'un," 21) to speculative "dialectics." For the question of "translation" in Malabou, *Plasticity at the Dusk*, cf. Martinon, *On Futurity*.

2. In *Plasticity at the Dusk*, Malabou remarks that Derrida's "Time for Farewells" ("a very subtle and generous response to my book") "clearly presents his philosophical resistance to plasticity," 74.

3. See Butler, *Psychic Life*.

4. Malabou and Derrida, *La contre-allée*; Malabou, *Counterpath*.

5. See esp. Derrida, "Marx & Sons," where, in replying to Negri, "Specter's Smile," Derrida wonders why, in the aftermath of deconstruction, what can

be labeled "postdeconstruction," "ontology" is to come back on the scene of a future philosophy, providing "restoration of order": "I agree, I agree about everything with the exception of one word, 'ontology'; why do you cling to that word? Why do you want to put forward a new ontology, after having duly noted the transformation that renders the Marxist paradigm of ontology obsolete? Why do you want to re-ontologize at all costs, at the risk of restoring everything to order, to the grand order, but to order?," 257.

6. Derrida, *Learning to Live Finally*.

7. Derrida, "Marx & Sons." "First of all, I believe, and have often emphatically stated, that deconstruction, which is affirmative right down to this conception of the messianic without messianism, is anything but a negative movement of nostalgia and melancholy . . . it is true that this has not prevented me from reflecting, just as insistently, on the work of mourning . . . without therefore relinquishing a certain gaiety of affirmative thinking," 259–61. See also Derrida, "Restricted to General Economy," devoted to the "laughter" (poetry, ecstasy) of George Bataille in the face of Hegel's "Absolute Knowledge."

8. For plasticity as "plasticage," see Malabou, *Plasticité*. In reference to the "difference" of plasticity from capitalistic "flexibility," Proctor, "Neuronal Ideologies," reads Catherine Malabou, together with Žižek, *Parallax View*, by affirming, "Contemporary capitalism might be characterized as a network society in which power is distributed across numerous nodes, but countering this model by advocating atomization, separation and extrication is surely not a viable political strategy. The process of healing need not equate to a forced reintegration into the existing status quo, but through the process of forging new connections, as the synapses are capable of doing, new languages and subjectivities may emerge that challenge the dominant political structures, creating alternative collective networks rather than leaving individuals stranded in hopeless isolation . . . Although her insistence on the potential explosivity of plasticity might differentiate it from flexibility, this annihilation of form results in profound alienation," 9, 10.

9. Cf. Malabou, "Eternal Return," 29.

10. The concept of *relève* plays a central role in setting the difference between plasticity and deconstruction: Malabou, *Plasticité*, refers to the translation, proposed by Derrida, of the Hegelian *Aufhebung* into *relève*—"maître du processus dialectique, qui signifie à la fois suppression et conservation" (10); but according to Derrida, from "Restricted to General Economy," "The notion of *Aufhebung* . . . signifies the *busying* of a discourse losing its breath as it appropriates all negativity for itself, as it works the 'putting at stake' into an *investment*, as it *amortizes* absolute expenditure," 257.

11. Derrida, "Paper or Me." For the work of the "im-possibility" in deconstruction, I refer to the special issue of *darkmatter* (8, 2012) devoted to "Impossible Derrida: Works of Invention."

12. The "guarantee" or "calculation" of the future is an undercurrent trait of the debate between Malabou and Derrida. In "Time for Farewells," Derrida thinks that, in interpreting the notion of future in Hegel, Malabou moves "from one farewell to the other. There is always more than a farewell, more than one adieu, in the farewell or the adieu; one renounces the future, the other hopes or promises, but the more it is assured or given (as the salutation inherent to salvation), the more the promise becomes a calculation, that is the more it is lost—as future," xl.

13. Derrida, "Marx, c'est quelqu'un," interprets Shakespeare's *Hamlet*: the play within the play (in dramatic terms and as *jeu*), in folding upon itself, brings the theatrical scene "outside" [*au dehors*] itself, towards the politics of our times; with this scene the French-Algerian philosopher associates, in its "essence," the ethical responsibility against all discriminatory acts of the other.

14. Derrida, "Time for Farewells," xlvii.

15. The question of "dialectic" is often emphasized by recent critics of Malabou. Patricia Pisters, "Plasticity and the Neuro-Image," who is appreciative of Malabou's work, notes: "Considering this trajectory of the concept of plasticity and its implication for the concept of difference, it seems to me that the consequence has to be that also dialectics is exploding. Yet, at other moments in Malabou's texts there remains a strong resistance to letting go of dialectics. In any case, one can wonder if difference as internal, immanent difference, and as salamander-like plasticity, is still a dialectical one." Galloway, "Catherine Malabou," who confesses his lack of "comprehension" of some plastic readings—"Like her Heidegger, I will admit that Malabou's Deleuze is not a Deleuze that I recognize" (10)—wonders ". . . what ideology proposes that everything should and must be mixed, that everything should be profaned? Plasticity to be sure, but is it more that that?" (11). He ultimately finds that "the thing most associated with change is the thing that does not change" (3).

16. Malabou, *Future of Hegel*, 55.

17. Esp. "Habit and Organic Life" and "The Proper of Man in Question" in Malabou, *Future of Hegel*, 57–74. In "Time for Farewells," Derrida remarks that "a profound thought or conception of animal life animates this entire book. It almost gives it its breath," xvii.

18. I mainly refer to Malabou, *Heidegger Change*; *Plasticity at the Dusk*; *New Wounded*; and "Eternal Return"; and Butler and Malabou, *Sois mon corps*.

19. For a different interpretation of the "trial," see Ronell, *Test Drive*.

20. Malabou, "Eternal Return," 28.

21. Butler and Malabou, *Sois mon corps*, 53. See, in "closed" circularity, the interpretation of Derrida, "Time for Farewells," of the question of the "abandonation" of time in Malabou's rethinking of Hegel. On a different critical interest, "In body if not in spirit: Malabou and Butler on Hegel" by Unemployed Negativity, stresses that the discussion on the "body" by Malabou and Butler

brings the elements of "death, work, and fear" back on the scene of public debate; this "return," associated with what Negri describes as a "post-humanist anthropology," "is both the challenge and the limit of their project: in some sense a posthumanist interpretation of "Domination and Servitude" is nearly impossible because it is precisely placing this section, with its drama of death, work, and desire, at the center of Hegel's thought that constitutes the humanist reading." http://www.unemployednegativity.com/2011/01/in-body-if-not-in-spirit-butler and_6182.html.

22. Derrida, "Paper or Me." For the genre of the "interview," its preestablished context, and the "dialogue" it stages, see Derrida, *Points*.

23. See Saghafi, "Derrida."

24. In Derrida's oeuvre, his impossible "trans-actions" were originally and extraordinary inscribed on the Hegelian page—see Derrida, *Glas* (1974). For the dialogue that deconstruction itself establishes with contemporary science, Derrida's "trans-actions" inform the "intra-actions" as elaborated by physician Karen Barad, "Quantum Entanglements."

25. For an "unmetaphorical" outcome of the "program of the baseless," it is interesting to note that, in the year of the quoted interview, Derrida gave the speech "Manquement du droit" at the Théâtre des Amandiers in Nanterre, during the event organized in support of Parisian "*sans-papiers.*" Derrida began his talk by saluting the chance of the "gathering," the opening of the theatre to its political vocation, affirming that its "scene" can become the "just" habitat where, "without representation and without demagogy," it is possible to give hospitality to the chance of "word" of the other; in this case, the poetry, songs, and analysis of the ones who, having lived in France for many years, found themselves exposed to the French law of expulsion. The "clandestines," the "undocumented," the ones without the "dignity" of papers testifying their identity: Derrida knows that the "violation of justice" affects the *sans-papiers* in an unbearable way—it is "an inadmissible discrimination, a crying injustice, a repression that requires an answer in the general protest and universal fight," 83. At the same time, this violation announces something terrifying for everybody, for all the "sans" of the world ("without" work, "without" home, "without" degree. etc.). "Le manquement à la justice" represents a universal symptom, a "global" tragedy organized by a "sad, depressing, depressed, hopeless and inducing lack of hope, power," (86), determined to punish even the "host" who welcomes the other—"the crime of hospitality," indeed. In this sense, for Derrida, we must fight against all its implementations at local and worldly levels, everywhere it takes place, because its "threat" concerns the freedom of everybody—the *sans-papiers* and the *non-sans-papiers*. This fight must employ all material, symbolic, financial, legal, and juridical resources; all chances of civil disobedience must resist its "evil"; all critical and political movements must "change" the law, so as to be able to reinvent a future chance of justice: "a real other justice, both intelligent and generous, which

washes the shame and the infamy of the actual laws, a politic of the stranger, a right of strangers which is not a *manquement à la justice*. We must finally have the chance of living, speaking and breathing otherwise," 91; translation mine. The publication is the transcript of Derrida's intervention, Jan. 21, 1996: http://pharsic.blog.lemonde.fr/2010/11/09/ derrida-note-sur-manquements-du-droit-a-la-justice/. "Breathing otherwise," here associated by Derrida with justice, is taken as the emergence of the "feminine" in philosophy by Irigaray, *Forgetting of Air*. In this respect, Malabou, in Vahanian, "Conversation," 3, refers to Irigaray as "her mother philosopher," while affirming that a "female" philosophy would belong to a "constitutive outside" or an "excessive materiality" that "cannot be said to be something, otherwise it wouldn't be able to transgress ontology. It is then impossible to create or imagine what a feminine philosophical subjectivity might be. . . ." See Malabou, *Changer de différence*. The "female question" is in fact very complex, and it exceeds the limits of this chapter.

26. For Derrida, "Marx, c'est quelqu'un," 24, the sentence "God is dead" goes hand in hand with "Marx is dead" and with the necessity of "le travail of deuil en politique": "When you say 'Marx is dead,' this formula so often repeated, what do you say? . . . To say 'Marx is dead' echoes the formula 'God is dead,' it means to speak after Hegel but also after Christ and Luther, the Christ, himself, 'God is dead' and it has lasted, it lasts. Thus Marx is dead, this sentence, this slogan . . . is the symptom, the symptom of a labour of mourning in progress, with all its phenomena of melancholy, of maniac jubilation, of ventriloquism . . . What seems to me necessary today, is to transport with the necessary transformation, with the necessary translation, to transport the psychoanalytic concept of 'work of mourning,' which normally concerns the individual, the family, to transport it into politics," 25. In terms of the theatrical "scene" on which to play Marx *otherwise*, Derrida appeals to "another way of playing, of operating the *mise en oeuvre*, of making theatre. On the scene of the world, we will have to play Marx, again, to play him well, *to play otherwise*," 65; translation and emphasis mine.

27. Bouabdellah and Sans, *Soft Transgression*, 29.

28. See www.bankgalerie.com/content/pop/pagezoulikha/biozoul.php.

29. Malabou, *Plasticity at the Dusk*, 28–44, is devoted to Hegel, Heidegger, and Levinas on the "fantastic intersection," "visibility," "phantasia" and the "phantasma."

30. Derrida, "Time for Farewells," xiv. It is interesting to note that, in Malabou and Derrida, *La contre-alleé*, at the beginning and at the end of their common journey, one difference between Derrida and Malabou concerns interpretation of *écart*. In the discussion of the "journey" of Ulysses and his experience of *dérive* (as deviation or derivation), Malabou thinks that "Ulysses' path would therefore be a *derived drift* apart from yet toward a founding point. Deriving understood as indicator of provenance wins out over the drift that disorients,

inasmuch, precisely, as the origin itself remains immune from the drift that it renders possible: the origin does not travel. When drift as deviation happens, like some unforeseen catastrophe, it always arrives as an accident befalling an essence, and far from causing structural damage, reaffirms it rather," 5. From here, the philosopher "derives" that "Derrida ne dérive pas," 16. Derrida, in his turn, comes back to the classical text at the end of their "journey" by giving his ("poetic") vision of *écart* in connection with the question of "poetic filiation": "And the Odyssey. There is really there, in the infinite detour, another origin of the world, an impassable secret, and death on the path, the most irreducible other 'within' (not with-in, be careful, but 'within') the one who commands us through a transversal, transversified deviation: the poem of the absolute other. Because it is a question of the poem, a poem, their poem, they [his sons] know it before me, they know it all before me . . . ," 260.

31. In Derrida, "Unsense the Subjectile," the philosopher quotes Heidegger in this respect: "*Wahn* belongs to Old High German and means *ohne*: without. The demented person . . . is gifted with another sense . . . *Sinnan* originally means: to travel, to stretch forwards . . . to take a direction. The Indo-European roots *sent* and *set* mean path," 70.

32. In *Aporias*, Derrida articulates his "concept-figure" of the "Marrano": ". . . Marranos that we are, Marranos in any case, whether we want to be or not, whether we know it or not, Marranos having an incalculable number of ages, hours, and years, of untimely histories, each both larger and smaller than the other, each still waiting for the other, we may incessantly be younger and older, in a last word, infinitely finished," 81. See also Goldschmit, "Cosmopolitique" and www.jacquesderrida.com.ar/comentarios/marrane.htm.

33. Bouabdellah and Sans, *Soft Transgression*, 29. Recently, in "Set Me Free," Z.B. inscribes what Isabelle van den Eynde describes as "couples of giant colorful Arabic letters cut out of aluminium sheets or formed of flashing neon hang randomly on the wall in a playful and lighthearted manner. They are deceptively simple. The elements are familiar—strings of neon twisted to form colourful letters. Yet their unconventional positioning and movement mount a remarkably visceral spectacle, with the suggestive title *Hobb* (Arabic for love) functioning as an integral part of the beguiling ensemble." http://www.docstoc.com/docs/75806900/ZOULIKHA-BOUABDELLAH.

34. Malabou, *What Should We Do*, 40.

35. See http://zoulikhab.com.

36. Derrida, "Unsense the Subjectile," 145.

37. In "Silence d'or," in Bouabdellah and Sans, *Soft Transgression*, 13, Z.B. quotes Marcel Duchamp, explaining that "silence is the best production there is, because it spreads—it propagates."

38. Derrida, "Unsense the Subjectile," 141–42.

39. Derrida, "Unsense the Subjectile," 147.

40. Derrida, "Unsense the Subjectile," 147.

41. *Islamic Arts Magazine* online, "'Mirage' by Zoulikha Bouabdellah," 2011. For the "revolution" in Malabou, a direct reference can be found in *What Should We Do*, 66, where, as she explains, the "neuronal man," as a product of scientific "revolutions," understands the absence of "revolution" in his life: "And what do we get from all these discourses, from all these descriptions of the neural man, from all these scientific revolutions, if not the absence of revolution in our lives, the absence of revolution in our selves." On his part, Derrida, *Death Penalty*, concentrates on the material "revolution" required by the international "legal systems" (see also Saghaki, "Derrida"). The "neural man," "death penalty," and "Arab uprisings" might provide another "outline" of a revolutionary articulation of "philosophy," "politics" and "art."

42. *Islamic Arts Magazine* online, "'Mirage' by Zoulikha Bouabdellah," 2011.

43. *Islamic Arts Magazine* online, "'Mirage' by Zoulikha Bouabdellah," 2011.

44. Derrida, "Quelqu'un s'avance et dit," in Derrida, Guillaume, and Vincent, *Marx en jeu*, 65.

CHAPTER **8**

Insects, War, Plastic Life

Renisa Mawani

▪ In a brief essay appearing near the end of his widely read and acclaimed *Mythologies*, Roland Barthes ruminates on the mass production and quotidian uses of plastics in modern life.¹ Emphasizing their perilous and undesirable qualities—most recently echoed in contemporary concerns over plastics and their hazardous effects on human/environmental health in the global north—Barthes differentiates this engineered, synthetic, and artificial material from the sublime authenticity of nature. "In the hierarchy of the major poetic substances," he writes, plastic "figures as a disgraced material, lost between the effusiveness of rubber and the flat hardness of metal; it embodies none of the genuine produce of the mineral world: foam, fibres, strata." Rather, plastic "is a 'shaped' substance: whatever its final state, plastic keeps a flocculent appearance, something opaque, creamy and curdled, something powerless ever to achieve the triumphant smoothness of Nature."² Here, Barthes is clear that plastic, despite its malleability, can never achieve the exalted qualities or dynamic surfaces of the natural world. Yet its mutability, he cautions, its ability to assume multiple forms, opens the possibility that plastic might eventually surpass and even *replace* nature. The "whole world *can* be plasticized, and even *life itself* since, we are told, they are beginning to make plastic aortas."³ The mid-twentieth century onwards, Barthes predicted with palpable disappointment, was to be an era of plastic.

More recently, Catherine Malabou has also described the contemporary moment in terms of plastic.⁴ Echoing Barthes, affirming his foresight, while at the same time diverting from his dystopic views, Malabou draws attention to the multiplicity of plastics, their everyday circulation, and expanding consumption: "plastic wood, plastic money, plastic paint, and the dangerous plastic material of putty-like consistency that can be shaped by hand."[5] In sharp contrast to Barthes, however, she emphasizes the malleability and transformability of plastic—not as an artificial substance—but as "a new mode of being of form" and a new way of conceptualizing "this mode of being itself." For Malabou, plasticity is not a material or an object but rather a "*new* scheme," one that opens the potential for resistance at a historical juncture increasingly marked by closure.[6] Plastic and plasticity, in her account, do not signal the demise or end of nature, as they did for Barthes, but are situated *between* biology and history, *between* determination and freedom. "The very significance of plasticity itself appears to be plastic," Malabou contends, "opposed to form, describing the destruction and the very annihilation of all form—as suggested by the term 'plastic' explosive for a bomb."[7] Its mutability, which concerned Barthes, is for Malabou what weights plasticity with possibility: "For is not plastic the substitutable material par excellence? Can it not take the place of everything, can it not deconstruct every idea of authenticity, is it not always engaged in the process of its own disappearance? Is it not always beyond its very own form because it can change?"[8] In Malabou's formulation, plasticity's ability to continually re-create content and rupture form is what lends itself to political transformation amidst the expanding horizons of global capitalism where opportunities for resistance seem limited, if not impossible.

In this chapter, I read Malabou's "new scheme" of plasticity and especially her efforts to deconstruct the biology-history divide as a wider imperative to revisit the human/nonhuman distinctions that have repeatedly been unraveled and yet continue to persist with tenacity in critical theory.[9] In the voluminous literature on biopolitics, for example, inspired and developed from Foucault's writings and lectures, discussions of "life itself" continue to be rooted in anthropocentric understandings that privilege the human over the animal and life over death. Despite ongoing scientific pursuits aimed at manipulating and transforming life-forms and notwithstanding critical approaches directed at assessing and analyzing such developments, discussions of life in debates over biopolitics continue to center on anthropocentric accounts of "man-as-species."[10] Whereas Malabou draws attention to human stem cells and to neuroplasticity emphasizing the mutuality of biology, history, and politics, my own interest centers on plasticity as a life and death force that runs through, between, and across human and nonhuman divides.[11]

Specifically, I conceptualize plasticity as a set of deep entanglements of life-forms and forms of life as evidenced in the growing significance of insects globally. Approaching insects as plastic life, I consider how their ability to mutate and reinvent new forms has been absorbed and integrated into a global biopolitical regime integral to the futurity of human and nonhuman life and death. While these entanglements exceed and unsettle the human as a privileged ontology, the plasticity of insects is always already asymmetrically organized across global terrains, nurturing life-forms and ways of life in the global north while producing regimes of death in other regions, not limited to or contained by the global south.[12] By reading plasticity through biopolitical concerns and through insect life, I situate its potentiality ambivalently *between* the dystopic views offered by Barthes and the emancipatory visions proposed by Malabou. Placed in the contemporary conditions of global war, the ability of plastic to form, transform, and explode its own plasticity, I suggest, cannot be lauded as a foreseeable opening to political transformation. The global contemporary is not only a moment of closure but one produced through uneven circuits and circulations of power. Thus, the "ontological combustion" of plasticity harbors the potential to explode its own possibility, reinforcing existing geopolitical divides while also producing new ones that ultimately constrain and even eliminate itineraries for emancipatory politics.[13]

In what follows, I develop this argument in three parts. Beginning with entomology, I consider the plasticity of insects and their ability to change, mutate, and explode form. Insects have figured prominently in philosophical and literary writings. Most significantly, anticolonial, postcolonial, and critical race theorists have drawn attention to the ways in which the native and colonized have been dehumanized as insects, justifying regimes of racial-colonial violence and ultimately death.[14] Informed by and building upon these metaphorical discussions of animality, part two considers the *materiality* of insect forms and asks how the plasticity of insects has been harnessed and mobilized by the US military as emergent and embedded technologies of surveillance and war.[15] As both killable species and model prototypes—expendable species well suited to kill prospective terrorists and enemies presumed to be threatening Western forms of life—insects have become a critical dispositif in the US-led war on terror. Their incorporation into tactics of war point to the expansion of a biopolitical regime that exceeds the human, highlights the interpenetration of human life and insect death and thus demands a fundamental rethinking of life itself. In the final section, I return to consider the political potentiality that Malabou ascribes to plasticity. Drawing from the work of Henri Bergson, I suggest that the political and ethical possibilities of plasticity do indeed lie in its "ontological combustion," a combustion that must explode the species differentiation which continues to persist, most noticeably in biopolitical conceptualizations of life and death. Plasticity, as I conceptualize it, is not merely a synthetic material, as Barthes claims. Nor is it situated between biology and history, as it is for Malabou. Plastic and plasticity, I argue, are vital impulses *animating, interrelating,* and *exploding* the uneven terrains of human and nonhuman life and death, thus rendering its political potentiality all the more ambiguous.[16]

PLASTIC INSECTS

Insects are not commonly regarded as companion species.[17] Unlike dogs, cats, and other domestic and nondomestic animals, they are small in size, deemed insignificant in effect, while defying the bounds of human recognition. Yet they are everywhere—in our bodies, beds, and food. They are consequential to human survival. Still, we do not often notice them. And when we do, we see them not as companions but as pests. At the levels of corporeality, consciousness, and affect they appear to have little affinity with human life. Even social insects, such as honeybees, are unfamiliar. They may have language and the capacity to distinguish colors, they carry olfactory receptors that allow them to intelligently locate feeding places, and they exhibit forms of memory, as Karl von Frisch, the Austrian ethologist, famously observed.[18] But honeybees and other insects cannot speak.[19] They communicate in languages that humans cannot understand, via pheromones and strange movements, including "waggle dances," modes unrecognizable to human consciousness and understanding.[20] Insects become palpable only when they impinge upon or disrupt human lives, when they are in places we do not want them to be, when they are doing things we do not want them to do. Then they become killable species.

Unlike other animals, insects in all their inscrutability exceed the grasp of human control. They defy attempts at regulation. They resist domestication. They do not obey. They "are radically different to anthropocentric norms," they "perform a *feral charisma* that is in stark contrast to the anthropomorphic cuddly charisma" commonly associated with cats, dogs, and other domestic animals.[21] Unsettling and unfamiliar, abject and disgusting, we cannot see ourselves in them. "The more we look," writes Hugh Raffles, "the less we know. They are not like us. They do not respond to acts of love or mercy or remorse." This lack of responsiveness "is worse than indifference. It is a deep, dead space without reciprocity, recognition, or redemption."[22] There are too many of them, fecund, proliferating. They are constantly moving. They do not go away. Because they are foreign and not like us, they can be killed without consequence. Not surprisingly, insects have been a recurring *racial* trope in acts of mass colonial and postcolonial violence. The racial and abject, transformed into insects, can be killed with impunity. Native vermin, Tutsi cockroach, Jew lice.[23]

To the ordinary observer, insects may appear strange, incomprehensible, insignificant, and even killable, but to entomologists they are remarkable in all their species diversity, richness, and multiplicity. It is in their fecundity, ferality, and inscrutability that insects vividly display the plasticity of life. Insect species are constantly evolving, transforming, and innovating. Their mobility of life exceeds established modes of intelligibility and regimes of regulation.[24] According to entomologists, insects are the multicellular organisms that have diversified most successfully on this planet; of the 1.4 million species identified to date, insects constitute 1 million.[25] In many, a single genome displays a remarkable capacity to accommodate a wide range of disparate phenotypes responsive to changes in environmental conditions.[26] This plasticity is especially vivid in holometabolous insects that fully metamorphose, including bees, butterflies, and moths, enabling these species to successfully alter their morphology, physiology, and behavior. The result has been twofold: the production of new insect life-forms on the one hand and an unprecedented resilience of existing insect forms, allowing survival in the face of hostile conditions, on the other. Whereas global climate change has held devastating effects for many animal species, it has presented new opportunities for insects to divide, differentiate, and evolve. This is not to suggest that insects should be regarded as indefinitely plastic. For entomologists, plasticity can be both adaptive and nonadaptive, generating new forms of life and death.[27] Honeybees, for example, have been devastated by global ecological changes, including the spread of diseases and the use of agricultural pesticides. As one-third of the world's crops depend on bees for pollination, the growing collapse of bee colonies and the resulting decline of bee populations hold significant implications for human and nonhuman life, significantly affecting global food supplies in years to come.[28]

Plastic and plasticity, as I have said, carry multiple and even opposing meanings: as synthetic and artificial, as biological and neuronal, as oppressive and transformative. Given these disparate conceptualizations, in what ways might insects be considered plastic? All organisms, from the most elementary to the most complex, exhibit some degree of plasticity, an ability to change, transform, and explode in response to internal changes and external stimuli. In Malabou's characterization, plasticity is the ability to give and receive form while also holding the "capacity to annihilate the very form it is able to receive or create." *Plastique*, she explains, "from which we get the words *plastiquage* and *plastiquer*, is an explosive substance made of nitroglycerine and nitrocellulose, capable of causing violent explosions."[29] In the terms of neuroplasticity, which forms a central focus in her elaboration, the brain draws its vitality, its life, from its "perpetual change in plasticity (which is also to say a plasticity of change itself)."[30] This ever-changing brain holds a potentially explosive capacity, as Malabou elaborates in her efforts to politicize neuroscience. This possibility comes from an awakening of the brain, an explosion "against a certain culture of docility" that can provide openings for another world.[31] In the context of insect life, plasticity is certainly the ability to give, receive, and annihilate form as evidenced in the process of metamorphosis, for example. However, the changes effected by plasticity are often difficult to specify and isolate. Although many insects do have plastic brains, they also manifest other forms of plasticity. Hymenoptera, including bees and wasps, exhibit a plasticity that is developmental, morphological, and phenotypical.[32] Given this wide range, the meanings of insect plasticity have themselves changed and can no longer be limited to the brain and its development alone.[33] Rather, plasticity might more accurately be regarded as an integral force animating insect life and death.

For critical vitalists, including Henri Bergson, the explosion of form is not something to be commanded, as in the case of awakening the brain. Rather, what Bergson calls vitality and what we might also term plasticity is more fundamentally the very essence of life itself. "*Life is like a current passing from germ to germ through the medium of a developed organism*," Bergson maintains.[34] The explosion of life, its creative bursts and its continual transformations, signal more than life's mutability. It demonstrates the ceaseless change, invention, creation, and emergence of life (and death) unfolding on a path that is successive but has no telos and thus pointing to life's inherent uncertainty and unpredictability. "The circumstances are not a mold into which life is inserted and whose form life adopts . . . There is no form yet, and life must create a form for itself, suited to the circumstances which are made for it."[35] For Bergson, this is the vital impulse of life; the explosive aspect of movement, the lack of a predetermined program, the unforeseeability of the future.[36]

Departing from Darwin and Lamarck, Bergson identifies this vitality of life, its plasticity, as further evidence that life does not merely adapt to its environment but alters and aspires to move beyond itself, creating new forms and species in the process.[37] Although all life-forms—human, animal, plant—are plastic and undergo continual change through the birth and death of cells, for example, these interior changes, Bergson suggests, do not often capture the attention of science or philosophy. Change is happening continuously in life, whether we see it or not. But we are opposed to this, writes Bergson; against this idea of continual change, "our whole intellect rises in revolt."[38] Where such internal and continual changes are visually and corporeally apparent is in the life cycle of insects. The plasticity of insects affords them the ability to alter their phenotype and morphology, not merely as adaptation but as *reply* to internal and external factors.[39] The mushroom bodies of honeybees, for example, have undergone noticeable transformations in volume encouraged through ecological changes, experience, and the social organization of hives.[40] The vivid materialization of plasticity in insects is partly what has rendered them enigmatic and compelling figures, sources of wonderment that mark the limits of the human in Western philosophy and literature.[41]

Although plasticity spans insect life cycles, it is most visually apparent in the process of metamorphosis. Metamorphosis is regarded as an age-related and thus developmental rite of passage that occurs in certain species, most notably holometabolous insects. Here, eggs become larvae, pupae, and eventually adults. Throughout this process, form is simultaneously emergent and eradicated. A bee larva reconstructs itself at the pupal stage and has little resemblance to an adult bee.[42] Metamorphosis has long been understood to be a genetic process, inevitable and thus predictable. Recently, entomologists have argued that these transformations are deeply influenced by external and environmental conditions and changes. In the case of honeybees, behavioral differences and the socially determined division of labor are now believed to be influenced by environmental stimuli. Whether the bee will become a worker or a queen, the division of labor into reproductive and nonreproductive phenotypes, as well as the shift from brood care to foraging that occurs amongst adult bees, has now been attributed to external influences at the larval stage.[43] Metamorphosis has been identified as a key developmental change in insect forms. Yet for entomologists, it is difficult to draw clear distinctions between metamorphosis and plasticity. The primary difference is that the latter affords insects the ability to innovate in the face of changing internal and external conditions, qualities that might intensify during the process of metamorphosis but that extend and continue beyond it.

Never referencing entomology explicitly, Bergson questions whether the mutability of life, its continual emergence in both insects and humans, can so easily be compartmentalized as predictable life changes. Puberty and menopause "in which the individual is completely transformed are quite comparable to changes in the course of the larvae or embryonic life," he observes.[44] For Bergson what is "properly vital in growing old is the insensible, infinitely graduated, continuance of the change of form."[45] Metamorphosis, puberty, and menopause, he contends, might be age-related and thus successive processes, but they are not teleological. They do not follow a predetermined plan but are merely spikes, evidence of the continual and ongoing change that is life. Evolution, Bergson argues, "has actually taken place through millions of individuals on divergent lines, each ending at a crossing from which new paths radiate, and so on indefinitely."[46] The markers of corporeal development occur at particular moments but are not easily plotted along familiar lines of growth.

For entomologists, metamorphosis and plasticity each point to changes in neuronal, morphological, and phenotypical development. While they intersect and interrelate, they remain differentiated processes. The former occurs at a certain point in the insect life cycle. Plasticity, by contrast, is thought to be ongoing and continual, allowing insects, at various points in life to respond to environmental change and to innovate in their surroundings, allowing escape from predators, for example. In *The Future of Hegel*, Malabou contends that the relation between plasticity and metamorphosis is not yet fully developed, "appearing here as synonyms rather than distinct processes."[47] In a world with no outside, metamorphosis, she argues, can open possibilities for transformation. "To think of the formation of a way out in the absence of a way out, within the closure, is to think about an immanent disruption, a sudden transformation without any change of ground, a mutation that produces a new form of identity and makes the former one explode."[48] Thus, for Malabou, metamorphosis is not a mythological or fictive reality but an "ontological essence."[49] In insect worlds, it is plasticity rather than metamorphosis that signifies the ontology of life, one that provides the impetus for continual and constant change, one that becomes a possible line of flight. While insect plasticity has facilitated richness in phenotypical diversity and has reduced the likelihood of extinction for some species, it has held varied effects. For some insects, transformation has extended life while in others it has produced death. Still in others, it has enabled "plastic species to be successful colonizers."[50]

What might this brief foray through entomology and the plastic life of insects offer to a wider discussion of plasticity and its ethicopolitical possibilities? To begin, plasticity must be conceived as both a life and death force, facilitating the creation of new life-forms and the destruction of others. Second, we must remember that the immanent disruption that Malabou lauds as holding potential for sociopolitical transformation and change is embedded within and is the product of unequal configurations of globality. Both of these forces are evident in the growing concern surrounding insects. Recently, the plasticity of insect life has become of interest to scientists, the United Nations, and US military personnel.[51] Insects have been newly mobilized and deployed in changing constellations of global biopolitics, demonstrating the mutual vulnerability of human and nonhuman life-forms. Growing concerns over global climate change and eco- and bioterrorism and their interconnections, for example, have rendered humans increasingly susceptible to the forces of nature. The natural world, including insects, has been regarded as essential to the futurity of human life and death. According to recent reports, insects will figure prominently in initiatives aimed at prolonging and saving human life in the global north. To begin, the world's ever-expanding population has created a scarcity in meat proteins that has generated particular concern in the West. Insects, scientists have argued, are highly efficient in converting vegetation and leaves into edible proteins.[52] In the face of anticipated food shortages, many have predicted that insects will be key agents in the production of resource-efficient foods and are also to become staples in Western diets.[53] Unlike meat production, which requires a large territorial base, insects are equally high sources of protein and can be easily farmed on small tracts of land. Unlike cows, they do not produce the same level of greenhouse gases and thus are friendlier to the environment.

Insects have other roles to play in the survival of Western and human life. The plasticity of insect life has garnered close attention from the US military as bees and other insects have been hailed as potential collaborators in the contemporary war on terror. Not yet "companion species," insects are newly becoming what I call "companions of war." Although insects have been deployed in military battles since antiquity, more recently and as a result of their plasticity, various types of insects have been harnessed as potential agents of surveillance enlisted to protect Western ways of life against the putative and uncertain threats of (Islamic) terrorism.[54] While the olfactory senses of honeybees are being trained to locate dangerous chemicals, including those found in landmines, snails and cockroaches are becoming "animal/machine hybrids," experiments aimed at harnessing their natural sensors and energies in pursuit of microsurveillance. Insect forms have also been appropriated as military prototypes embodied in drones and new nanotechnologies.[55] Taken together, what these military and technological developments signal is that plasticity is not only the ability to give and receive form but also its explosion and annihilation, a point that Malabou emphasizes in her references to nitroglycerine and nitrocellulose.[56] The plasticity of the bee and the entomology of war as combustion and explosion are tightly entangled and vividly condensed in the words *bomb* and *bombard*. They derive from the Greek *bombos*, which carries a double meaning, both signifying the bee and intimating a humming, buzzing, and booming, onomatopoeically reflecting the sounds of bees *and* bombs.[57] These entanglements gesture to the ambiguities of plasticity, its ability to produce new forms and conditions, but ones that may not necessarily be emancipatory and/or transformative in the ways predicted or anticipated. Although the effects of plasticity may not be determined in advance, what these recent US military appropriations highlight are the crucial interconnections between human and insect life and death and the need to rethink their form and substance.

BIOPOLITICS AND THE REFIGURING OF LIFE ITSELF

The plastic qualities of insects, their mutability and malleability, allow them to be easily trained and conditioned. Honeybees, for instance, demonstrate a considerable plasticity in spatial memory, facilitating the vital storage of information such as the location and position of new nests.[58] Their antennal lobes are covered with chemoreceptors, triple those of insects such as mosquitoes and moths, enabling them to easily distinguish between flowers, locate pollen, and engage in social communication. Olfaction is the sensory modality that allows bees to retain memory. Because of their plasticity, including this heightened and malleable sense of smell, bees can easily be taught to associate the onset of light, smoke, or airflow with reward.[59] The adaptability of honeybees has been lauded and harnessed, rendering them prospective and promising wartime companions.

For over a decade, the Defense Advanced Research Project Agency (DARPA) has actively mobilized the plasticity of honeybees in the advancement of military technologies. Through its various research sites in the United States, most notably Los Alamos, DARPA has been training bees to detect hazardous chemicals commonly found in explosives.[60] Because of their heightened olfactory senses and the sheer number of chemoreceptors on their antennal lobes, the training process is swift: with a sugar and water reward, bees can rapidly and effectively be taught to ignore pollen and to smell and locate chemicals instead. By placing explosives near food sources, DARPA has successfully been training bees in labs. The objective is to use honeybees and other insects on the front lines in war, replacing "companion species," including dogs. According to recent reports, many of the dogs deployed in Afghanistan and Iraq to aid US soldiers in finding landmines and other explosives are—like human military personnel—also affected by posttraumatic stress disorder.[61] Because of their inscrutability, insects—unlike dogs—do not evoke the same ethical crisis over loss of life.

This growing interest in bees is not limited to their individual and corporeal capacities alone. Rather, honeybees as a collectivity and as an aggregate in hives have also been a source of investigation and inspiration for scientists and military personnel. The architecture of the hive and the organization of bees offer valuable insights into the shifting configurations of global capitalism and (anti)terrorism. In *What Should We Do with Our Brain?*, Malabou observes that sovereign command, like the brain, no longer operates through a centralized system. Instead, it works through an organizational agility, a suppleness that is held together through a multiplicity and dispersion of centers.[62] In the contemporary moment, the horizon of global capitalism is ever expanding, drawing in the peripheries and incorporating the most marginal populations from the global south.⁶³ Malabou limits her observations largely to capitalism. However, this decentralized model of command is also operative in current conditions of war in which sites of putative threat and danger are also alleged to be scattered and dispersed.

Shortly after the September 11 attacks, the US government under George W. Bush claimed that the war on terror would be a new type of war—not a war fought between sovereign states but between the West and a new enemy that defied territorial boundaries. Reflecting on these changes, Zygmunt Bauman has argued that in the post-9/11 era the "global space has assumed the character of a frontierland."⁶⁴ Here, threats and responses are increasingly diffuse rather than centralized, alliances are constantly in flux, and extreme violence is legitimated in a fight against enemies believed to have no clear or identifiable borders. The enemy has become increasingly difficult to determine, the US government has argued, rendering the dangers of terrorism uncertain, unpredictable, and perilous. Not only have the conditions of war changed in the last decade, but this new "planetary frontierland" has interconnected the world's regions in unprecedented ways.⁶⁵

Entwined with global capitalism, these new conditions of global war can also be mapped through the reticular organization of the bee colony. As a social and collaborative species, honeybees cannot survive individually and/or beyond their hive. They are interdependent. Despite their seemingly hierarchical and caste-based structure, the hive reflects an *absence* of hierarchy and a *lack* of centrality.⁶⁶ Each hive comprises a queen, female workers, and male drones. However, the queen is chosen by her workers and maintains sovereignty only over reproduction, laying thousands of eggs to ensure the futurity of the hive but exercising little control over its operation and organization. Bees depend on one another. Their collectivity and division of labor is central to their survival. This is not to suggest that the geopolitical global order is one without hierarchy. Just as there remains a clear order of civility and sovereignty among nation-states, the putative newness of this continual war and the intensities of violence it has made possible are described through *a lack of centrality*. The United States and its allies claim that they have been responding to the diffuse networks of terrorist cells, their absence of visibility, and their self-organizing structure, all of which demand tactics and strategies that are resonant with and echo the reticular design of the hive.⁶⁷ Perhaps unsurprisingly the plasticity of the individual bee and the population has been appropriated and re-created by the US military, as it mobilizes the honeybee as a potential agent of this new war and mimics its corporeal and collective qualities via drones. Although bee training has not yet been actualized in battle, drone warfare has proliferated under the Obama regime.[68] As scientists, entomologists, and military personnel continue to conduct research and assess the feasibility of deploying insects in a world of uncertain and unpredictable threat, insect plasticity has become pivotal to the production of new forms of surveillance in the pursuit of national and global security.[69] As the insect becomes a dispositif in contemporary biopolitics, the biopolitical requires a rethinking of life itself.

Since the publication of Foucault's *History of Sexuality, Volume 1*, and more recently with his newly translated lectures, his formulation of biopolitics has fomented a vibrant site of debate in critical theory and political philosophy. Amidst claims of the growing biologization of politics and the politicization of biology largely attributed to technological innovations rapidly changing the meanings of life, Foucault's fragmented and unfinished thoughts have been reinvigorated as holding crucial insights into changing configurations of power from the eighteenth century to the contemporary moment.[70] Arguing that the rise of biopower in the eighteenth century lent a "vitalist character" to the existence of individuals as political subjects and to populations as sites of management and intervention, Foucault famously and contentiously claimed that biopower emerged as a new modality of government that seized life through a radically different configuration of dynamic forces.[71] The emergence of this new mode of power, many have interpreted Foucault as saying, eroded the centrality and significance of sovereign command.[72] In the first lecture of *Security, Territory, Population*, Foucault famously defines biopower as "the set of mechanisms through which the basic biological features of the human species became the object of a political strategy, of a general strategy of power." From the eighteenth century onwards, he claims, "modern Western societies took on board the fundamental biological fact that human beings are a species."[73]

Foucault's many critics and interlocutors have raised important questions regarding his formulations of biopower and biopolitics, alleging that his conceptualizations are vague and inconsistent and that his periodization and geographical focus are Eurocentric and parochial.[74] Several have also questioned his formulations of life. For Robert Esposito, it is because Foucault was so focused on questions of power that he "never sufficiently articulated the concept of politics" or the contours of "life."[75] Although Foucault described life "analytically in its historical-institutional, economic, social, and productive nervature," Esposito insists that in Foucault's analytic, life remains insufficiently problematized "with regard to its epistemological constitution."[76] Foucault's schematic, I add, does not adequately address the ontology of life. The formulation and politicization of life in Foucault's writings and lectures is narrowly premised and established upon the anthropocentric claim that "life" is human life and nothing more.

Amid these pressing critiques of Foucault's conceptions of biopower and biopolitics, there has been a growing concern with explicating, expanding, and specifying the contours of life. Whose life and which life has newly become the object of power? In what ways have life and death been/become integrally linked as political strategies of the state, global capitalism, and war? How has the vitality and investment in some forms of life in colonial states and in late liberal democracies been possible through death? Put differently, how have the deaths of the racial, colonial, abnormal, diseased, and dangerous figured in struggles over (Western) life?[77] The interpenetration of life and death that have been central to late nineteenth- and early twentieth-century vitalisms and that animate Foucault's own vitalist understandings of biopolitics gesture to the ambiguities in his own thinking and to the narrow interpretations of his writings and lectures. Sovereign power and death were never displaced by biopower and life, as some have read Foucault as saying. Rather, biopolitical regimes often operated through sovereign command, rendering some lives worthy of economic and scientific investment and others inhuman, wasted, and expendable.[78] These debates have pointed to the limits of Foucault's conceptualizations while opening new ways of moving beyond and expanding his analytics. Despite the rich insights and developments in this literature, one thread remains constant: life continues to be understood as human life and man-as-species.[79]

To be clear, Foucault's formulations of the biopolitical have been revised and expanded to address the animalization of life, most notably in the work of Giorgio Agamben.[80] Yet even in his distinctions and differentiations between *zoë* and *bios*, animalization persists as *metaphor* rather than materiality. Thus, while the *bios* in biopolitics, following in part from Agamben, has come under increasing scrutiny of late, it remains tightly tethered to Foucault's "man-as-living-being."[81] Under contemporary conditions of war, as my discussion of insects has thus far intimated, life can no longer be conceived through an anthropocentric focus on the figure of the human. While tactics of war have always encompassed more-than-human life-forms, including microbes and environmental conditions, what has changed is that the futures of human life and death (as instantiated by Western life), whether in the context of global food or global war, have become increasingly intertwined with the agentive force of insects. How might a recasting of the biopolitical through a *bios* that accounts for this mutuality and thus erodes the ontological distinctions between human and nonhuman life open new analytic and political possibilities for rethinking life in the global present? As a force no longer contained within the human body or population but as plasticity, a vital and creative burst that runs through and interconnects human and nonhuman life.[82]

Recent efforts to conceptualize the war on terror provide some generative openings in this regard. Writing on war and the weather, Brian Massumi explicitly questions the *bios* of biopolitics through a compelling analysis of nature and war. "The figure of today's threat," he writes, "is the suddenly irrupting, locally self-organizing, systematically self-amplifying threat of large-scale disruption," a threat that is not only "indiscriminate but indiscrimin*able*. Its continual microflapping in the background makes it indistinguishable from the general environment."[83] Hurricane Katrina, he argues, was the "meteorological equivalent of the improvised devices then exploding on the scene of the US war effort in Iraq," rendering war and the weather equally unpredictable and indiscernible.[84] Here, Massumi begins his meditations by raising a question that Foucault poses in *The Birth of Biopolitics*: "does power's becoming-environmental 'mean that', politically, 'we are dealing with natural subjects?'"[85] Acknowledging that Foucault's observations were specific to a particular historical moment, Massumi's objective is to elaborate and expand these insights to the present context. It is where "Foucault's question ends" that we must begin, he insists, "in light of how the recomposition of power, whose dawning he glimpsed in 1979, has since played out."[86] Can this new configuration of environmental power, in which war and the weather are closely interconnected, still be considered an expression of biopolitics, Massumi asks? Beginning with the *bios* in biopolitics, Massumi argues that the current configuration of global power is an *environmental* and not a *biopolitical* one. What we are newly witnessing, he argues, is environmental power as ontopower, "a power through which being becomes . . . not a force against life" but "a positive force. It is positively productive of the particular form a life

Insects, War, Plastic Life 173

will take next."[87] For Massumi, what places this constellation of power outside the biopolitical is that environmental power, in his formulation, is a preemptive power that operates not on a territory but on a prototerritory in which life becomes unlivable.[88]

In his lectures at the Collège de France, Foucault does not fully or clearly distinguish between environmental power and biopolitics. Indeed, in "Society Must be Defended," he emphasizes their interface. "Biopolitics' last domain," Foucault explains, is operative through the "control over relations between the human race, or human beings in so far as they are a species in so far as they are living beings, and their environment, the milieu in which they live."[89] For Foucault, biopolitics "includes the direct effects of the geographical, climatic, or hydrographic environments," including swamps and epidemics that became objects of state concern and intervention in the nineteenth century.[90] Although he continues to privilege the human as living being, Foucault's brief gestures to the environment as a biopolitical force thus highlight, albeit momentarily, the possible interpenetration and interrelation of human and nonhuman life. That "the problem of the environment . . . has been created by the population and therefore has effects on the population" provides a small opening to rethink the *bios* in biopolitics as a vitality that exceeds "man-as-species," a problematic that Massumi raises but ultimately does not pursue in his juxtaposition of war and the weather.

The distinctions that Massumi draws between the biopolitical and environmental on the one hand and his claims that the global contemporary has witnessed a "major shift" in the exercise of power via the environment on the other can be advanced only if the protracted histories of colonial violence commanded by European powers are successfully ignored and obfuscated. Critics have long noted that the colonial remains a palpable absence in Foucault's corpus of lectures and writings, an absence we might conceive as replicated in Massumi's analysis.[91] In the colonies, the biopolitical and environmental were never fully separate domains. Colonial violence acquired its force and gained traction through their interpenetration. The domestication of nature, including the death of the colonized, who were always already resigned to the natural world, were sites of struggle over the meanings and value of human, nonhuman, and inhuman life. The machinery of colonialism, its taxonomizing impulse, was aimed at categorizing and classifying different "species" of humans and of flora and fauna while distinguishing the lives that should live, that were in need of protection, from those that should die and that demanded annihilation.[92] Fanon, like some of his contemporaries, was well attuned to the environmental entanglements of human and nonhuman life-forms: "The Algerians, the veiled women, the palm trees, and the camels make up the landscape, the *natural* background to the human presence of the French . . . Hostile nature, obstinate and fundamentally rebellious, is in fact represented in the colonies by the bush, by mosquitoes, natives, and fever, and colonization is a success when all this indocile nature has finally been tamed."[93] For Fanon, life in the colonies was inevitably bound up with a hostile, forceful, and indiscriminate nature, indocile and rebellious, requiring a preemptive and violent expression of force to domesticate and eliminate the threats that *nature* posed to white European life.

Under current conditions of war, the world of nature, to paraphrase Foucault, has become a "dense transfer point for power," a terrain on which struggles over human and nonhuman life and death continue to unfold.[94] The plasticity of insects, as I have suggested, renders them ideal companions of war, producing conditions in which war, nature, life, and death are inseparable. Over the past decade, commentators have routinely observed that the war on terror is both a response to and the product of a new and unprecedented battle, requiring a preemptive and intensifying violence that has legitimated the creation and imposition of new juridical regimes with little or no recourse to international law.[95] This is a new world, we are reminded, where the terrains of war are not easily legible, where distinctions between friend and enemy have become increasingly difficult if not impossible to delineate.[96] The enemy is alleged to be hidden throughout the tissues of a global population, traversing familiar divides between north/south, east/west, and foreign/domestic. The global war machine is no longer the domain of nation-states but includes private contractors, mercenaries, and extraterritorial organizations.[97] The targets are "suspects," the military techniques, including the use of drones, are preemptive.

Preemptive power, as Massumi explains, averts disruptive events before they occur. These are tactics that do not forbid or proscribe behavior. They do not target the body but work on the environment and its modification, shaping the possible fields of action.[98] This preemptive power, I suggest, incorporates and operates through nonhuman agents as environmental forces. Efforts by the US military to train honeybees could be regarded as the development and deployment of preemption: bees sniffing chemicals, detecting explosives and landmines before they detonate, preventing large-scale disruptions before they occur, protecting against the loss of Western life through the death of terrorism and those identified as "terrorists." Insects as material form and prototype have informed US military technologies and tactical plans, dramatically reconfiguring the battlefield via the development and expanded use of drones and other insect-inspired technologies. Through the deployment of drones, those *suspected* of terrorism can now be identified, targeted, and assassinated in the interests of *prevention*, hundreds and even thousands of miles from the battlefield and through computer controls that are situated even farther from war zones.[99] Drones, swarms, and other military technologies, including nanos, have been closely modeled on the insect form, opening further possibilities for preemptive strike. By 2025, the US military estimates that nanos, which operate collaboratively like social insects (including honeybees), will be routinely deployed in combat operations. With an unlimited and unrestrained mobility to fly, crawl, adjust position, and navigate increasingly confined spaces, these machinic insects have been hailed as a prototype for the future, aimed at altering the environment and ultimately preventing threats and disruptions to Western ways of life.[100]

In the contemporary war on terror, insects have become what Foucault has termed a dispositif, a nonhuman agent incorporated into the "heterogeneous ensemble consisting of discourses, institutions, architectural forms, regulatory decisions, laws, administrative measures, [and] scientific statements," all assembled to address the urgent need of global security.[101] In the current geopolitical context, the biopolitical as a global regime of life and death must be redefined beyond the individual/population and *zoë/bios* distinctions that have persisted in critical theory and political philosophy. The mutuality of insect and human life and death demands a conceptualization of life as a plastic and circulating force that exceeds "man-as-species" and highlights the interrelationality of the human/nonhuman.[102] By way of conclusion, let me elaborate this point on plasticity as life force through what I term political vitality.

POLITICAL VITALITY

Plasticity's "native land" may well be the field of art, but it cannot be reduced or limited to art and aesthetics alone.[103] For Malabou, the promise of plasticity is to be found in its ethical and political potentiality. Plasticity, as she conceives it, is a kind of "metabolic power" that holds the ability to explode and *"order transformation."*[104] It is the "mutability of beings," our plasticity, she insists, that "opens a future in the absence of any openness in the world."[105] Stem cell plasticity is for Malabou a vivid example, "perhaps the very paradigm of the 'open' meaning of plasticity."[106] This openness is the ability to harness the vitality of the brain and thus to change one's destiny, a capacity that we hold and inhabit, she insists, but that we have not yet recognized. "What we are lacking," Malabou contends, "is life, which is to say: *resistance*. Resistance is what we want," plasticity unleashes its possibility.[107]

Plasticity is not solely a human potentiality. Rather, its capacity resides in all living things. Neuronal creativity, Malabou explains "is already at work in the most rudimentary nervous systems," including the most elementary levels of animal life.[108] Insects, as I have suggested, demonstrate the breadth and possibilities of plasticity. Their ability to incite transformation in the face of internal, environmental, and ecological changes are evident in metamorphosis and in other phenotypical and morphological changes. Insect plasticity has enabled various species to survive by opening lines of flight and by producing modalities of endurance in an increasingly hostile world. Yet in the case of insects, it is precisely their plasticity, their ability to give, receive and annihilate form, that has rendered them easily appropriated, trainable, and adaptable as companions of war in the global war on terror. If plasticity, as I have intimated thus far, is generated and embedded in uneven distributions of power and is cultivated in global capitalism and perpetual war, what is its potentiality for change? Can plasticity be conceived as a creative burst that transforms nature into freedom? Is the radical potentiality that Malabou ascribes to plasticity as resistance to flexibility and as refusal of form sufficient for political transformation?[109] If plasticity is a current that runs through all forms of life, connecting bees, bombs, human life, and insect death, can it not be both a site of liberation *and* subjection?

Bergson's vitalism, which he develops most fully in *Creative Evolution*, provides some generative opportunities through which to consider these questions. Bergson's formulations of life as creative burst, so I claim, can be conceived in terms of plasticity.[110] Life, as an animating force, does carry plastic qualities: its ever-changing conditions open the possibility to form, transform, and respond to change itself. It is here that Bergson provides some useful intimations on the ethicopolitical possibilities of plasticity. Undoing the dualisms instantiated by modernity (science/

philosophy, nature/culture, and human/nonhuman), he points to the unceasing and indefinite creation of life as force that not only exists in all forms of life but runs through and across them. "The idea of transformation," he claims, "is already in germ in the natural classification of organized beings."[111] In the "animal and vegetable world," he continues, we see this ongoing interrelation "between the generator and the generated." As Bergson explains: "on the canvas which the ancestor passes on, and which his descendants possess in common, each puts his own original embroidery. True, the differences between the descendant and the ancestor are slight, and it may be asked whether the same living matter presents enough plasticity to take in turn such different forms as those of a fish, a reptile and a bird."[112]

It is in this context that Bergson explicitly identifies plasticity as life force and expands it not solely as *continuity* but as the *unity* of animal, plant, and human life. Up to "a certain period in its development," he writes, "the embryo of the bird is hardly distinguishable from that of the reptile, and that the individual develops, throughout the embryonic life in general, a series of transformations comparable to those through which, according to the theory of evolution, one species passes into another." Daily and "before our eyes, the highest forms of life are springing from a very elementary form."[113] Several pages later, in a brief footnote Bergson elaborates accordingly: in "the domain of life the elements have no real and separable existence."[114] There is no life "which does not contain, in a rudimentary state," he continues, "the essential characters of most other manifestations."[115] Thus, plasticity, as Bergson adumbrates here, is a force that animates and permeates human and nonhuman life-forms, connecting the most elementary to the most complex. It interconnects and unifies these forms of life, unraveling their distinctions and hierarchies, and all the while demonstrating that evolution is successive but never linear or predetermined. In Bergson's formulation, this creative capacity of life, its ability to evolve along divergent lines, is what repudiates the mechanistic and teleological understandings of life and what opens possibilities for creative bursts and transformations.

Bergson further develops this unity of matter, its immanent relationality, in his famous discussion of instinct and intelligence. Like evolution itself, instinct and intelligence cannot be perceived as successive states. Nor can they be viewed as privileging the superiority of the human (via intelligence) over the animal (via instinct). Instead, Bergson formulates these as opposing, complementary, and interrelated ways of knowing.

"There is no intelligence in which some traces of instinct are not to be discovered, more especially no instinct that is not surrounded with a fringe of intelligence."[116] For Bergson, instinct and intelligence are "tendencies" as opposed to "things," and neither can be rigidly defined, hierarchized, or fully separated from the other.[117]

Drawing on the horsefly and the wasp as his examples, Bergson attends to the difficulties in distinguishing instinct from intelligence and insect and human ways of knowing: "When the horse-fly lays its eggs on the legs or shoulders of the horse, it acts as if it knew that its larva has to develop in the horse's stomach and that the horse, in licking itself, will convey the larva into its digestive tract. When a paralyzing wasp stings its victim on just those points where the nervous centers lie, so as to render it motionless without killing it, it acts like a learned entomologist and a skillful surgeon rolled into one."[118] Here, Bergson concludes that instinct and intelligence are not to be ascribed an order or value but must be regarded as different ways of approaching, understanding, acting in and on the world. Whereas the former is a knowledge of matter, he explains, the latter is a knowledge of form, and neither can be fully separated.[119] "On the one hand, the most perfect instinct of the insect is accompanied by gleams of intelligence, if only in the choice of place, time, and materials of construction," he writes. Bees, for instance, "build in the open air, invent new and really intelligent arrangements to adapt themselves to such new conditions."[120] Thus, intelligence, he cautions should not be considered superior to instinct, as "intelligence has even more need of instinct than instinct has of intelligence." The power "to give shape to crude matter involves already a superior degree of organization, a degree to which the animal could not have risen, save on the wings of instinct."[121]

Life, for Bergson, is clearly situated beyond the anthropocentricity of human life. The creative impulses that animate and penetrate all living things are always in a process of becoming and follow paths that are never willed by human agents alone. Plasticity, therefore, already exists, traverses, and connects and thus does not require an awakening, as Malabou suggests.[122] Rather, plasticity as creative life force is immanent to the vitality of human and nonhuman life, emerging in part through their interconnections and interrelationality. By formulating life as more-than-human and as interpenetrating, Bergson offers useful possibilities to rethink the *bios* of biopolitics beyond "man-as-species." I am calling this conception of plasticity *political vitality*. By taking nonhuman life seriously he aims to erode the ontological separation between nature/culture, human/nonhuman, a process of disentanglement that Bergson begins in his analysis of instinct and intelligence. This is an ethicopolitical position that moves away from conceptions of life as solely human but that also rejects the anthropomorphizing of animals and plants by granting them rights, for example.[123] It is a conception of life and an ethicopolitical project that highlights the mutual relationality, vulnerability, and dependency of living things as evidenced by the insect as dispositif. In so doing, such conceptualization emphasizes that plasticity itself is never beyond power, and while it might open "the form of another possible world," as Malabou anticipates, plasticity as a product of asymmetrical geopolitics can also be generative of other dystopic worlds always already situated within uneven distributions of life and death.[124]

Conceptualizations of life, Bergson argues, can never be separated from theories of knowledge. Thus, life itself offers an ontoepistemological critique. "A theory of life that is not accompanied by a criticism of knowledge," he cautions, "is obliged to accept, as they stand, the concepts which the understanding puts at its disposal."[125] Formulations of life and knowledge, he argues, "should join each other . . . as a circular process" that should "push each other unceasingly."[126] Entangled global futures of climate change, food shortages, and everyday wars demand a different conception of life, one that moves beyond the Western and/as the human. In *Insectopedia*, Hugh Raffles compellingly points to the mutual and growing entanglements between humans and insects:

> There is the nightmare of the military that funds nearly all basic research in insect science, the nightmare of probes into brains and razors into eyes. . . . These are the nightmares that dream of coming wars, of insect wars without vulnerable central commands, forming and dispersing, congealing and dissolving, decentered, networked; of netwar, of network-centric warfare, of no causality wars (at least not on our team). . . . These are the nightmares of invisible terrorists, swarming without number, invading intimate places and unguarded moments. The nightmares of our age, nightmares of emergence, of a hive of evil, a brood of bad people, a superorganism beyond individuals. . . . Where are the bees now? Collapsing in their colonies, gliding through their plastic mazes, sniffing out explosives . . . Keeping us safe. Helping us sleep at night.[127]

These nightmares are not of a disturbing past already lived but dwell in the threat of the present and the future to come, a present and future in which the differentiations that have for so long aimed to circumscribe life as the principal domain of the human can no longer persist or endure. The global and interspecies biopolitical regimes in which humans and nonhumans are enlisted thus demand a rethinking of life as more-than-human through its plasticity, its mutual relationality and vulnerability. The contemporary moment is indeed an era of plastic, as both Barthes and Malabou predicted. Not as imitation, synthetic and artificial, but as a more-than-substance, a creative impulse, that penetrates, circulates, and interconnects in ways that might rupture those racial oppositions (human/nonhuman, north/south, east/west) through which life and death continue to be understood and (de)valued.

NOTES

I want to thank the participants at the "Plastic Materialities" workshop held at Goodenough College, London, November 2011. In particular, I thank Brenna Bhandar, Jon Goldberg-Hiller, and Catherine Malabou. I am also grateful to Thomas Kemple and Sherrie Dilley for conversations that pushed me to develop the ideas presented here and to Barnor Hesse and Minelle Mahtani for comments and suggestions. Please direct all correspondence to renisa@mail.ubc.ca.

1. Barthes, *Mythologies*.
2. Barthes, *Mythologies*, 98.
3. Barthes, *Mythologies*, 99. First emphasis is in original, second emphasis is mine.
4. Catherine Malabou formulates plasticity in a series of books. Those translated into English include *Future of Hegel*; *What Should We Do*; and *Plasticity at the Dusk*.
5. Malabou, *Plasticity at the Dusk*, 67.
6. Malabou, *Plasticity at the Dusk*, 57; emphasis in original.
7. Malabou, *Plasticity at the Dusk*.
8. Malabou, *Plasticity at the Dusk*, 74.
9. These distinctions have been most vigorously undone in posthumanist and animal studies. Donna Haraway's work has been central in both literatures. See Haraway, *Simians*, and *When Species Meet*.
10. "Man-as-species" is drawn from Foucault, "Society Must be Defended," 247. The focus of contemporary biopolitics, I argue throughout, has maintained the human as a privileged ontology. Although Agamben dwells at length on the animalization of human life as *homo sacer*, his discussion emphasizes

animality in metaphorical rather than material terms. See Agamben, *Homo Sacer*. The more recent literature that engages biotechnologies and/or animal life has emphasized how the human has been transformed by biotechnologies, as opposed to approaching the nonhuman animal as an agent in and of itself and/or how humans have been governed as animals. On the latter, see Pandian, "Pastoral Power," 85–117. See also Chen, *Animacies*; Shukin, *Animal Capital*. For a recent collection that begins expanding the biopolitical to include a critical evaluation of human and nonhuman relations, see Livingston and Puar, "Interspecies."

11. My interpretation of plasticity here is drawn from entomology and is also informed by the work of Henri Bergson, who viewed life as a creative burst that aimed to move beyond itself. See Bergson, *Creative Evolution*. I expand and elaborate this view in the final section of this chapter.

12. It is important to remember that north/south and east/west divisions have always been constituted in racial terms. For a fascinating discussion of the global terrain as marked by the racial, see da Silva, *Global Idea of Race*. The targets in the global war on terror—Afghanistan, Iraq, Palestine, Pakistan—while also configured racially, put north/south divides in question.

13. The term "ontological combustion" comes from Malabou's reflections on Hegel's discussion of birth as both blossoming and explosion. See Malabou, *Future of Hegel*, 187.

14. See, for example, Césaire, *Discourse on Colonialism*; Fanon, *Wretched of the Earth*; Mbembe, *On the Postcolony*.

15. My discussion of insects and war is especially informed by the recent work of Kosek, "Ecologies of Empire," 650–78, and Raffles, *Insectopedia*.

16. Although Bergson does not address plasticity beyond one brief mention in *Creative Evolution*, I read his conceptualization of vitality as a plasticity of life. Importantly, his work is also useful in developing a more-than-human view of plasticity. Bergson undoes the human/nonhuman dualism by emphasizing the (inter)relationality and connectivity of human, plant, and animal life forms. My arguments here build on and expand from Bergson, as I am interested not only in human/nonhuman life but also in the interrelations of human/nonhuman death.

17. The term "companion species" comes from Haraway, *Companion Species Manifesto*. Haraway distinguishes between "companion species" and "companion animals," explaining that the former cannot be reduced to the latter, although they often are. Yet "companion species" in her own work tend to include dogs (specifically her dog, Ms. Cayenne Pepper), as well as baboons, as opposed to insects, fish, and other species that seem distant from human lifeforms. See Haraway, "Encounters," 97–114. Insects, I suggest here, are not only antithetical to humans but are opposed to these sentient animals and thus are not often regarded as "companion animals" or "companion species."

18. See Raffles, *Insectopedia*, 171.

19. For a brilliant analysis of the mosquito that cannot speak, see Mitchell, *Rule of Experts*, ch. 1.

20. On waggle dances, see Wenner, "Sound Production," 79–95.

21. Lorimer, "Nonhuman Charisma," 920.

22. Raffles, *Insectopedia*, 44.

23. On colonialism, insects, and annihilation, see Césaire, *Discourse on Colonialism*; Fanon, *Wretched of the Earth*; Mamdani, *Victims*; Mavhunga, "Vermin Beings," 151–76. On Jew lice see Mavhunga, "Vermin Beings," esp. "Jews," 141–61.

24. For Bergson, life is "mobility itself." See Bergson, *Creative Evolution*, 128.

25. Moczek, "Phenotypical Plasticity," 594.

26. Moczek, "Phenotypical Plasticity," 594.

27. Nylin and Gotthard, "Plasticity," 63–83.

28. Kosek, "Ecologies of Empire," 650.

29. Malabou, *What Should We Do*, 5.

30. Malabou, *What Should We Do*, 66.

31. Malabou, *What Should We Do*, 66, 80.

32. See Groh and Meinertzhagen, "Brain Plasticity," table 1.

33. According to Groh and Meinertzhagen, "Brain Plasticity," 280, the plasticity of insect brains no longer falls neatly within existing categories but overlaps with other forms of plasticity and is thus difficult to distinguish/isolate.

34. Bergson, *Creative Evolution*, 27; emphasis in original.

35. Bergson, *Creative Evolution*, 58.

36. Although Bergson says little of death, he does speak of aging, which he describes as an inevitability. Inevitability and teleology are not the same, however. In his critique of Leibniz, Bergson rejects teleology as the realization of a program already determined. Death may be an inevitability, but the course of life is not programmed to end in death in a familiar or predictable path. Life, for Bergson, is filled with ceaseless change that renders predictability and development to be impossible. See Bergson, *Creative Evolution*, 39.

37. Bergson, *Creative Evolution*, 128.

38. Bergson, *Creative Evolution*, 29.

39. Bergson's famous quote is: "adapting is not *repeating*, but *replying*." Bergson, *Creative Evolution*, 58; emphasis in original.

40. Groh and Meinertzhagen, "Brain Plasticity," 279.

41. In *Creative Evolution*, many of Bergson's references are to insects and insect forms. Another famous discussion of insects appears in Franz Kafka's short story "The Metamorphosis." See Kafka, *Metamorphosis*.

42. See Winston, *Honey Bee*, esp. ch. 3.

43. Groh and Meinertzhagen, "Brain Plasticity."

44. Bergson, *Creative Evolution*, 18–19.
45. Bergson, *Creative Evolution*, 19.
46. Bergson, *Creative Evolution*, 53.
47. Malabou, *Future of Hegel*, 24.
48. Malabou, *Future of Hegel*, 67.
49. Malabou, *Future of Hegel*, 68.
50. Moczek, "Phenotypical Plasticity," 596.
51. The UN has been encouraging the introduction of insects into global diets. See White, "US Food Advisor."
52. BBC Food Blog, "Why Not Eat Insects."
53. BBC News Europe, "Dutchman Urges World."
54. On the deployment of insects in war, see Lockwood, *Six-Legged Soldiers*. For a fascinating ethnography of the US military's deployment of honeybees, see Kosek, "Ecologies of Empire."
55. See, e.g., Gorman, "Snails of War."
56. Malabou, *What Should We Do*, 5.
57. See Lockwood, *Six-Legged Soldiers*, 24. Lockwood makes this point with respect to the etymology of "bombard," which is also cited in Kosek, "Ecologies of Empire," 654.
58. Robinson and Dyer, "Plasticity of Spatial Memory," 311–20.
59. Wenner and Johnson, "Simple Conditioning," 154–55.
60. See Kosek, "Ecologies of Empire," 655–57.
61. The *New York Times* published a series of articles on the prevalence of post-traumatic stress disorder in dogs working in Iraq. See Dao, "More Military Dogs."
62. Malabou, *What Should We Do*, 33.
63. Pheng Cheah offers a critical and very useful discussion of how biopower has produced and changed in the international division of labor. See Cheah, "Biopower," 179–212.
64. Bauman, "Reconnaissance Wars," 81–90.
65. Bauman, "Reconnaissance Wars," 81–90.
66. Horn, *Bees in America*, 8.
67. Malabou argues that contemporary capitalism "rests on a delocalization and a reticular suppleness in the structures of command." One could make a similar argument regarding the organization and deployment of war, which has become increasingly delocalized and reticular, shifts made possible by arguments about the war on terror as a new type of war that requires novel techniques and technologies of violence that work through distance and decentralization, including drones and nanotechnologies. See Malabou, *What Should We Do*, 33. It is now commonplace for critics to observe that the war on terror has been described as a new war. One of the earlier arguments to this effect is made by Bauman, *Society under Siege*, esp. ch. 3.

68. See www.cnn.com/2012/09/05/opinion/bergen-obama-drone/index.html.

69. On research and bee training, see Kosek, "Ecologies of Empire," and Lockwood, *Six-Legged Soldiers*.

70. On the biologization of politics and the politicization of biology, see Rabinow and Rose, "Biopower Today," 195–217; Rose, *Politics of Life Itself*.

71. On the vitalist character that Foucault ascribes to biopower and biopolitics, see Rose, "Politics of Life Itself," 1.

72. This claim has been placed into doubt especially through Europe's colonies, where sovereign command, violence, and death were ongoing and also continue to persist, albeit in different ways. See esp. Mbembe, "Necropolitics," 11–40.

73. Foucault, *Security, Territory, Population*, 1.

74. See, e.g., Stoler, *Race and the Education*.

75. Esposito, *Bios*, 44.

76. Esposito, *Bios*, 44.

77. For colonial engagements with Foucault and biopolitics, see Mbembe, "Necropolitics," 11–40; Mawani, *Colonial Proximities*, esp. the introduction; Stoler, *Race and the Education of Desire*.

78. Mbembe, "Necropolitics," 11–40. See also Braun, "Biopolitics, 6–28.

79. Again, notable exceptions are Chen, *Animacies*, and Shukin, *Animal Capital*.

80. See Agamben, *Homo Sacer*.

81. "Man-as species" comes from Foucault, "Society Must be Defended," 242. Esposito has been one of Foucault's sharpest critics, yet he does not extend the question of life beyond the human. See Esposito, *Bios*.

82. Not writing specifically about biopolitics or plasticity, Thacker, *After Life*, advances a similar challenge by arguing for a philosophy of life through the nonhuman and unhuman.

83. Massumi, "National Enterprise Emergency," 154.

84. Massumi, "National Enterprise Emergency," 154.

85. Foucault, *Birth of Biopolitics*, 261.

86. Massumi, "National Enterprise Emergency," 155.

87. Massumi, "National Enterprise Emergency," 168.

88. Massumi, "National Enterprise Emergency," 168.

89. Foucault, "Society Must be Defended," 245.

90. Foucault, "Society Must be Defended," 245.

91. The most famous of these critics is Stoler, *Race and the Education of Desire*.

92. On colonial categorization, see Pratt, *Imperial Eyes*.

93. Fanon, *Wretched of the Earth*, 250; emphasis in original.

94. Foucault, *History of Sexuality*, 103.

95. See Hussain, "Beyond Norm and Exception," 734–53.
96. Bauman, "Reconnaissance Wars."
97. Mbembe, "Necropolitics," 32.
98. Massumi, "National Enterprise Emergency," 156.
99. Shaw, Graham, and Akhter, "Unbearable Humanness," 1–20.
100. US Army, *Eyes of the Army*, 11.
101. Foucault, "Confession of the Flesh," 194.
102. In an interesting essay, Eugene Thacker argues that one of the "primary challenges" to biopolitics is *"how to acknowledge the fundamentally unhuman qualities of life as circulation, flux, and flow, while also providing the conditions for its being governed and managed."* Here, Thacker argues that biopolitics is not simply about the governance of bodies as individuals and aggregates but as "vital forces" that are "at once 'above' and 'below' the scale of the human." Thacker's project coincides with my concerns here except that he draws his inspiration on vitality and life from Aristotle's *psyche*. By contrast, my interest in vitality, as I mentioned earlier and discuss in the following section, is drawn from the philosophy of Bergson, who offers a sustained critique of Aristotle for his failure to consider time and for his linear and successive approach to evolution. See Thacker, "Shadows of Aetheology," 134–52. All of the quotes above are from 136. For Bergson's critique of Aristotle, see *Creative Evolution*, esp. 149.
103. Malabou, *Future of Hegel*, 8.
104. Malabou, *Plasticity at the Dusk*, 21.
105. Malabou, *Plasticity at the Dusk*, 78.
106. Malabou, *What Should We Do*, 17.
107. Malabou, *What Should We Do*, 68; emphasis in original.
108. Malabou, *What Should We Do*, 7–8.
109. Malabou sees plasticity as resistance and explosion. While she describes plasticity as resistance to flexibility, she also describes it as "energetic discharges, creative bursts that progressively transform nature into freedom." See Malabou, *What Should We Do*, 68, 74.
110. Although Malabou is critical of Bergson's formulation of the brain, she does acknowledge his influence on her formulations of plasticity. See Malabou, *What Should We Do*, 72.
111. Bergson, *Creative Evolution*, 23.
112. Bergson, *Creative Evolution*, 23.
113. Bergson, *Creative Evolution*, 24.
114. Bergson, *Creative Evolution*, 29n.
115. Bergson, *Creative Evolution*, 106.
116. Bergson, *Creative Evolution*, 136.
117. Bergson, *Creative Evolution*, 136.
118. Bergson, *Creative Evolution*, 146.

119. Bergson, *Creative Evolution*, 149.

120. Bergson, *Creative Evolution*, 142.

121. Bergson, *Creative Evolution*, 142.

122. Malabou, *What Should We Do*, 78.

123. Jane Bennett offers compelling reasons for anthropomorphizing that have nothing to do with rights. See Bennett, *Vibrant Matter*.

124. Malabou, *What Should We Do*, 80.

125. Bergson, *Creative Evolution*, xiii.

126. Bergson, *Creative Evolution*, xiii.

127. Raffles, *Insectopedia*, 203–4.

CHAPTER **9**

Zones of Justice: A Philopoetic Engagement

Michael J. Shapiro

INTRODUCTION: A JUSTICE DISPOSITIF

The initiating provocation for this essay is a long passage in Mathias Énard's novel *Zone* (2010).[1] The novel's protagonist, Francis Servain Mirković, is a French Croatian who had enlisted to fight in the ethnic purification–driven Croatian independence war, motivated by the neo-Nazi ideology he had absorbed as a youth. As one passage in the novel puts it, "the truth is that there were loads of neo-Nazis, hooked on the mythology of victory over the Serbs, on the mythology of the single 'independent' Croatian State scoured clean by the partisans."[2] The novel is structured as one sentence of reflections for 517 pages (there are no periods, only commas), narrated by Mirković while on a train trip from Milan to Rome to deliver an archive of the war crimes that had occurred in the "zone" (an area comprising Mediterranean nation-states) to the Vatican. The passage that inspires my analysis contains his recollection of the day he saw his former Croatian commander, Blaškić, at his war crimes trial, a "multilingual circus of the ICJ." "Blaškić [is]:

> in his box at The Hague among the lawyers the interpreters the prosecutors the witnesses the journalists the onlookers the soldiers of the UNPROFOR who analyzed the maps for the judges commented on the possible provenance of bombs according to the size of the crater determined the range of the weaponry based on the caliber which gave rise to so many counter-arguments all of it translated into three languages recorded automatically transcribed ... everything had to be explained from the beginning, historians testified to the past of Bosnia,

Croatia, and Serbia since the Neolithic era by showing how Yugoslavia was formed, then geographers commented on demographic statistics, censuses, land surveys, political scientists explained the differential political forces present in the 1990's . . . Blaškić in his box is one single man and has to answer for all our crimes, according to the principle of individual criminal responsibility which links him to history, he's a body in a chair wearing a headset, he is on trial in place of all those who held a weapon. . . . [3]

In this remarkable passage, Énard's protagonist, Mirković, describes a justice dispositif, where a dispositif, as Michel Foucault has famously elaborated it, is "a thoroughly heterogeneous ensemble consisting of discourses, institutions, architectural forms, regulatory decisions, laws, administrative measures, scientific statements, philosophical, moral and philanthropic propositions . . . the said as much as the unsaid . . . the elements of the apparatus."[4] Methodologically, to evoke a justice dispositif rather than attempt to simply define justice is to analyze the historical conjunction of emerging practices rather than focus on an isolated concept (where the latter is empiricism's practice, in which concepts are translated into measurement protocols to set up and test explanations of the causes of justice/injustice). Analyzing justice as a dispositif allows for a dense mapping of an emerging world of forces that justice, as part of an ensemble of knowledge practices and complex interagency relations, references. In short, "justice," as articulated in Mirković's recollection, is a complex historical event ("the concept speaks the event" as Gilles Deleuze and Félix Guattari suggest).[5] Mirković's recollection is a radical *interpretive* event in that it gestures toward an altered spatiotemporal world. In the analysis that follows, I draw on two genres of spatiotemporality—philosophical and literary—in order to pursue the insights that Mirković's recollection evokes. Adopting Énard's spatial trope, the "zone," I propose an approach to justice that emerges through a reading of Énard's novel by exposing the text's literary tropes to philosophical concepts.

A POLITICALLY PERSPICUOUS PHILOPOESIS

With its emphasis on a particular zone of violence, the literary geography of Énard's novel offers an alternative "ideology of space."[6] It challenges both the state-centric map of European nation-states and the dominant narrative that locates European politics in a progressive story of negotiated economic and political integration. Rather than the traditional geopolitical cartography that features and legitimates centers of policymaking, the space of the novel is an axiologically rendered map that both identifies and abjures spaces of violence. However, to grasp the ethicopolitical force of *Zone*, it's necessary to "interfere" with its literary content by engaging it with philosophical concepts, an interference that Cesare Casarino renders as philopoesis: "Philopoesis names a certain discontinuous and refractive interference between philosophy and literature."[7] Casarino's concept of "refractive interference" is predicated on Deleuze and Guattari's classification of the functioning of genres, in which philosophy is an "art of forming, inventing, and fabricating concepts," and artistic texts are "bloc[s] of sensations . . . compound[s] of percepts and affects."[8] It also draws inspiration from Deleuze's way of conceiving philosophy's interference with artistic texts: "Philosophical theory is itself a practice, just as much as its object. It is no more abstract than its object. It is a practice of concepts, and it must be judged in the light of the other practices with which it interferes."[9] In sum for Casarino, philopoesis-as-method is deployed by staging an encounter between philosophical concepts and literary texts.

The novel's governing spatial trope, the zone, provides a propitious opening to articulate philosophy with literature in this way because both have zones. In the case of philosophy, the zone becomes its main spatial trope when we heed Deleuze and Guattari's analysis of philosophy as a concept-creating practice; they treat concepts not in terms of their referents (through the use of "coordinating definitions," as is the case in empiricist modes of analysis) but in terms of the territoriality of their connections with other concepts. Concepts, they point out, have overlaps with other concepts, both temporarily ("every concept relates back to other concepts, not only to its history but in its becoming") and spatially ("each [concept] . . . has a zone of neighborhood [*zone de voisinage*]").[10] In the case of Énard's novel, its geographical setting, the zone, is the spatial imaginary that frames the dynamic shaping of the identity of the novel's protagonist or aesthetic subject, Mirković. However that subject cannot emerge fully as a political and ethical subject until he is brought into an encounter with another zone, a set of philosophical concepts whose proximities constitute a conceptual zone. The interference between the genres (an interzonal engagement) provides for a political discernment of the contemporary justice dispositif, not only because that interference opens up "emergent potentialities that disrupt the status quo of the history of forms"[11] but also because the philosophical concepts themselves challenge the already conceptually invested political status quo.

PLASTICITIES: CHEZ MALABOU AND BAKHTIN

Plasticity is a primary concept for both the philosopher Catherine Malabou and the literary theorist M. M. Bakhtin. However, although Malabou's primary genre is philosophical discourse and Bakhtin's is literary discourse, neither is a pure type. Literary tropes and examples are abundant in Malabou's texts, and philosophemes abound in Bakhtin's. As Casarino suggests in his elaboration of philopoesis-as-method, political discernment derives from the mixing of idioms. He points out, for example, that both Marx and Melville inquire into the "political nature of being" precisely because the former "found it necessary to depart from the practice of philosophy" [as is the case for Malabou] and the latter "from the practice of literature in order to experiment with whole new worlds of writing and thought"[12] [as is the case for Bakhtin]. Perhaps most significantly, both Malabou and Bakhtin share a philosophical perspective on the writing subject. Malabou applies her concept of plasticity to herself, rendering her "conceptual portrait as a *transformational mask*"[13] as she rehearses her changing conceptual history throughout her various writings on philosophers. And Bakhtin sees the writer as a mobile subject; his "authors" are open to themselves by seeing themselves as "unconsummated," as subjects who are always becoming, who are, as he puts it, "axiologically yet-to-be." That mode of self-recognition articulates itself through how they fashion the "lived lives" of their protagonists as dynamics of accommodation to a complex, changing world.[14]

Spatially, Malabou's version of plasticity is constituted as a zone of concepts that exists in the interstices of the philosophical idioms of Hegel, Heidegger, and Derrida: dialectics, destruction, and deconstruction, respectively. Drawn initially from Hegel's use of the concept and intended ultimately to replace Derrida's writing-predicated "motor scheme" (a tool or "image of thought" with which "the energy and information of the text of an epoch"[15] is garnered), plasticity for Malabou involves the self- and world-shaping work of "productive imagination."[16] Committed to a "*symbolic rupture between the plastic and the graphic components of thought*,"[17] Malabou constructs a mode of subjectivity that emphasizes mutability rather than mimesis or representation. For example, in one application, as she connects philosophical and neuroscientific discourses, she notes that "plasticity, far from producing a mirror image of the world, is the form of another possible world. To produce a consciousness of the brain thus demands that we defend a biological alterglobalism."[18] Malabou thus articulates her plasticity model of philosophical consciousness with brain science, suggesting that we recognize the plasticity of the brain because thought is part of organic nature: "the mental is not the wise appendix of the neuronal."[19]

In contrast with Malabou, Bakhtin locates plasticity in the narratological structure of genre rather than in the dynamics of mentality. "The novel," he argues, "is plasticity itself" because "it is a genre that is ever questing, ever examining itself and subjecting its established forms to review."[20] In this sense, Bakhtin shares with Malabou a version of plasticity that privileges a future-oriented temporality, a commitment to the mutability of forms and to the ways in which changing forms attain greater proximity than fixed frameworks to the changing realities of the lifeworld. Evoking the concept of the zone, Bakhtin notes that the novel as a genre "structures itself in a zone of direct contact with developing reality."[21] Crucially for purposes of my analysis, throughout his discussion of novelistic genres Bakhtin's analyses of space and temporality provide appropriate models for the way Énard's protagonist/aesthetic subject, Mirković's movements (both his traveling and his identity changes) disclose aspects of his contemporary world. In particular, Bakhtin's analyses of some versions of the bildungsroman apply very well to Énard's *Zone*, especially one type, the "travel novel": "[In] *The Travel novel*: The hero is a point moving in space. He has no distinguishing characteristics, and he himself is not the center of the novelist's artistic intention. His movement in space—wanderings and occasional escapade-adventures . . . enables the artist to develop and demonstrate the spatial and static social diversity of the world (country, city, culture, nationality, various social groups and the specific conditions of their lives)."[22]

In his treatment of another type, the "novel of emergence," Bakhtin captures the way the mutability of Énard's protagonist, Mirković, reflects the historical changes in the world. In some version of this type, the changes in the character are not the sole focus. Rather, "He emerges *along with the world* and he reflects the historical emergence of the world itself. He is no longer within an epoch, but on the border between two epochs, at the transition point from one to the other. The transition is accomplished in him and through him. He is forced to become a new, unprecedented type of human being. The organizing force of the future is therefore extremely great here—and this is not, of course, the private biographical future, but the historical future."[23]

Here, Bakhtin applies his concept of the chronotope to the way the text's temporal figuration orients his protagonist's changing character to reflect a reconfigured world. Similarly, in her conception of a future-oriented temporality, Malabou focuses on the way consciousness moves toward its future state: as it is involved in dialectically oriented transformative movement that is both form giving and form dissolving and as it shows "the capacity to differentiate itself from itself."[24] In what follows, I heed Malabou's approach to plasticity by conceiving Énard's Mirković philosophically as a changing "conceptual persona," a figure in a philosophical text.[25] And I heed Bakhtin's approach to plasticity by conceiving Mirković as a "hero" (Bakhtin's term for his protagonists; in my terms an "aesthetic subject")[26] in a literary genre, the novel, that privileges a process of self-fashioning responsive to changes in the sociopolitical arrangements of the lifeworld. I thus conceive Mirković as both a conceptual and aesthetic figure in a novel that is both philosophically profound and lyrical, as it seems to mimic the genre of a prose poem. In effect, Mirković enacts two different "powers," where "the difference between conceptual personae and aesthetic figures consists first of all in this: the former are the powers of concepts, and the latter are the powers of affects and percepts."[27] Jacques Rancière provides a model of the politics of literature that captures both effects and applies well to Énard's novel: "Literature does not 'do' politics by providing messages or framing representations. It 'does' so by triggering passions, which means new forms of balance (or imbalance) between an occupation and the sensory 'equipment' fitting it . . . It is the politics of literature—that is, the politics of that art of writing—which has broken the rules that make definite forms of feeling and expression fit definite characters or subject matters."[28]

ZONE

> Between the upsurge and explosion of form, subjectivity issues the plastic challenge.
> —Catherine Malabou[29]

> I'm changing my life my body my memories my future my past
> —Mathias Énard's Mirković

Much of the complexity of Énard's novel derives from one of the primary aspects of its form, its framing as an epic: Homer's *Iliad*. Like the *Iliad*, its 517 pages are broken up into twenty-four chapters, and as Énard attests, "I wanted to do a contemporary epic."[30] At times the other Homeric epic, the *Odyssey* is also evoked. The mixing of the two genres, novel and epic (which Bakhtin sharply distinguishes, seeing the novel as "the sole genre that continues to develop" and the epic as a genre that "has not only long since completed its development, but one that is already antiquated"),[31] enhances *Zone*'s critical effect, for as Bakhtin also suggests, "The novel parodies other genres (precisely in their role as genres); it exposes the conventionality of their forms and their language; it squeezes out some genres and incorporates others into its own peculiar structure, reformulating and re-accentuating them."[32]

Among the critical effects of the novel's epic framing is the juxtaposition of postwar fates that are afforded by the intermittent evocation of the adventures of Homer's heroes. Ulysses returns home to recover his domesticity, while Mirković is involved in radical transformation as he heads off toward a future that bears no resemblance to his origins. Accordingly, in its "reformulating" of the epic form, the novel lends philosophical weight to Mirković's type of journey. For example, at one point in the novel, one of Mirković's fellow soldiers, Antonio, is described as one who would avoid Ulysses' fate: "Antonio back from the Eastern Front runs through the countryside to escape the fate of Ulysses, his sewing wife, the good hunting dog who will sniff between his legs, he flees the future that he guesses at" (a return to mundane domesticity).[33] Malabou, as she involves herself in her philosophical journey, "deriving and arriving," also evokes Ulysses' path because of how freighted with significance his mythical journey is. Referring to "the paradigmatic value accorded in the West to a certain form of voyage: the Odyssey," she writes, "In one way or another, the Western traveler always follows the steps of Ulysses."[34] It's a philosophical or symbolic voyage, which has for her (and Derrida, whom she accompanies), a "phenomenological motif," a type of symbolic drifting (a *"derived drift"*).³⁵

Énard's Mirković also summons the concept of drift, comparing the violent topology of his journey to Stratis Tsirkas's fictional trilogy *Drifting Cities* (1974),³⁶ a saga of the drift toward chaos of three cities—Jerusalem, Cairo, and Alexandria—which are headed towards chaos as World War II recasts allegiances and enmities in the same "zone," the Middle East. Like the subjectivity effect in Malabou's philosophical-territorial journey, Mirković's renders him a plastic subject as he purposively undergoes transformation (as he strives to reshape his world's self-understanding). To repeat the section's epigraph, "I'm changing my life my body my memories my future my past. . . ."³⁷ Like Malabou, who takes a territorial and philosophical journey with Derrida, Mirković combines the two modes; he is on both a territorial and symbolic journey.

To summarize: Mirković, a French Croatian, joins the Croatian independence movement after being influenced by Yvan Deroy, his neo-Nazi childhood friend. Subsequently, he exits from his combat vocation and becomes a French secret agent whose zone is the Mediterranean area between Barcelona and Beirut. After being appalled by photos of the atrocities in the Westerbork concentration camp, he takes on a five-year task of compiling an archive of atrocities in the zone. Throughout the novel, his entire temporal trajectory is narrated as recollections while he is on a train from Milan to Rome, carrying his archive in a suitcase he plans to sell to the Vatican. His ultimate goal is to disappear after the sale with the woman, Sashka, with whom he wants to spend the rest of his life. Throughout the journey he reveals himself to be a quintessential plastic subject inasmuch as he is involved in erasing past selves, fashioning new ones, and creating a new form (in effect repartitioning the sense of the world he is and has been in). For example at one point he states, "Francis Servain Mirković disintegrated in the same way Paul Ricken did [an SS man who assembled a secret photo archive of atrocities], maybe I too wanted to document the journey, disappear and be reborn with the features of Yvan Deroy."³⁸ And at another point he imagines himself dissolving into the archive in his suitcase: "I think little by little I left my identity behind in those pseudonyms, I split myself up, little by little Francis Servain Mirković dissolved into a single one. . . ."³⁹

However, while one narrative thread focuses on Mirković's transformations, another rearticulates the history of atrocities in the zone and speculates about the vagaries of bringing the perpetrators to justice in a world in which those who carried out the atrocities are minor players whose violence is aided and abetted by others, especially those who are involved in the exchange of commodities. Recalling Bakhtin's observations about how the hero or aesthetic subject in the travel novel "emerges along with the world and . . . reflects the historical emergence of the world itself. He is no longer within an epoch, but on the border between two epochs, at the transition point from one to the other. The transition is accomplished in him and through him";[40] there is a telling moment as Mirković is observing some of his fellow passengers on the train. There are "Egyptian, Lebanese, and Saudi businessmen all educated in the best British and American prep schools, discretely elegant, far from the clichés of colorful, rowdy Levantines, they were neither fat nor dressed up as Bedouins, they spoke calmly of the security of their future investments, as they said, they spoke of our dealings, of the region they called 'the area,' the zone, and the word 'oil' . . . some had sold weapons to Croats in Bosnia, others to Muslims."[41]

Here Mirković's observations are not about himself but about a changing imaginative cartography of the zone. The map of cultural difference is being supplanted as persons from diverse national cultures become assimilated as predatory entrepreneurs in a world in which global capitalism is profiting from ethnonational enmities. As a result, warring bodies are treated not in terms of national and cultural allegiances but as human capital, as a clientele, and fates are determined by a network of initiatives in which violence is a consequence rather than an intention. As Mirković adds, "our businessmen from the Zone didn't see the threat behind the outstretched hand, the deadly games that would play out in the course of the years to come. . . ."[42] Achille Mbembe addresses succinctly the necropolitical consequences of the money flows that restructure perceptions of human capital in diverse zones of violence: ". . . the controlled inflow and the fixing of movements of money around zones in which specific resources are extracted has made possible the formation of enclave economies and has shifted the old calculus between people and things. The concentration of activities connected with the extraction of valuable resources around these enclaves has in return, turned the enclaves into privileged spaces of war and death."[43]

How can we therefore conceive the novel's justice pedagogy? At a minimum, in addition to the specific connections the novel provides—for example, that between capital flows and violence—what it says about the atrocities and the issue of justice is radically entangled with the form of its expressions. Its one-sentence structure, which moves the reader through rapid juxtapositions of information and imagery, mimes Mirković's train ride, in which the rider witnesses rapid changes in the landscape. For example, jumping into one passage we join Mirković on his train while he narrates information about the forced train transfers of Jews from the zone to concentration camps in 1944:

> ... the German administration [in Italy] went to the trouble of organizing convoys, transports for the partisans and the last Jews from Bologna or Milan, to Fossoli then Bolzano and finally to Birkenau.... Birkenau, where all the tracks join, from Thessalonica to Marseille, including Milan, Reggio, and Rome, before going up in smoke, my train has windows ... the Jews from Prague, the Greek Jews who even paid for their ticket to Poland, they sold them a ticket to death, and the community leaders negotiated bitterly over the price of the journey with the German authorities, strange cynicism of the Nazi bureaucrats, Eichmann, Höss, Stangl, calm men, quiet family men whose tranquility contrasted with the virile belligerent hysteria of Himmler or Heydrich, Franz Stangl loved flowers and well-ordered gardens, animals.... [44]

Here, as elsewhere in the novel, rather than merely supply information or offer an explanation, Énard creates ironic tropes and striking incongruities—in this case referring to the cynicism of "calm men" arranging the deaths of others—all located within a symbolic contrast between different kinds of train trips (the trains with blacked-out windows that carried victims to concentration camps and Mirković's with windows that allow for observation as he carries the reader through a zone of atrocities, headed in the opposite direction). On the one hand, Énard's Mirković speculates conceptually about justice, agency, historical memory, and changes in the administration of justice, in this sense functioning as a conceptual persona. On the other hand, his observations affect us with percepts and affects, as he also functions as an aesthetic subject, bringing us through the zone in a way that repartitions the political sense of European space. Simon O'Sullivan provides some appropriate language for how we are affected. Énard's Mirković challenges our "world of affects, this universe of forces [which is] our world seen without the spectacles of habitual subjectivity [and his dizzying ride through the zone, as he prepares to deliver a historical archive of horrors helps us] . . . to remove these spectacles, which are not spectacles at all but the very condition of our subjectivity."⁴⁵

The subjectivity to which O'Sullivan is referring is our traditional political subjectivity, our absorption into a world of separated sovereignties, on the basis of which we are located on the contemporary geopolitical map. Énard's passage thus disrupts the cartography of our traditional citizen subjectivity, moving us to reflect on our responsibility to a space and history of victimization. It shifts our focus from the archive of national consolidation ("the storing and ordering place of the collective memory of [a] nation or people")⁴⁶ to the archive of atrocities and injustice that contains the historical record of the violence in the zone. Ultimately, then, the "archive" emerges as an essential component of the justice dispositif.

ARCHIVES ABOUND

There are effectively three archives in Énard's *Zone*. The most explicit one is the archive of atrocities residing in Mirković's suitcase. Within the narrative of the train journey, Énard provides an oblique commentary on the politics of the archive. To secure that archive, Mirković handcuffs the suitcase to a bar on his seat. That gesture, along with the convenient symbols supplied by the train's destination, Rome's Termini station, and the suitcase's destination, the Vatican, implies that once they are situated in the archives of political or religious authorities, the records are sealed, locked up, immune from modification, because those authorities (archons) administer "the law of what can be said."⁴⁷ However, as the novel's construction of its plastic aesthetic subject, Mirković (as he goes "backwards toward his destination")⁴⁸ shows and its testimony to the fragility of historical recollections and allegiances to which his journey indicates, the archive is never finally secured. However institutions and bureaucracies may try to hold onto words and meanings (e.g., reifying them in the architectural sites and icons in the Vatican), they will ultimately be modified or supplanted. Despite Mirković's desire to terminate both the archive he carries and the selves he has embodied, they will continue to be part of an uncertain, continually modified future.

Apart from what is in Mirković's suitcase, the novel contains a literary archive—those who inspire the novel's unusual form: Apollinaire, Butor, Homer, Joyce, and Pynchon; the canonical fictional responses to war and atrocities by Joseph Conrad, Ernest Hemingway, Ezra Pound, and others who jostle for space in the narrative along with the perpetrators of the atrocities; and other literary figures, many of them writers who had personal connections with the zone and had been personally affected by the violence that has transpired there. However, Énard does more than merely mention them. For some of them, he retraces journeys, both actually and symbolically. In this sense, his novel is reminiscent of Sven Lindqvist's trip to Africa, in which the author follows the route that inspired Joseph Conrad's fictional anti-imperialist text *The Heart of Darkness*. To tell the story of the extermination of much of Africa's native population by Europeans in the nineteenth century, Lindqvist fashions *himself* as an aesthetic subject. He enacts a travel story as he visits the extermination sites to reflect on the violent nineteenth-century European-African encounters while at the same time interspersing archival material to rehearse the rationales used to justify the slaughters. Rendering his investigation as a "story of a man [Lindqvist] traveling by bus through the Sahara desert while simultaneously traveling by computer through the history of the concept of extermination,"[49] he provides a view of Europe's violent encounter with Africa that is largely fugitive within traditional geopolitical narratives. In small, sand-ridden desert hotels, his investigation is driven by one sentence in Joseph Conrad's *Heart of Darkness*: "Exterminate all the brutes." Textually, Conrad accompanies Lindqvist in his travels through the many references Lindqvist provides from the story of the famous novel. Conrad also accompanies Mirković, who recalls his "passion for reading" Conrad's *Nostromo* and *The Heart of Darkness*, among others, as a device to erase himself, "to forget myself,"[50] as he puts it. Moreover, in his mentioning those Conrad novels, the fictional Mirković, like the ethical traveler Lindqvist, summons a literary archive of violence.

The third archive enacted in *Zone* is the novel itself. Like Lindqvist's archive of the exterminism visited on Africa, which names perpetrators and the perverse thought models that encouraged their genocidal violence, Énard's novel provides a survey of the zone's atrocities, names the key perpetrators, and (also like Lindqvist) refers to those thinkers and activists who sought to either mitigate the violence or bring it to public attention. Both texts are in effect addressed to the justice of the historical archive. They refocus perceptions of the history of the territories whose violent encounters they narrate. Instead of such banal geopolitical concerns as "regime change" (a preoccupation of both politicians and political scientists), they focus on both the perpetuation of atrocities and the relatively anemic attempts of various agencies, national and international, to provide justice for the victims. With respect to this latter dimension, *Énard plays with the trivia evinced in war crimes trials and speculates about the clashes of temporality involved in the contemporary justice dispositif*:

> .... in the Great Trial organized by international lawyers immersed in precedents and the jurisprudence of horror, charged with putting some order into the law of murder, with knowing at one instant a bullet in the head was a legitimate *de jure* and at what instant it constituted a grave breach of the law and customs of war . . . peppering their verdicts with flowery Latin expressions, devoted, yes, all these people to distinguishing the different modes of crimes against humanity before saying *gentlemen I think we'll all adjourn for lunch . . . the Chamber requests the parties to postpone the hearings planned for this afternoon until a later date, let's say in two months*, the time of the law is like that of the church, you work for eternity. . . . [51]

AN ALTERNATIVE JUSTICE DISPOSITIF:
THE ETHICS AND POLITICS OF THE ARCHIVE

In a treatment of the relationship between archives and justice from a South African perspective, Verne Harris narrates a version of the justice dispositif that contrasts with the one narrated in Mirković's observations about the trial of his former commander, Blaškić, which moves the justice process toward a judgment rather than an open-ended process of collective reflection. Committed, Harris writes, to "A World Whose Only Horizon Can Be Justice," he sees the justice dispositif as both contested and political: "In this space archivists—together with the creators of records, and a host of other players—narrate the meanings and significance of 'the record' in an open-ended and contested process. The record, then, is always in the process of being made. And all of us who narrate its meanings and significances, whether we do it in a togetherness of hospitality or in a separateness of insularity, are record makers . . . The harsh reality is that the shape (and the shaping) of record-making is determined by relations of power."[52]

Heeding the contestability of the South African archive of colonial violence, and recognizing that the past must be open to the future, Harris suggests that the archives that contain "the memory of the nation" should be rendered as a file open to new voices, new types of archivist vocations, and new technologies of inscription, so that "over time the file will be expanded or revised, and it will be made available in different ways and contexts . . . as it is migrated forward to new generations of technology." Structured in this way, the archive, as Derrida would have it, "opens out of the future."[53]

Among the implications of Harris's transformative approach to the archives of violence and atrocity (he sees the archive as plastic, being shaped and in turn having a shaping effect) is an encouragement to consider "an ethics of time."[54] Considered within an ethics of temporality, the archives of atrocity would tend to summon what commentators of Walter Benjamin refer to as a "guilt history," a history imagined in terms of "debt and payback," contextualized within "the time of the law . . . in which the unavoidable incurring of guilt is atoned in an equivalent penance that is just as unavoidable."[55] However, reacting against this model of history as guilt and atonement, which imposes a "uni-directionality [narrative] . . . of what occurs," Benjamin famously juxtaposes "divine history," which resists such a unidirectional temporality (which he deems "a 'completely improper temporality' ") and allows for "morally meaningful action" within a model of "genuinely historical time,"[56] which stands as an implicit critique of guilt history. From the poetry of Hölderlin, Benjamin derives what he calls a "plastic structure of thought,"[57] a "temporal plasticity"[58] or time "wholly without direction."[59] Temporal plasticity accords well with Benjamin's view of a history that permits new beginnings instead of being seen as "a sequence of events like the beads of a rosary."[60]

Benjamin's "plastic temporality" model of history, which extricates ethical thinking from a unidirectional guilt history, is congenial with Harris's transformational model of the justice of the archive in which the archive is assembled within a complex and shifting dispositif—new technologies of inscription, increasingly different archival vocations, new forms of media exposure of the record-making process, and new contestations about relevant content.[61] And as Harris (edified by Derrida)[62] points out, the temporal structure of the archive itself is plastic inasmuch as although aspects of the past shape it, the very form of the record keeping in turn reshapes the way the past is understood.[63]

Ultimately, *Zone* articulates well with Harris's model of archival openness because it provides a countereffectuation of a juridically oriented justice dispositif. Although Énard's Mirković is headed toward Termini station (symbolically a termination of his task and thus an end to the assembling of his archive) to deliver his archive to an institution, the Vatican, not known for open-ended ethical negotiation, much of the novel's text suggests that what constitutes a just encoding of the atrocities in the zone is contestable. Although the form of the novel rushes the reader toward the termination of Mirković's journey, the passages reflecting on those whose pasts made them eligible for war crimes trials suggest alternative archival modes—for example, the treatment of the self-archiving Paul Ricken, "Professor of art history" (and commander of the Mauthausen prison camp), who took "hundreds of self-portraits . . . documenting his own moral collapse."[64] And as many of the passages in the novel suggest, what has gone on in the ICJ in The Hague barely touches on the complex of forces that have created the conditions of possibility for atrocity. As noted in an earlier section, Mirković's former commander, Blaškić (an actual historical person, a Croatian commander who served eight years for war crimes), whom he sees on trial in The Hague "in his box [is] . . . one single man [who] . . . has to answer for all our crimes, according to the principle of individual criminal responsibility that links him to history."[65]

Here as in other parts of the text, the implication is that a juridical model commands a very limited part of the ethical and political issues surrounding the zone's atrocities. To put it concisely, the juridical response must end in a judgment (e.g., the one that led to the actual Blaškić's prison sentence). However, the novel gestures toward a more critical analytic and a different ethos, one that accords with Deleuze's Spinoza-inspired approach to ethics, which "overthrows the system of Judgment" and substitutes an evaluation of alternative qualities of life for moral injunctions.[66] As I have put it elsewhere (heeding an application of Deleuzian ethics), "morality as traditionally understood is about deriving imperatives from fixed moral codes, while ethical imperatives are invitations to negotiate meaning and value, given situations of either competing and incommensurate value commitments and/or alternative perspectives on what is the case."[67]

To illustrate such alternative perspectives and thereby to offer a nonjuridical justice of the archives, we can imagine an opening up of the US National Archives to voices that, both at their inception and continuously, provide critical commentaries on the founding documents (the *archai* of the archives). Taking as an example the Declaration of

Independence, we can imagine turning it from a sealed document to a Talmudic text, the exemplar of a text that is open to continuing commentary, a text whose history "is the history of its effacing . . . a special effacing that is not necessarily the effacing of the text . . . it takes place through the adding of . . . additional texts . . . there is effacing of the control of the discourse, of the violence perpetrated by the discourse."[68] For this purpose, I suggest three commentaries that could be affixed to the Declaration's margins in order to efface its discursive singularity by addition. One is David Walker's 1829 "Appeal . . ." not only to "the Colored Citizens of the World" but also "and very Expressly to Those of the United States of America."[69] Walker, an African American abolitionist, did not achieve a substantial readership. "Published privately in Boston and often confiscated and suppressed during its dissemination, Walker's appeal refers to the 'disparity' between the condition of people of African descent in the United States and the 'inalienable rights' and republican principles laid out in the Declaration of Independence."[70] Another is the nineteenth-century commentaries of the Pequot philosopher William Apess, who, in his autobiography, "Son of the Forest,"[71] and his "Eulogy on King Philip,"[72] appropriates the language of white founders (often Thomas Jefferson) and urges Euro-Americans to apply the principles in their founding documents equally to "Indians." In the "Eulogy," Apess's "rhetorical strategy . . . effectively seeks to disable white Americans' ready assumption of a seamlessly glorious and singular American story."[73]

For a more contemporary critical commentary, we could add Jamaica Kincaid's observations on the Declaration of Independence. Kincaid, an émigré from Antigua, a place whose ethnoscape was shaped by an enterprise, the sugar plantations, that brought in coerced labor and who was herself a bonded servant when she first came to the United States, viewed the portrait of the signing of the Declaration of Independence, Jefferson et al.'s democratic initiative, differently from those who celebrate it as the inauguration of American's unimpeachable democratic experiment. Ignoring the lofty rhetoric of the document and instead heeding what she sees, Kincaid ponders the occupational infrastructure of the studied ease of the white men assembled in "Independence Hall" and speculates about those whose labor has provided the condition of possibility for the enactment of "freedom" by the signers. She writes: "America begins with the Declaration of Independence . . . but who really needs this document. . . . There is a painting in Philadelphia of the men who signed it.

These men looked relaxed; they are enjoying the activity of thinking, the luxury of it. They have time to examine this thing called their conscience and to act on it . . . some keep their hair in an unkempt style (Jefferson, Washington), and others keep their hair well groomed (Franklin), their clothes pressed . . ." She then refers to those who have worked to prepare the men for the occasion: "the people who made their beds and made their clothes nicely pressed and their hair well groomed or in a state of studied dishevelment."[74]

Ironically, right-wing Republicans in the American Congress recently did their own effacing commentary on another founding document. Recognizing and wanting to conceal the "founding violence"[75] of the US Constitution, they skipped the three-fifths clause (referring to the enumeration of slaves) during an oral reading of the text "on the House floor."[76] That gesture was not the critical one of effacing by addition; rather, it subtracted in order to deny the darker side of the American founding and, in effect, to depoliticize the American archive by negating a violent event in the history of the making of the African American subject. This is not the place to rehearse the many ways in which African Americans have engaged in effective counterhegemonic, archive-challenging modes of self-making in treatises and in a wide variety of artistic genres. However one work to which I call attention stands out as an important and underappreciated counterarchive: Duke Ellington's musical history of the African American experience: *Black, Brown, and Beige: A Tone Parallel to the History of the American Negro*.

Ellington's *Black, Brown and Beige* effects an African American right to participate in a dissonant way in the archive of American history by restoring what the dominant Euro-American historical markers have tended to efface. It adds the experience of another America to the archive. Ellington was well aware of that effect. As he puts it, "Negro music is America . . . developed out of the life of the people here in this country."[77] In Ellington's composition, as in many other parts of the African American sound world, what are articulated are the disjunctures in the American archive, the modes of separation in the midst of belonging that "founding violence" and "preserving violence" have wrought.[78] As a result, as Ellington puts it, "dissonance is our way of life in America. We are something apart, yet an integral part."[79] Ultimately, as Ellington's important composition shows, an effectively politicized and ethical archive is one that cannot be sealed; it operates within a "temporal plasticity," which, as I have noted, derives from a model of history

Zones of Justice   205

that extricates ethical thinking from a unidirectional guilt history and promotes a transformational model of the justice of the archive. It is a model in which the archive is assembled within a complex and shifting dispositif that is hospitable to contestations about relevant content. Returning to the insights derived from Mirković's archival adventure, we can recognize that national archives, as textual zones of citizen subjectivity, are an essential part of the justice dispositif. To the extent that we unseal and continue to alter the archives of national consolidation ("the storing and ordering place of the collective memory of [a] nation or people"),[80] we provide an alternative to traditional citizen subjectivity, opening up participation in a transformative text that continually reflects on the violence of law making and law preservation.

NOTES

1. Énard, *Zone*.
2. Énard, *Zone*, 145.
3. Énard, *Zone*, 72–73.
4. Foucault, "Confession of the Flesh," 194.
5. Deleuze and Guattari, *What Is Philosophy?*, 21.
6. Moretti, *Atlas of the European Novel*, 22.
7. Casarino, "Philopoesis," 86.
8. Casarino, "Philopoesis," 67.
9. Deleuze, *Cinema 2*, 280.
10. Deleuze and Guattari, *What Is Philosophy?*, 19.
11. Casarino, "Philopoesis," 86.
12. Casarino, "Philopoesis," 79.
13. Malabou, *Plasticity at the Dusk*, 2.
14. Bakhtin, "Author and Hero," 13.
15. Malabou, *Plasticity at the Dusk*, 14.
16. Malabou, *Plasticity at the Dusk*, 33.
17. Malabou, *Plasticity at the Dusk*, 3.
18. Malabou, *What Should We Do?*, 80.
19. Malabou, *What Should We Do?*, 81.
20. Bakhtin, "Epic and Novel," 39.
21. Bakhtin, "Epic and Novel," 39.
22. Bakhtin, "*Bildungsroman* and Its Significance," 10.
23. Bakhtin, "*Bildungsroman* and Its Significance," 23.
24. Malabou, *Future of Hegel*, 16.
25. Deleuze and Guattari, *What Is Philosophy?*, 61–83.

26. Shapiro, *Time of the City*, 7.
27. Deleuze and Guattari, *What Is Philosophy?*, 65.
28. Rancière, "Afterword," 278–79.
29. Malabou, *What Should We Do?*, 82.
30. Everson, "Introduction," ix.
31. Bakhtin, "Epic and Novel," 3.
32. Bakhtin, "Epic and Novel," 5.
33. Énard, *Zone*, 251.
34. Malabou, *Counterpath*, 4.
35. Malabou, *Counterpath*, 6.
36. Tsirkas, *Drifting Cities*.
37. Énard, *Zone*, 104–5.
38. Énard, *Zone*, 212.
39. Énard, *Zone*, 207.
40. Bakhtin, "*Bildungsroman* and Its Significance," 23.
41. Énard, *Zone*, 21–22.
42. Énard, *Zone*, 23.
43. Mbembe, "Necropolitics," 33.
44. Énard, *Zone*, 174–75.
45. O'Sullivan, *Art Encounters Deleuze and Guattari*, 50.
46. Brown and Davis-Brown, "Making of Memory," 17.
47. Brown and Davis-Brown, "Making of Memory," 129.
48. Énard, *Zone*, 127.
49. Lindqvist and Tate, *Exterminate the Brutes*.
50. Énard, *Zone*, 150.
51. Énard, *Zone*, 75.
52. Harris, *Archives and Justice*, 5.
53. Derrida, *Archive Fever*, 15.
54. Hamacher, "Guilt History," 82.
55. Hamacher, "Guilt History," 81.
56. Hamacher, "Guilt History," 84, quoting Walter Benjamin.
57. Benjamin, "Two Poems," 31.
58. Benjamin, "Two Poems," 34.
59. Fenves, *Messianic Reduction*, 3.
60. Benjamin, "Concept of History," 397.
61. Harris, *Archives and Justice*, 13.
62. Derrida, *Archive Fever*.
63. Harris, *Archives and Justice*, 13.
64. Énard, *Zone*, 21.
65. Énard, *Zone*, 73.
66. Deleuze, *Spinoza*, 23.
67. Shapiro, "Slow Looking."

68. Oaknin, *Burnt Book*, xiv–xv.
69. Walker, *Appeal*.
70. Shapiro, *Deforming*, 7.
71. Apess, *On Our Own Ground*, 1–90.
72. Apess, *On Our Own Ground*, 277–310.
73. O'Connell, "Introduction," xxi.
74. Kincaid, "Little Revenge," 70.
75. Benjamin and Demetz, *Reflections*.
76. Hunter, "Antebellum Myth," A21.
77. Tucker and Ellington, "Interview in Los Angeles," 51.
78. Benjamin and Demetz, *Reflections*.
79. Tucker and Ellington, "Interview in Los Angeles," 150.
80. Brown and Davis-Brown, "Making of Memory," 17.

CHAPTER **10**

Law, Sovereignty, and Recognition

Brenna Bhandar and Jonathan Goldberg-Hiller

In *Plasticity at the Dusk of Writing*, Catherine Malabou employs Claude Lévi-Strauss's descriptions of indigenous masks as an analogy for the concept of plasticity.

> These masks are plural, composed of multiple faces—masks of masks, if you like. As Lévi-Strauss explains, "they opened suddenly like two shutters to reveal a second face, and sometimes a third one behind the second, each one imbued with mystery and austerity." These composite creations are known as transformational masks. Transformational masks never reveal the face they mask. They are ill suited to the human face and never marry the model, nor are they designed to hide it. They simply open and close onto other masks, without effecting the metamorphosis of someone or something. Their being lies essentially in the hinge that divides them in half, which is why they are sometimes called "articulated masks." . . . By showing the transformational relations that structure any face (opening and closing onto other faces) rather than disguising a face, the masks reveal the secret connection between formal unity and articulation, between the completeness of form and the possibility of its dislocation. . . . The secret, primitive connection that bonds transformation and substitution, metamorphosis and replacement, contrast and functional relation marks the impossibility for figure or form to be self-identical, to coincide purely and simply with itself.[1]

These masks orient the reader towards the hinged aspects of Malabou's philosophical movements, staging the encounters between three systems of thought: deconstruction, destruction, and dialectic. They also echo Lévi-Strauss's own recuperation of the primitive, that universal human condition that infused early structuralism and that Malabou has drawn upon in her own return to biology.[2] Where biology has revealed a conserving metamorphosis of the primitive in organismic development (consider, e.g., Haeckel's famous dictum that "ontogeny [is a] recapitulation of phylogeny,"[3] as well as the arguments for *neoteny* in natural selection[4]), so Malabou's philosophy reveals "a childhood to come in the text, the promise of a primitive stage in the text."[5]

The promise of the "primitive" is simultaneously a permanent condition of possibility and its constantly agitated supersession. Preserved in the art of the transformational mask and in what Lévi-Strauss called the savage mind, the primitive is made available for an overcoming of its very condition through Western scientific concepts and systems of thought that can harness its potential in the creation of a universal theory of knowledge. Yet this intellectual framework of primitivism parallels the imperial ideology of colonialism that justified saving people from their own "savagery" and the gloom of their perpetual childhood through religion, science, and law. Although colonialism was historically advocated as a triumph over savagery, its institutions also preserved—even as they masked—an anachronistic other in the play of symbolic difference, a "savage" that could make potent the intellectual, cultural, legal, and military projects of "civilization" and modernity.[6] The philosophical investment in and recuperation of the primitive (along with poverty, dispossession and exploitation)[7] raises significant questions about its interplay with imperialism on the ground, that "largely obscured boundary with the colonial past"[8] that Lévi-Strauss—and early structural anthropology—masked by saying very little.[9] As the anticolonial critic Edward Said wrote in a review of Lévi-Strauss's *Savage Mind*, his structuralism "seems either to require total rejection, which would probably involve the creation of a whole new system that ought to supplant his, or a kind of slavish paraphrase. This kind of problem is characteristic of the best systematic thought, though it is always possible to have nothing to do with the system by ignoring it. My contention is that Lévi-Strauss is too important and fascinating for that."[10]

Indeed, as Malabou has tacitly agreed, Lévi-Strauss's structuralism is too fascinating and significant to ignore. Yet while Lévi-Strauss's often fleeting encounters with indigenous communities the world over are deployed in the service of philosophical systems that argue that so-called primitive modes of thought are in fact a product of a universal desire for order,[11] he could not account for the ways in which colonial encounters, political repression, and resistance—the very stuff of history—shaped indigenous knowledges, languages, and art forms. For instance, Lévi-Strauss never wrote that objects such as transformational masks might demonstrate the limits of knowledge, accessible neither to the native nor the anthropologist searching for their signification, perhaps due to cultural dislocations, as some native artists have disclosed.[12] To undertake Said's alternative of the "creation of a whole new system . . . to supplant his" would require a painstaking deconstruction of his thought, whereby the very analytical categories he utilizes and his presumptions about indigenous communities would have to be taken apart with an intellectual toolkit constituted by indigenous philosophies and forms of thought.

We don't attempt this complete deconstruction here, not least because we do not write from an indigenous locus of enunciation. But we do wish to focus on elements of Malabou's return to structuralism from the vantage point of colonial critique. We do this by examining the status of the primitive as a structural problematic within colonialism. Patrick Wolfe has argued that settler colonialism should be seen not as a singular historical event but as an ongoing structure whose logic is one of replacement of indigenous peoples in an effort to secure their land.[13] While genocide is one replacement strategy, as Wolfe and others have argued,[14] legal, cultural, and political forms of elimination often conserve and conscript the role of indigenous peoples as a more insidious form of control over land.

This ambivalence between replacement and conscription plays, we think, upon the gap between the primitive and modern. Thus, primitivism operates akin to the floating signifier which lends meaning to the colonial enterprise. The floating signifier suggests to Lévi-Strauss, who coined it from his reading of Jakobson, "the disability of all finite thought," condensed in such Polynesian terms as *mana*—that ineluctable power of leadership—that organize the symbolic by serving as "a symbol in its pure state, therefore liable to take on any symbolic content whatever."[15] This pure symbol organizes language, social relations, and art—as well as their interrelations—but it also mobilizes these structures. Levi Bryant has written that the floating signifier indicates "the possibility of a void point within structure, a point of complete indetermination, marking a space where both the social might be transformed and where the subject might exist as something more than a patient or object of social forces."[16] Malabou argues in her chapter "Will Sovereignty Ever Be Deconstructed" that the gap between the biological and the symbolic is this void, serving as both the hidden dimension of sovereign discourse and its point of rupture and plastic transformation. Can sovereign formations in the settler colony be challenged by a deconstruction that places the biological, as an inherently plastic force, at the forefront of its mode of thinking? If "primitive" thought serves as both the structuralist insight and as one symbolic point around which colonialism patterns its own structures of symbolic meaning and violence, in what ways is it vulnerable to plasticity?

We pursue these questions by focusing on the form of colonial law. We inquire whether law that is deployed to further indigenous cultural and territorial dispossession—a law that once sustained the division between savage and civilized and today codifies multicultural social relations that reduce indigenous peoples to one equivalent identity among many—may be vulnerable to anticolonial efforts.[17] In this chapter, we examine two aspects of the legal form in order to assess its plasticity, its resistance to and deformation by anticolonial efforts. First, we turn to an analysis of the limits of indigenous recognition. The recognition of indigenous peoples has implications for the boundaries of community and the form in which that community can represent itself and is frequently one response to government efforts at reconciliation for past colonial violence against indigenous peoples. To what extent does a rethinking of recognition permit a conceptual challenge to the legal foundations of settler colonialism built on suppressing and reforming the primitive other? We then turn to a discussion of colonial biopolitics through which the juridical negotiates its own limits. In this discussion, we examine the intermixture of science and law regulating territorial communities. We illustrate our arguments with examples drawn from Canada and Hawai'i, two settler colonial societies.

INDIGENOUS RIGHTS AND RECOGNITION'S FAILURES

While efforts to secure indigenous claims in settler colonial contexts (such as Canada, Australia, the United States of America, South Africa, and many other places) have always incorporated a plethora of strategies and tactics of resistance, they are often discursively framed as struggles for recognition and for rights. Political claims for land, citizenship rights, self-government, and a range of other civil and political rights have been articulated in the idiom of recognition, in part, as Fanon diagnosed so acutely,[18] because the colonial space is one that is constituted through and by the mis- and nonrecognition of indigenous subjects.

It is important from the outset to mark the limits and also the seeming inescapability of the recognition framework. While resistance to settler colonialism takes many forms, there is a long-standing tendency within the political terrain of the liberal democratic settler state towards the juridification of politics. Many scholars have analyzed the political pitfalls inherent in utilizing legal strategies in the struggle for equality and freedom from discrimination and oppression.[19] While this tendency might be ascribed to a range of political struggles for freedom from various forms of subjugation and subjection, aboriginal communities have out of necessity turned to the law for the protection of their land and resources, often because legal policies of the settler state further the forms of indigenous dispossession and because rights are sometimes offered as a means of reconciliation. More than this, however, the framework of recognition is difficult to simply cast aside for two other reasons. First, the notion that we can only "persist in [our] own being . . . on the condition that we are engaged in receiving and offering recognition"[20] with others in a scene imbued with social norms is compelling if we consider what it means to live a life without recognition of our humanity, a condition faced by many indigenous peoples in the early phases of colonialism (as we explore later in this chapter). Second, the philosophical framework of recognition presents a means of thinking about the effects of language on the constitution of the subject.[21] The ways in which linguistic tropes are imbricated with social norms and political-economic relations and work to produce the subject is vitally important when considering the effects and uses of the enduring language of indigeneity, aboriginality, and primitivism in settler colonial contexts. Where indigenous status and citizenship align and differ is often of material consequence in settler colonies, particularly where norms of multiculturalism mute the historical demands for self-determination under regimes of racial and ethnic nondiscrimination.

While recognition extends the promise of respect and reconciliation, are we "bound by recognition" and its "cunning" character as several recent critiques have asked?[22] Can legal recognition permit the subject to be as it desires, or does it reproduce the self-same subject compatible with dominant cultural norms? Do indigenous rights promise anything more than the empty promises of an ideal of justice that has historically upheld colonial power?

There is reason for skepticism when we look to the law. The form of aboriginal subjectivity that has been recognized by settler colonial courts has been characterized as one that remains caught in a primordial, premodern past.[23] More than this however, the legal subject historically constituted through the appropriation and ownership of native land remains undisturbed by aboriginal challenges to existing structures of ownership and control over resources. As we explore here, recognition takes place, and both the proper subject of law or, to put it somewhat more succinctly, the "proper(tied) subject"[24] and the aboriginal legal subject who has been cast outside of the domain of modern legal relations remain more or less intact and distinct. We examine this persistent gap as one of the prime instances of recognition's failure, its inevitable, structural inability to allow for decolonization.[25] We also consider whether this gap might to some degree become a site of plasticity, open to new forms of recognition, legal relations, and politics.

In 1982, the newly patriated and reformed Canadian constitution included the recognition and protection of aboriginal rights, contained in section 35. For the first time in Canadian history, existing aboriginal and treaty rights received constitutional protection. An aboriginal person or community seeking the recognition of its land rights or rights to hunt, fish, or trade under section 35 must demonstrate that the practice, activity, or custom has a 'reasonable degree of continuity with the practices, traditions, or customs that existed prior to contact' with nonaboriginal settlers. The test as reiterated in Mitchell v. Minister of National Revenue (2001), a case involving an aboriginal rights claim to import goods across the US-Canada border, is worth quoting:

> The practice, custom or tradition must have been "integral to the distinctive culture" of the aboriginal peoples, in the sense that it distinguished or characterised their traditional culture and lay at the core of the people's identity. It must be a "defining feature" of the aboriginal society, such that the culture would be "fundamentally altered" without it . . . This excludes practices, traditions and customs that are only marginal or incidental to the aboriginal society's cultural identity, and emphasises practices, traditions and customs that are vital to the life, culture and identity of the aboriginal society in question.[26]

The dispossession that is continually reiterated through an aboriginal rights jurisprudence developed on the basis of cultural difference, one rooted in both an essentialist concept of aboriginal identity and a notion of culture devoid of economic dimensions, has been quite profound. A close analysis of one amongst many section 35 cases that illustrate this point follows here.

In 2005, the Supreme Court of Canada released its judgment in R. v. Marshall; R. v. Bernard, [2005] 2 S.C.R. 220, two cases heard jointly on appeal before the Court. Both of these cases involved members of the Mi'kmaq First Nation on the east coast of Canada. In Marshall, the thirty-five accused had been convicted in the lower court of illegally cutting timber, while in Bernard the sole accused had been convicted of the unlawful possession of logs cut from Crown land. In the appellate courts, the convictions were overturned. The Supreme Court of Canada upheld the appeal by the Crown and restored the convictions.

In the case of R. v. Marshall, thirty-five Mi'kmaq Indians were convicted of cutting timber on Crown lands in Nova Scotia without authorization. In R. v. Bernard, one Mi'kmaq man was convicted of the unlawful possession of spruce logs, which had been cut from Crown lands in New Brunswick. At stake was the right asserted by the Mi'kmaq people in Nova Scotia and New Brunswick to harvest timber on Crown lands on the basis of their treaty rights or, alternatively, on the basis of their aboriginal title to the land pursuant to section 35 of the Canadian Constitution Act, 1982. Ultimately, the Supreme Court of Canada rejected both of these claims.

The treaty rights that the Mi'kmaq relied upon derived from the Peace and Friendship Treaties of 1760 and 1761, which the British Crown concluded with the Mi'kmaq upon the British defeat of the French colonists. The treaties were intended to ensure a mutually exclusive trading relationship between the Mi'kmaq and the British (R. v. Marshall; R. v. Bernard, [2005] 2 S.C.R. para. 7). The Mi'kmaq claimed a right to harvest logs outside of provincial regulation on the basis that at the time the treaty was concluded, they used wood from their lands to make products which they traded for other goods from the Europeans, such as canoes, snowshoes and toboggans (R. v. Marshall; R. v. Bernard, para. 34). On this basis, they claimed the right to harvest logs from their ancestral lands in order to "obtain a moderate livelihood." The Court, however, found that commercial logging is not an activity that has "logically evolved" from a "traditional activity" of the Mi'kmaq (R. v. Marshall; R.

v. Bernard, para. 16) and thus denied their claim that it was protected by a treaty.

The Court made a distinction between "traditional" activities and "modern" ones. The majority found that in order for activities to be protected by the treaty, they must be one of the "trading activities that were in the contemplation of the parties at the time the treaties were made" but also can be "modern activities that can be said to be their logical evolution" (R. v. Marshall; R. v. Bernard, para. 16). However, even in allowing for the "modernization" of traditional aboriginal activities (after all, as the Court points out, "modern peoples do traditional things in modern ways"), the Court found that the "activity [claimed as a right] must be *essentially* the same [as the traditional practice]" (R. v. Marshall; R. v. Bernard, para. 25; our emphasis). The contemporary activities that are protected are "'types of things "gathered" by the Mi'kmaq in a 1760's aboriginal lifestyle' like 'fruits and berries'" (R. v. Marshall; R. v. Bernard, para. 24, quoting from Marshall 2, para. 19–20).

Because the harvesting of trees was not the object of a commodity trade between the Mi'kmaq and the Europeans until the late eighteenth century, the Court concluded that the treaty does not protect this activity. There is an explicit distinction between aboriginal practices that are traditional and "European" (and subsequently, Anglo–Canadian) practices that are modern. The aboriginal litigants are constructed as *essentially* "premodern," primitive in a sense, and while their rights find modern counterparts due to technological innovations, the essential core of the activities that are protected are defined and constituted as those belonging to a "traditional aboriginal lifestyle," untainted by contact with Europeans.

In this linear narrative of the nation's history, aboriginal peoples are defined by their cultural practices as they existed before the colonial assertion of sovereignty. The colonial assertion of sovereignty, in the eyes of the Court, inaugurated the modern juridical foundation of the nation-state. Although they were the prior occupants of the land, contemporary courts presuppose that the subject of aboriginal rights has always already been subsumed within the bounds of colonial sovereignty. The time prior to the assertion of colonial sovereignty constitutes a sort of prehistory from which courts can divine the ahistorical essence of aboriginal cultural difference. While the recognition of aboriginal rights heralds a movement towards a postcolonial era and a time of reconciliation, the presumed absence of aboriginal sovereignty and presumed legitimacy of colonial sovereignty produces a paradox: the work of recognition in this putatively postcolonial era reproduces a subject of aboriginal rights that is proper (in qualities, characteristics, and practices) to the juridical and territorial boundaries of a colonial settler state and its historical and ongoing economic and political imperatives.

In relation to claims for aboriginal title, the priority of the Crown is to preserve private property relations based on a unitary and underlying Crown sovereignty, and thus other ways of owning and using land—subjectivities shaped through irregular, nomadic, or nonexclusive use of the land—fall out of the bounds of intelligibility. For instance, in R. v. Marshall; R. v. Bernard, the Mi'kmaq also asserted the right to harvest logs on Crown land on the alternative basis of aboriginal title. Their claim on this basis similarly failed. The majority on the Court found that the Mi'kmaq did not have aboriginal title to the areas claimed because there was insufficient evidence to show that the Mi'kmaq, prior to contact with Europeans, occupied the cutting sites regularly or often enough to constitute possession; nor did they possess the desire or capacity to exclude others from this territory. Aboriginal title is defined according to the hallmarks of the modern law of private property ownership devised by the British. The subject of contemporary aboriginal rights is in fact trapped, temporally speaking, in a time prior to European settlement because the core or essence of aboriginal rights is defined in relation to the moment that colonial sovereignty was asserted.[27]

Since 1982, when the acknowledgement and protection of existing aboriginal and treaty rights were enshrined in the Canadian constitution under section 35, the Supreme Court of Canada has devised the tests for establishing aboriginal rights and the content of those rights. The recognition of aboriginal rights on the basis of aboriginal peoples' prior occupation of the land must be reconciled, according to the objectives of section 35 delineated by the Court, with the assertion of Crown (colonial) sovereignty. This creates contradictions and disjunctures that have been resolved, thus far, by establishing criteria for the proof of aboriginal rights and title to land that limits the rights to "activities, customs or practices" that were central, defining features of the community's culture prior to contact with the Europeans. The nature of recognition in the settler colonial context of Canada has done little to restore First Nations' self-determination or to incorporate indigenous understandings of the land into defining the contours of aboriginal rights.

PLASTIC POTENTIALITY

The gap between the "primitive" aboriginal subject, conceived without and beyond colonial history, and the modern settler subject seems vast and persistent in these examples from Canadian jurisprudence. What is the potential for mutual recognition and reconciliation? The dialectic of recognition as first articulated by Hegel in *The Phenomenology of Spirit* has become a means to comprehend how subjects come into being and transform themselves through a process of mutual interpellation that is situated within social norms, political-economic relations, and psychoanalytic frames. Judith Butler argues, "It is important to see that the struggle for recognition as it is staged in the *Phenomenology* reveals the inadequacy of the dyad as a frame of reference for understanding social life. After all, what eventually follows from this scene is a system of customs (*Sittlichkeit*) and hence a social account of the norms by which the reciprocal recognition might be sustained in ways that are more stable than either the life and death struggle or the system of bondage would imply."[28] Several hundred years after encounters among settlers and indigenous peoples, the social norms for reciprocal recognition are, despite some claims,[29] nowhere in sight. Nonetheless, the desire for law, legal rights, and the promise of reconciliation and equality is unabated.[30]

As already explored, the figure of the primitive or, at least, the premodern reappears at the heart of aboriginal rights law. The law is enfolded within the social norms and economic relations that structure recognition in manifold ways: laws governing desire, repressive laws (which, in Althusser's infamous example, enacts a mode of subjection through the voice of the police officer who commands the attention of an individual by hailing him on the street), and within the colonial context, a law of subjection that is based on a racial system of property appropriation.

It is in the work of Fanon that socioeconomic relations and the psychic contours of nonrecognition in the colonial context, saturated with a discourse of primitivism and biologically grounded racism, find their most acute diagnosis. Writing incisively about the "atmosphere that offers not the slightest outlet"[31] from the scientific, economic, metaphysical, and ideational construction of the "Negro," Fanon finds recognition in the colonial context to be an impossibility. Mutual recognition, for Fanon, would require the shattering of worlds—psychic, economic, metaphysical—and nothing short of a revolutionary breakage of property relations built on racially based dispossession. Many of Fanon's critiques of the impossibilities of recognition remain pertinent to the legal dimensions of settler colonialism today. For instance, a concept of race that was grounded in the biological notion of "blood quantum" continues to inform the logic governing Indian status in the Canadian context.[32] To take another example, an explicitly ethnoracial nationalism in the Israeli-Palestinian context informs citizenship laws that were imposed on the Palestinians in 1948 and again in 1967 in order to prevent the reunification of Palestinian families living across the borders.[33]

In a passage that seared itself on the brains of many Marxist anticolonial intellectual migrants in New York, Oxford, London, and similar places in the 1960s and 1970s, largely because it often mirrored their own experiences upon arrival in the "metropole,"[34] Fanon recounts a moment in which he is hailed as a "Negro" by a white boy passing him on the street: "'Mama, see the Negro! I'm frightened! Frightened! Frightened!' . . . I made up my mind to laugh myself to tears, but laughter had become impossible. I could no longer laugh, because I already knew that there were legends, stories, history, and above all historicity, which I learned about from Jaspers. Then, assailed at various points, the corporeal schema crumbled, its place taken by a racial epidermal schema."[35] The child, often associated with the primitive, has been the focal point for the inculcation of racial knowledge central to colonial nationalisms.[36] Here, it is not Althusser's police officer who engages in an act of interpellation but the white child, reminding Fanon that the child's fear was an inheritance of a temporal-political conjuncture that combined a notion of the primitive with biological racism.

Racist ideologies that have biological effects, manifest in what Fanon describes as the epidermalization of a sense of inferiority and biochemical reactions to European racism,[37] draw our attention to the body, and his inclusion of the child suggests the significance of temporality. Might temporality and the body provide a way out of recognition's impossibility? While Malabou identifies recognition explicitly as a political concern in *What Should We Do with Our Brain?*, her rethinking of the Hegelian dialectic that exposes the plasticity inherent in the temporal dimensions of his philosophy and her consideration of the place of the body in Hegel's dialectic of recognition offer a space for rethinking the limits of recognition.

In *The Future of Hegel: Plasticity, Temporality and Dialectic*, Malabou uncovers the plasticity in Hegel's dialectical logic that breaks with the reception of Hegel's thought as effecting ontological closure. She does this, as we have mentioned in the introduction, by contesting the idea that there is a mechanical inevitability to this formulation of the dialectical logic and the emergence of the subject who arrives at the end point of a long struggle for recognition. Her argument for a "future" time that exists within Hegelian thought rethinks the subject "as a structure of anticipation, and, by the same token, a structure of temporalization."[38] In other words, the Hegelian subject is in some sense structured by its capacity to temporalize itself. Does this present a way of conceiving how subjects exist in multiple temporalities at once? Malabou's conceptualization of temporality uncovers a structure in Hegel's thought that permits, on a conceptual level, a mode of understanding how subjects confined to particular *historicities* survive, psychically speaking, by thinking, acting, and living according to a temporality that exceeds and perhaps even contradicts the confines of sovereign orders.

The question of temporality, insofar as it relates to historicism, has been a central concern of anticolonial scholars and postcolonial critics. Whether it is the theologically inflected state of nature that informs aboriginal rights jurisprudence, the infamously Hegelian relegation of Africa to a space and time outside of history, or the Eurocentric historicism of various Marxist traditions, challenges to historicism(s) that capture indigenous Asian, African, and other non-European peoples in the elsewhere of a "homogenous empty time"[39] are at the core of subaltern, postcolonial, and indigenous theorizations of temporality. Malabou's deconstruction of Hegel's thought in a more purely philosophical register rather than one of literary theory or history similarly explodes these confines.

The capacity to exist in two times at once also has a spatial dimension, about which Malabou has jointly written with Judith Butler in *Sois mon corps* and "You Be My Body for Me: Body, Shape, and Plasticity in Hegel's *Phenomenology of Spirit*."[40] In this dialogue, Butler and Malabou explore the body smuggled into Hegel's argument about self-consciousness. The emergence of the body in the master/slave dialectic occurs as a moment of alienation. As the slave comes to recognize himself in the constant threat to his autonomy that the expropriation of the objects of his labor present, the self recognizes itself but also recognizes that it is not itself. Butler has referred to this as the "I redoubled";[41] the self becomes conscious of its existence as both an 'I' who is present—*here*—and yet is also *there* in the shape of an Other who is never wholly independent of me, and vice versa.

> The "I" is a bounded shape, but it finds itself reduplicated, at which point substitutability counters the specificity of this body here as the defining characteristic of the "I." Both seem to be true, and paradoxically so: this body here constitutes my life; but that body there is also me. This means that I am at once here and there, and that whatever certainty I may gain about the truth of this "I" will be one that accepts this spatial vacillation as its precondition. That other shape is not me, if "I" am understood only as this body here. But it turns out that my shape only gains its shape through being differentiated from that other shape, and so I am bound to that other. *For a body to be a body, it must be bound to another body.*[42]

In the settler colonial context, the bodies of the settlers and the indigenous are bound in similarly complex ways. Settlers have used indigenous bodies and ways of life to promote national sovereignty (as in the Boston Tea Party), to enact environmental policies, to name their sports teams, and to advance tourism. Whether it is the everyday racism that informs the structural and sometimes lethal violence aboriginal bodies are subjected to[43] or discursive constructions of the primitive native subject, the power relations inherent in settler-indigenous interrelationality remain steadfast. But the bodies that emerge in Butler's and Malabou's retelling of the dialectic of recognition need not be limited to dominant notions of the body. Many indigenous peoples maintain philosophies of the body that are not limited to the human form and that value the recognition gained among many life forms. In addition, the body is often understood as a collective being in contrast to the individuality assumed within much Western legality and culture.[44] As we explore below, anticolonial resistance to the colonial legal form based in indigenous ontologies has succeeded on some occasions in disrupting some norms of property ownership. We also argue that the affinity between indigenous philosophies and activism, on the one hand, and the particular concept of plasticity developed by Malabou, on the other, have interesting points of contact when considering indigenous struggles for psychic, material, and social survival.

COLONIAL BIOPOLITICS

Malabou argues that one of the philosopher's tasks today is to deconstruct biopolitical deconstruction that has hitherto masked a persistent gap between biology and the symbolic, a synapse around which sovereignty persistently organizes itself. "Such a task," she writes, "requires that we situate the point where biology and history, the living subject and the political subject, meet or touch."[45] In this section, we trace three historical aspects of the contact between the political subject and the living subject within settler colonies: the problem of the humanization of native peoples, the constitution of indigenous identity as race, and the regulation of natural resources. In the previous section we examined the manner in which the form of legal recognition exacerbates the gap between the living and political subject. Here, we are attentive to law and its extrajuridical limits, the "state of exception" that Agamben—who has ignored the colonial and imperial histories of biopolitics—has aptly called the "floating signifier."[46] We argue that the juridical limits created by the exception in the settler colony—in the same manner as recognition—mediate but never resolve the tension between the "primitive" and the modern. The complex colonial interplay of biology and law that defines the conditions of life for native peoples raises significant questions about the uneven forms of access to the biological that organize the concluding parts of this section. If "the symbolic still *colonizes* all discourses in human sciences,"[47] according to Malabou, and if the biological should be embraced as the plastic site of a new symbolic, what kinds of meaningful and legal access to the biological are available to native peoples? And what indigenous analogs to conceptualizing biological matter might offer a form of plasticity adaptive to undoing colonial biopolitics?

One barrier to the biological has been that native peoples have been historically identified with nature and against culture in the colonial context. Fanon famously generalized, "when the colonialist speaks of the colonized he uses zoological terms,"[48] and Achille Mbembe has echoed, "in the eyes of the conqueror, savage life is just another form of animal life."[49] Arriving in Hawai'i in 1832, the Rev. William P. Alexander wondered upon his first encounter with native Hawaiians, "Can these be men and women? Are they not mere animals?"[50] a question whose rhetorical force was repeated throughout Pacific and African colonial encounters. Alexander's prescription for humanizing native Hawaiians was a steady dose of Christianity, but religion also called upon the corrective of the law. As Sally Merry[51] has explained, the divinity and *mana* associated with the Hawaiian *ali'i*, or rulers, seeped slowly into the influence of Christian morality and, by 1840, was absorbed into the authority of the Western law. The law brought with it a patina of civilization but at the cost of suppressing the "animal" in the human: sexuality, dress, and dance were regulated with the threat of imprisonment in the hope that law could "confer sovereignty even upon a female monarch with brown skin when white masculinity seemed the essential badge of rule."[52]

The project of annulling the animal was never fully completed in Hawai'i and elsewhere. Samera Esmeir has explored the Benthamite emphasis on mitigating the suffering of both prisoners and agricultural animals that infused British colonial governance of Egypt in the late nineteenth century.[53] The constrained treatment of prisoners and draft animals were sites for the production of "juridical humanity," that claim to "civilized" political life under the law that could protect the colonized from biopolitical alternatives that would otherwise let them die.[54] Like colonial Egypt, Hawai'i instituted policies of massive native incarceration to civilize and to reinvent the "savage"[55] (an overincarceration of native peoples that persists to this day), and the law, as early as 1850, penalized cruelty to animals, convictions for which were relatively common.[56] Despite these efforts to enforce colonial humanity through the humanization of Hawaiians, the association of natives with the nonhuman has persisted ever since. At times of native Hawaiian political resurgence following the overthrow of Queen Lili'uokalani in 1893, animal imagery was deployed to dampen threats to colonial sovereignty. For instance, in 1901, the surging Home Rule Party, predominantly composed of native Hawaiians agitating for their interests, was ultimately excoriated for an attempt to eliminate a tax on dogs, which some Hawaiians ate. This won their majority the synechdochal moniker "lady-dog legislature," a reminder of a poorly concealed native savagery unfit for democratic politics.

The association of Hawaiians with animals reached a symbolic climax in 1959, the year that Hawai'i became a state of the United States following a plebiscite. In response to a deadly shark attack on a young surfer several months before the vote, the territorial legislature organized a massive culling of sharks.[57] Nearly 600 sharks were killed, and some of their bodies paraded through the streets of Honolulu in a demonstration of sovereign power. As Noenoe Silva and Goldberg-Hiller have argued, the violence against these animals at a time when the territory was being considered for statehood demonstrated the state's capacity to defend its society against external threats, symbolized by a creature whose Western association with the terror of dismemberment[58] analogizes a primary sovereign concern for bodily and territorial integrity. Because some native Hawaiians have another historical association with sharks, one that accepts these animals as members and protectors of the family, the shark kill was also a symbol of the suppression of the native, whose absence as a distinct voting bloc on the statehood plebiscite contravened United Nations protocol.

Today sharks are no longer killed after an attack but instead are protected, in some cases in the name of Hawaiian values.[59] The explicit embrace of indigenous ways of life to legitimate the scientific management of natural resources is nonetheless ambivalent. On the one hand, it symbolizes a changing internal dynamic in which Asian and American settlers acknowledge and assimilate Hawaiian cultural values to create a "rainbow" society. On the other hand, the recognition that Hawaiians maintain a special relationship to sharks and to the land generally and the conscription of this romantic ideal for state policy reinforce an immiscible primitive otherness that augments dispossession of indigenous lands and their resources. The scientific-ecological state has empowered scientists, rather than Hawaiians, to conserve and restore the collateral damage of the colonial economy and to position science as a sovereign exception to juridical power. Scientists' authorization to determine endangered species and prohibit human interference with "nature" superficially hearkens back to the power of the Hawaiian monarch to establish the *kapu*, or taboo, prior to the adoption of Western law. Among other things, the kapu prohibited the harvesting and even the touching of some creatures, much the way green sea turtles are today managed by scientists, who, like the monarchs of old, are the only ones permitted the exception of touch. Yet rather than managing the land and ocean bounty to preserve valued ways of life, the scientific state leaves few options for native peoples to assert a specific relationship to organisms with significant cultural relationships. Indeed, scientists often have no way to integrate history with ecology. They make few conceptual distinctions for "alien" plants and animals; the pig, for example, which was brought to the islands more than a millennium ago by Polynesian voyagers and is still actively hunted for subsistence by some Hawaiians, is now condemned as disruptive to the ecology.[60]

Historical claims to preserve ways of life are also inhibited by racial policies. Foucault has argued that the biopolitical control over populations today relies more upon an "analytics of sexuality" than a sovereign "thematics of blood."[61] Yet as Ann Stoler has noted, the colonial context is distinctive, and "the notions of a 'population' and a 'people' often were being crafted by administrators *cum* ethnographers at the same time."[62] Blood quantum is still calculated for some native Hawaiian entitlements to homestead land. As Kehaulani Kauanui has argued,[63] the legal legacy of blood quantum reinforces the idea that native peoples are an always dying race. Indeed, such legal rules ensure it. Blood quanta minima, established to regulate government entitlements in Hawai'i, were first instituted as a means to preserve the last few authentic native Hawaiians; only later, following intermarriage, which diluted native blood, did such policies extinguish rights in the same manner they did for North American Indians and First Nations peoples: protecting a few while warranting the dispossession of many others.

Race is also used to block some efforts to strengthen native governance in the name of multicultural cosmopolitanism. In 2000, the US Supreme Court ruled against native-only voting for the Office of Hawaiian Affairs, which supervises some native entitlements, on the grounds that this was an unconstitutional racial imposition on the right to vote.[64] Nine years later, the Court dismissed the preamble to the 1993 apology resolution, which acknowledged US involvement in the overthrow of the Hawaiian kingdom, symbolically nailing shut the legal doorway through which native Hawaiians could be recognized as a political rather than racial group.[65] The legal definition of who is a native Hawaiian reinforces this ambivalent gap between the primitive and the modern that defines the colonial legal form. The requirement to trace one's ancestry to a Hawaiian living at the time of Captain Cook's 1778 visit, a time before the advent of the civilizing Western law, ambivalently renders the native forever suspect and sovereign.

Theories of biopolitics suggest to us that native peoples do not suffer alone from racism, scientific management, or civilizing projects of these sorts. But because the raison d'être of colonial power is the dispossession of native peoples from the land (and historically from their culture, language, and family traditions), colonial biopolitics has created an unusually pernicious regime under which native peoples are positioned closer to nature than culture.[66] If there is value in rethinking the symbolic within biology, as Malabou insists, then the extreme alienation from the scientific and legal dispositifs that have cooperated with the colonial state makes this symbolism both essential and fraught. It is not that native peoples necessarily reject the validity of scientific knowledge; it is rather that when natural history, biology, genetic research, and scientific management practices dispossess native peoples from their land and cultural traditions, plasticity and its promise of the other of legal and sovereign forms may have to be located elsewhere.

One significant source for this alternative thinking is what was once abjected as a primitive and timeless metaphysics: the indigenous ontologies that extol the often metamorphic interrelationships of humans with animals, plants, and landforms.[67] These indigenous conceptions of a vibrant matter have much deeper roots than those of a contemporary new materialism, but they have (often unacknowledged) parallels. In their approach to a symbolic within the Western realm of the biological, they also offer a potential critique and pathway of resistance to colonial biopower. If plasticity orients us to political spaces located between history and biology, then the cultural meanings of struggles informed by these indigenous ontologies seem infused with a plasticity in a new key with self-reinforcing potentials. Consider the following engagements.

In 2005, the University of Hawai'i was discovered by Hawaiian activists to have patented, three years previously, several varieties of *kalo* (taro) that had been genetically engineered. University scientists claimed they were motivated to eliminate diseases in the crop, diseases that could crash what limited production remained, and they had not consulted Hawaiian farmers because patenting the engineered hybrids was necessary under their union contract.[68] Citing Hawaiian cosmologies in which kalo, as Hāloa, is the metamorphic elder sibling of humans, the opponents argued that the manipulation and patenting of the plant was akin to genocide: "The owning and selling our *mana* or life force. Mana is the spiritual force that comes from our knowledge and intricate relationship with nature. Part of mana is what westerners call 'biodiversity.'"[69] While biodiversity has been a key concept justifying the scientific management of state resources, this reference to biodiversity specifically draws negative attention to what the growing industrial commitment to GMO technology means for Hawaiian survival. In an unprecedented action, the university relinquished the patents, agreeing to turn them over to a Hawaiian entity. But the activists, stressing that they could not own their ancestor, destroyed them instead.

The ancestral claim in the kalo controversy challenged the technical manipulation of genes in several ways. Metonymically, it contested the idea that a Hawaiian individual (e.g., kalo, as elder sibling) could be technically created and, by analogy, that the extension of legal rights to this individual—or to an indigenous people within a cosmopolitan scheme of governance—could effect a politically relevant metamorphosis. Since bioengineering is also a speculative capitalist venture oriented towards the mitigation and control of future risk, a risk that underwrote the value for the patent holders, opposition to kalo's genetic manipulation also reoriented kinship within different temporal frames. One frame could be seen from within the body of the kalo itself. Hawaiian kalo farming depends upon replanting the *huli*, or green sprout, after harvesting the corm. Thus, Hawaiian kalo is reproduced as a clone; the selfsame being lives at once as ancestor and again as the following generation.

Malabou argues that, even in Western philosophy, clones are not identical replicas, and as such they challenge some aspects of genomic thinking.

> The fact that it's possible to become daughter of your daughter, to be simultaneously older and younger than yourself, to auto-clone yourself in some way, effectively . . . produces difference not in the sense to which we've become accustomed by good old DNA and other such kinds of code—a difference between individuals—but a difference *between code and message.* . . . We might not ask ourselves anymore if clones are really twins, but instead how the phenomenon of cloning allows us to take twinness as the model of truth. Plasticity, from the perspective of such an investigation, [would be linked] to the eruption of a reversibility between before and after that modernizes posterity by giving new forms to atomized, nuclear sameness.[70]

Replanting kalo intervenes in the plant's life cycle in order to assure a clone that also moves from field to field, identical yet different, creating the semantic possibilities of new messages based on an ancient lineage.

One new semantic possibility emerges in the potential interjection of history into an otherwise ahistorical scientific regulation of the land and its biological diversity. The argument that ecological science can designate and control destructive and often "alien" species has its analog in the political claims that species diversity is both an appropriate policy and a reflexive value by which the multicultural human society sees itself in nature and its management, including paternalist protections for those (flora, fauna, and people) considered primitive and ill fitted to survive into this modern cosmopolitanism.[71] And yet that which is alien has rarely been understood from an indigenous standpoint. Hawaiians have many stories and chants identifying the sources of plants and animals brought to the islands on their transoceanic voyages of trade and settlement across the Pacific, and like the pig, many of these are essential to subsistence and have integral places in native cosmogonies.[72] The pig god Kamapuaʻa is revered in literature as a troublemaker with the metamorphic capacity to assume various body shapes, useful for avoiding punishment.[73] The defense of the pig's place in the Hawaiian ecology echoes these stories, as it relates ambivalently if not metamorphically to the law-backed science that has ranked the pig as one of the most destructive pests. The need for pig control provides an adequate legal basis for Hawaiians to access otherwise restricted lands, whether for hunters who work to control pig populations or for others who protect endangered native plants on culturally significant lands controlled by the military and so normally off-limits to Hawaiians. This bending of the legal property form to the interest of some indigenous practices creates small spaces for Hawaiian stewardship of the land.

If plasticity orients us towards the philosophical imperative of a symbolic within the biological, one that might disrupt the biopolitical mask of sovereignty, then perhaps we should see plasticity emerging in alternative conceptions of living matter where the symbolic has long been rooted, especially in colonial societies where indigenous peoples have been most abjected as nature out of place. Thinking through these ontologies reveals—against most notions of the primitive—a history that is mobilized to embrace multiple temporalities and complex interrelationships among humans and nonhuman others whose possibilities permit new forms of survival. For some, the narratives of the many beings on the land are key tropes for reconceptualizing a jurisprudence that is less committed to the Western legal form. Christine Black, a Yugumbeh scholar in the territory of Australia, has argued that it is not the Western colonial keystones of property and recognition but the land, made accessible through the stories that have grown up around it, that forms an appropriately indigenous source for the law. "My mother taught me to 'notice' nature. In so doing she taught me the Law of the Land . . . The best in the Indigenous jurisprudential tradition, with its blending of legality and narrative contains a subjectivity that ensures the predominance of *feeling*: a continuous feeling for the web of interconnected relationships that patterns humans into their environment. . . . Through the dialogic [encounter with these narratives], the story of law is able to continue to flux through time."[74]

A law that is in dialogue with the land and its many interconnected inhabitants invests in the symbolic character of a nature too often made arid or inaccessible by settler colonial biopolitics. Like the return to biology, this is a plastic conception of the law, one that reinforces and repairs that which is most threatened by colonial power.

NOTES

1. Malabou, *Plasticity at the Dusk*, 2, 4; citing Lévi-Strauss, *Way of the Masks*.

2. On the role of universalism in Lévi-Strauss's thought, see Montag, *Althusser*, 4. On the role of primitivism in French cultural thought after World War II, see Sherman, *French Primitivism*.

3. Haeckel, *Evolution of Man*, 1. Haeckel's point is that early morphological structures can be located in some stages of embryonic development.

4. See Gould, *Ontogeny*. Neoteny is the survival of juvenile traits into adulthood, one means of evolutionary development.

5. Malabou, *Plasticity at the Dusk*, 54.

6. Byrd, *Transit of Empire*; Fitzpatrick, *Modernism*; Merry, *Colonizing Hawai'i*.

7. Malabou writes in ch. 2, "Poverty, dispossession, exploitation are the points of departure of philosophical thinking, not because they would constitute objects or topics for philosophers, but because practice and theory both owe their energy, the power of their dynamism to their originary absence of determinate being," 57.

8. Sherman, *French Primitivism*, 3.

9. One exception is Lévi-Strauss, "Anthropology," 124–27. But see discussion of Lévi-Strauss's fight with Georges Baladier over the latter's insistence on the relevance of colonialism: Dosse, *History of Structuralism*, 264ff.

10. Said, "Totalitarianism of Mind," 257.

11. Lévi-Strauss, *Savage Mind*, 10.

12. Chris Friday, who collaborated with the famous indigenous artist and mask maker Lelooska, writes, "For fleeting moments, readers get glimpses into an inner life, but all too quickly the masks slam shut, leaving only the outer shell visible, that form we expect to see. We know there is more behind the mask once we have glimpsed it, but it is difficult, even impossible, to truly know all of a story or to present it as the story." Friday, *Lelooska*, 19.

13. Wolfe, *Settler Colonialism*.

14. Wolfe, "Settler Colonialism"; Barker, *Native Acts*.

15. Lévi-Strauss, *Marcel Mauss*, 63–64.

16. Bryant, *Democracy of Objects*.

17. It is interesting to note in this context Homi Bhabha's argument that multiculturalism has itself become a key floating signifier, as well as Stuart Hall's argument for race in that role. Both candidates, we suggest, hide the plight of indigenous peoples in settler colonies. See Bhabha, "Culture's In-Between"; *Race*. For an analysis of whether law can be utilized to create legal-political ruptures in the colonial context, see Bhandar, "Strategies of Legal Rupture."

18. Fanon, *Black Skin*.

19. See, e.g., McCann, *Rights at Work*; Goldberg-Hiller, *Limits to Union*; Stychin, *Law's Desire*.

20. Butler, *Undoing Gender*, 31.

21. The constitution of (the Hegelian) subject through language (subtended by social norms, political economy, and history) is a core and common theme in the work of Fanon and Butler and can be understood in part as a reaction to and engagement with the inheritance of the French reception of Hegel in the work of Hyppolite, Kojève, and Sartre. Elena Loizidou discusses the centrality of language to the becoming of the Hegelian subject in the context of Butler's ethics. Loizidou, *Judith Butler*, 69.

22. References to Markell, *Bound by Recognition*; Povinelli, *Cunning of Recognition*. See also Barker, *Native Acts*; Klopotek, *Recognition Odysseys*; Den Ouden and O'Brien, *Recognition*.

23. Bhandar, "Resisting the Reproduction"; Borrows, "Frozen Rights."

24. For an elaboration of the concept of the "proper(tied)" subject, see Bhandar, "Plasticity."

25. See Coulthard, "Subjects of Empire."

26. Mitchell v. Minister of National Revenue, 1 S.C.R. (Canada) 911, para. 12 (2001).

27. See Delgamuukw v. British Columbia, ¶147. See also Borrows, *Recovering Canada*; Bhandar, "Resisting the Reproduction."

28. Butler, *Giving an Account*, 29.

29. Taylor, *Multiculturalism*.

30. See, e.g., Merry, *Colonizing Hawaii*; Milner and Goldberg-Hiller, "Feeble Echoes"; Goldberg-Hiller, "Reconciliation."

31. Fanon, *Black Skin*, 11.

32. Palmater, *Beyond Blood*.

33. Masri, "Love Suspended."

34. Stuart Hall, e.g., recounts this very passage in the film *The Stuart Hall Project* when reflecting on his experiences as a young Jamaican immigrant in Oxford in the 1960s. See also Bannerji, *Thinking Through*, where she relays the feelings of alienation and estrangement that she experienced when arriving in London from Calcutta in the 1960s, despite having been thoroughly accultur-

ated to English sensibilities, literature and history through a classical English education in West Bengal.

35. Fanon, *Black Skin*, 84.
36. Levander, *Cradle of Liberty*.
37. Fanon, *Black Skin*, 12.
38. Malabou, *Future of Hegel*, 130.
39. Chakrabarty, *Provincializing Europe*, 12.
40. Butler and Malabou, *Sois mon corps*; Malabou and Butler, "You Be My Body."
41. Malabou and Butler, "You Be My Body," 630.
42. Malabou and Butler, "You Be My Body," 631.
43. Razack, "Making Canada White," 159; Razack, "Gendered Racial Violence," 91.
44. Rifkin, "Indigenizing Agamben."
45. Malabou, ch. 1, 37.
46. Agamben, *State of Exception*, 37.
47. Malabou, ch. 1, 40.; emphasis added.
48. Fanon, *Wretched of the Earth*, 7.
49. Mbembe, "Necropolitics," 24.
50. Alexander, *Mission Life in Hawaii*, 168.
51. Merry, *Colonizing Hawai'i*.
52. Merry, *Colonizing Hawai'i*, 8.
53. Esmeir, *Juridical Humanity*.
54. A. Pandian has argued that "a close examination of the government of animals by humans is vital for an anthropology of biopolitics: for an understanding, that is, of the many ways in which humans themselves have been governed as animals in modern times." Pandian, "Pastoral Power," 86.
55. The reference is to Luana Ross, *Inventing the Savage*. Ross has argued that imprisonment of American Indians plays this dual role. For a similar argument in Hawai'i, see Keahiolalo-Karasuda, "Colonial Carceral and Prison Politics."
56. See discussion by Bird, *Hawaiian Archipelago*, 451.
57. See Goldberg-Hiller and Silva, "Sharks and Pigs."
58. Lane and Chazan, "Symbols of Terror."
59. Recent proposed legislation to ban shark cage tours acknowledged sharks "carry great cultural, historical, and spiritual significance for many native Hawaiians, native Hawaiian practitioners, and others who value the Hawaiian culture." Legislation that bans shark finning has been premised on a similar claim.
60. For a study of scientific taxonomies in relation to native interests, see Helmreich, "How Scientists Think."
61. Foucault, *History of Sexuality*, 148.

62. Stoler, *Race and the Education of Desire*, 39; see also generally Wolfe, *Settler Colonialism*.

63. Kauanui, *Hawaiian Blood*; see also, generally, Barker, *Native Acts*.

64. Rice v. Cayetano, 528 U.S. 495 (2000).

65. Hawaii v. Office of Hawaiian Affairs, 129 S. Ct. 1436 (2009).

66. On the Western and colonial history of this distinction, see Descola, *Beyond Nature*.

67. Moreton-Robinson, "I Still Call Australia Home," esp. 32ff.; Bignall, "Potential Postcoloniality," 267ff.; Goldberg-Hiller and Silva, "Sharks and Pigs"; Allewaert, *Ariel's Ecology*.

68. Schlais, "Patenting," 581.

69. Ritte and Freese, "Haloa," 11. See also Goodyear-Kaopua, "Kuleana Lahui."

70. Malabou, "Following Generation," 32–33. See also Franklin, *Dolly Mixtures*, 41. Michael Marder has provocatively suggested that "the meaning of vegetal being is time." Marder, *Plant-Thinking*, 95.

71. Consider this statement by Edward O. Wilson on mass extinctions, the causes of which include "especially on the Hawaiian archipelago and other islands, . . . the introduction of rats, pigs, beard grass, lantana, and other exotic organisms that outbreed and extirpate native species." Wilson, *Nature Revealed*, 241. On the politics of biological designations, see Gould, "Evolutionary Perspective"; Subramaniam, "Aliens Have Landed!"

72. This is true of some other indigenous cultures as well. See Trigger, "Indigeneity." See also Goldberg-Hiller and Silva, "Sharks and Pigs."

73. Charlot, *Kamapuaʻa Literature*; Kameʻeleihiwa, *He Moʻolelo*.

74. Black, *Land Is the Source*, 6, 11, 12.

CHAPTER **11**

Something Darkly This Way Comes:
The Horror of Plasticity in an Age of Control

Jairus Grove

The only laws of matter are those which our minds must fabricate, and the only laws of mind are fabricated for it by matter.
—J. M. Maxwell (February 1856)

The Brain That Changes Itself: this recent book's title expresses, via neural plasticity, the very situation of the philosopher today. A brain that changes itself. That is exactly what "I" am.
—Catherine Malabou (2008)

Don't you see Peter? I'm not safe. It's my mind. Ever since the pieces of my brain were reimplanted, it's been changing me back to the man I was before. Bit by bit, I'm losing the man that you helped me become.
—"Walter Bishop," character in *Fringe*

In J. J. Abrams's genre-bending masterpiece *Fringe* the lead character, Walter Bishop, is confronted with his double from a parallel universe. In this twisted version of the twin paradox it is not the speed of light that marks the difference between the Walters but a single decision decided differently by each Walter. The Walter of the quotation experienced a moment of shock when he discovered that he almost destroyed the entire universe by traveling between dimensions. In this brief moment of humility, reminiscent of J. Robert Oppenheimer's response to the atom bomb test, Walter decides to make himself dumber.

Walter compels his best friend to give him a selective lobotomy in hopes that his hubris will be restrained and his ability to achieve such scientific feats will be safely limited. Evil Walter (Walternate) from the parallel universe is genetically identical, and his history is also identical in almost every way. However, a slight difference causes Walternate to embrace his intellect and confidence. The result is an unmatched brilliance but one that no longer has any regard for human life, as every cost can be rationalized, thought to its final conclusion. The result of unfettered brilliance is a Walter that is sociopathic, maniacal, and almost unstoppable.

In order to counter the threat of Evil Walter the sweet and quirky lobotomized Walter must reimplant the lobotomized tissue. The caring and kind man who has grown attached to this world and its inhabitants is struck by the horror of plasticity. Despite his *choice* to cut out pieces of his brain and his *choice* to reimplant the lobotomized pieces, he cannot control his return to hubris and destruction. The man that cares about the world enough to risk becoming something he hates is becoming a man that will no longer care about the world. That is, the indexical value "care for the world," which distinguishes the two Walters, is lost in the moment of reimplantation. There is no going back; the man Walter will become *cannot* care that he is what he has become.

This is the paradox of modern morality. Malabou's question "What should we do with our brain?" is a real question, but the choices before us are not under our control. They are leaps and bounds, and where we land erases the point from which we leapt. This problem of a disappearing measure of change is a limit to plasticity not as a process but as a thinkable question. So the investigation of one's own plasticity is always a kind of thought experiment. When the process actually takes place, whether subtle or dramatic, it is often imperceptible. Like Walter, we have flashes of transition. Similarly, stroke victims and those suffering Alzheimer's become frustrated when they feel capabilities they once had but now seem cut off from. Schizophrenics have moments of pharmaceutical and nonpharmaceutical clarity in which they fear a return to the other cognitive order or sometimes regret the things they have done. In these more dramatic cases it is clear that something like psychoanalysis is well out of its league, as are any number of chemical treatments and mechanical interventions. Plasticity is a frustrating causal conundrum and is the real condition of our daily neuronal existence. "The self is synaptic" and vice versa.[1] And despite that maelstrom of operators in our daily neuronal life, most people still cling to the idea of their own determination, of being masters of their domain.

In presenting plasticity as both empirical fact and philosophical question, Malabou compels us to think something thought to be unthinkable and something that Malabou reminds us we do not know. There is an epistemological question about how the embodied brains we call scientists study other embodied brains we call objects of study. The question goes something like this: how can we make knowledge out of the condition of possibility of knowledge without reaching some kind of logical paradox? The knowledge of a thought in itself would either be merely a representation (say, an MRI image) or the idea of a thought in itself (the idea of that MRI image). Malabou's position has gotten support from many prominent neuroscientists championing neuroplasticity, as well as from political theorists like William Connolly and Brian Massumi, who see in neuroscience the terrain of contemporary political engagement. Further, the backlash against such positions has reached a screeching pitch pursued in the name of defending the dignity and uniqueness of the human. To address these concerns for the fate of man, I take Immanuel Kant's resistance to neurophilosophy as emblematic of the reactionary humanist position—the argument has changed little in the intervening 220 years—the hope being to lay out the philosophical landscape in which contemporary neuropolitics unfolds before thinking through the neuropolitical practices that have proceeded with little attention to the lack of philosophical consensus on its possibility.

In the preface to *Anthropology from a Pragmatic Point of View*, Immanuel Kant declares the investigation of "cranial nerves and fibers . . . a pure waste of time."[2] For Kant the brain as mind is noumenon, in the sense that it cannot be appreciated by the senses, and the brain as brain is phenomenon, to the extent that it can be appreciated by the senses but not known in itself. On this point I almost agree. However, there is no reason that Malabou's materialist adventure with the brain requires a naive realism in which things are self-evident and waiting only for sufficient scientific explanation. Malabou is not making an argument for material transparency. Instead, what is truly discomforting for Kant and provocative for Malabou is the insistence of the brain as matter, that which gives and receives form, to be thought.

Further, Kant's rejection of this kind of speculation goes much farther than the philosophical proof of the unreachable thing in itself. For Kant the problem of the brain is a threat to the very image of "Man" required by his thinking. Kant cannot deny the natural and physical nature of the human, but such a nature requires a difference in kind from the "irrational animals" of which he says one can do with "as one likes."[3] Kant accomplishes this task through a developmentalist account of human maturation.[4] The transition of early childhood to the possibility of a free human is for Kant the difference between "feeling one's self" and "thinking one's self," marked by the linguistic shift of speaking in the third person to the use of the "I" to describe one's actions.[5] The internal coherence of thinking rather than feeling is at the heart of Kant's disdain for brain science. According to Kant, the material problems of the brain's work must be fully under the dominion of the thinking subject, or man is merely an animal. The sense data of sensation must then also be a purely passive stream of which thought is in command. Kant lays out the stakes of this view of cognition in a section he titles "Apology for Sensibility":

> Sensibility . . . monopolizes conversation and is like an *autocrat*, stubborn and hard to restrain, when it should be merely a *servant* of the understanding. . . . The inner perfection of the human being consists in having in his power the use of all of his faculties, in order to subject them to his *free choice*. For this is required that *understanding* should rule without weakening sensibility (which in itself is like a mob, because it does not think), for without sensibility there would be no material that could be processed for the use of legislative understanding.[6]

So Kant does not deny the materiality of consciousness; in fact, he insists upon it. However, the brain of the mind must remain a substrate under the command of the faculties. The substance of these faculties is elided by Kant's command-and-control model of consciousness by sleight of hand, not explicit argument.

In light of what is lost for Kant, if the brain is of serious importance to the question of thought leads me to think that the rejection of brain research as a "pure waste of time" is not the traditional Kantian epistemological problem. I want to read his rejection as an overreaction caused by the fear that the brain would unravel the *free choice* of human action. The faculties then are a kind of artifice to bridge a gap Kant would rather not think between the brain's ability to give and receive form. The thing that changes itself confronts Kant with the horror that the human is an animal among animals. We are an organism with moods, instincts, bodies, brains, nerves, perceptions, affects, encounters, lesions, tumors, headaches, hallucinations, parasites, ideas, interfaces, implants, desires, frailties, glasses, memory, recordings . . . So rather than an epistemological question we have an ontological question: "A brain that changes itself. That is exactly what 'I' am."[7] It is in this weird space of Kant's "mob," the melee of forming and being formed, that Malabou's questioning takes place. However, like Kant, many others find such questions not only a "pure waste of time" but a threat to what it is to be human.

Following Kant, somatic fundamentalists like Jürgen Habermas, some neo-Arendtians, self-described intentionalists, and humanists of various stripes see the recourse to the brain as the death of man. For these thinkers neuroscience is just the next normalizing discourse to follow psychoanalysis in a long line of expert power moves that seek to subjugate people through the naturalization of pathology and control.[8] Furthermore and somewhat contradictorily, they fear that the instrumentalization of the brain will lead to an objectification of the human, destroying the dignity and intrinsic value on which human rights are premised.[9] The image conjured is of a mechanistic world where freedom is abolished via genetic, surgical, educational, or pharmaceutical intervention. As Slavoj Žižek has rightly pointed out, the irony of holding both positions is that one affirms both the ideational view of the mind's autonomy and that the mind, dignity, or what you will are, while independent of material existence, directly threatened by its modification. According to Žižek, "It's not so much that we are losing our dignity and freedom with the advance of biogenetics but that we realize we never had them in the first place."[10] This is the affective horror that animates the reactionary position of Kant and other enfeebled humanists. Those that cling to intentionalism or a mind-dependent existence feel plasticity gnawing away at the certainty of their values.

At this moment, while I am writing about the problem of plasticity, 25 milligrams of sumatriptan are dissolving into my bloodstream. As the drug circulates through my body and finally passes into my brain, it will stimulate serotonin receptors. The purpose of the drug is to interrupt my pounding migraine headache. The theory is that migraines are caused by the swelling of blood vessels in the brain. Stimulating the receptors causes contractions that compress the swelling in hope of ending the headache. However, this very mechanical reaction is paralleled by the effect on my serotonin. As a serotonin agonist, the medication also blocks the signal of the pain caused by the migraine. Further, serotonin is a critical neurotransmitter for my sense of well-being. Well-being is something we code as a psychological state in humans, but in both humans and even simple invertebrates, serotonin signals both need and satisfaction regarding food, sex, and other basics.

I am feeling better already, and I have less pain. Is my change in mood because of the alteration of my internal brain chemistry? Is my internal brain chemistry changing because the drug has changed my sense of "well-being" or because I "feel better" from the pain relief? My mood has definitely improved, but I do not *know* why it has. And most importantly while I "chose" to pop a pill, it is difficult to say I "chose" to feel better. The epistemological morass does not, however, foreclose the ontological provocation. Instead the pill, my brain, my neurons, my serotonin, my general mood, are agents provocateurs of thought. Each alien yet intimate.[11]

Plasticity takes a darker turn away from the everyday when the cause of such a change is not a pill "I" popped but the intervention of the alea.[12] The relationship between plasticity and chance for Malabou takes the form of traumatic brain injuries, lobotomies, Alzheimer's disease, sudden shifts in hormones or other regulating neurological chemicals. The aleatory world of the brain puts the "I" in the potent grip of forces well beyond our control. However, unlike the more general confrontation with mortality, what Malabou calls "destructive plasticity" forces us to confront the fact that our identity, the I, is not essential. In fact, the horror of plasticity is that our life can go on without us. The "us" is changeable and can be lost without the cessation of life. Not only are our minds not autonomous or independent of our bodies, they can undergo metamorphoses that leave no trace of what we once were, erasing the consciousness of what we have become. This, for Malabou, is a critical element of plasticity. Unlike elasticity, plasticity has no promise of return. Both concepts suggest a limit point at which the system breaks. However, the change in each is different, as something elastic returns or can return to form after its change. Plasticity names an unredeemable metamorphosis. So the "I" and its attendant and mysterious "faculties," which are essential to moral freedom for Kant and others, always has the potential to explode and return to the mob of sensation only to reemerge as something altogether different.

This is the terror that keeps Jürgen Habermas up at night. What will we do if we discover our freedom is contingent, that our very nature can change?[13] The plan of the rest of this essay is to follow Malabou's provocation through to the heart of that terror. However, unlike Habermas and others, I hope to do so without the sentimental attachment to a humanity that never existed. Rather, I want to push Malabou's concepts farther. I want to consider what happens to plasticity and destructive plasticity when they are let loose in the wilds of politics. As knowledge of our formable and forming nature becomes not just known but made practical, the nightmare of humanists becomes real. Populations of human bodies without essential identities can be altered or, in the language of cybernetics, steered. Unlike understandings of power, even subtle forms of disciplinary power, plasticity on the scale of the individual and the polis represents the possibility of change without subjection; that is, without resistance. Rather than the relations of power that make subjects in the Foucauldian image, we have the possibility of designing or steering subjects that have no index of what they were before, such that something could resist. Instead, plasticity represents the possibility of a frictionless change—in the sense that one can imagine (and has imagined) the alteration of the brain or the assemblage of bodies-brains-semiotics-technics that is often called the social—that would leave no trace of what could be called an alternative. This is not the failure of resistance to produce an outcome, as in the case of the noncompliant prisoner who nonetheless remains imprisoned. Instead, plasticity raises the question of techniques that produce bodies that do not know that the "they" that they once were wanted to resist or even are imprisoned.

The incorporation of plasticity into politics raises the specter of Gilles Deleuze's "societies of control," in which individuals become "dividuals"[14]—humans as counters in a flexible and constantly "modulating" economy.[15] Control in this context is often read systemically, as if only the "society" views humans as counters but the "dividuals" themselves, like Robert Duvall's character in THX 1138, yearn to be free, to be unique. Confronting plasticity and its explosive potential to obliterate precursors poses a different dividual, a real dividual. Bodies stripped not just of their identity but of the desire to have an identity or to have an identity nonidentical to the identity that preceded it. Control represents the real possibility of order without the leverage or friction of ordering.

Normatively I do not disagree with Habermas and others that this reduction of freedom to an engineering problem is horrifying. The point of disagreement is that arguing against the existence of such a possibility will have an effect on the probability of this nightmare.[16] The attempt to safeguard humanity through the scapegoating of materialist thinking is self-defeating, as it insists that human freedom and dignity are independent of the brain while also decrying the possibility of each "becoming material." In its cruelest form this line of argument amounts to trying to cure someone with Alzheimer's by scolding her about the intrinsic dignity and rationality of humans. Lesions beat argument every time. So rather than take recourse to moralizing the horror of control, it is necessary to take seriously the possibility of control as a material configuration enabled by the inessential nature of humans: their plasticity. Furthermore, I ask the reader to affirm the horror of destructive plasticity rather than look away or flee into the arms of humanist sentimentality.

DREAMING OF CONTROL, OR THE FIRST AGE OF NEUROPLASTICITY

The generation of cyberneticists that came of age in the 1940s was inspired by the brain, in particular brain pathology. The now commonplace understandings of networks, feedbacks, chaos, self-organization, and complexity that organize the functioning and understanding of everything from the Internet to the global climate system come from this extravagant period of intellectual innovation. Nearly all of the influential thinkers of the period, save Norbert Wiener, started with the brain as inspiration and model for their new ontology of nature and science.[17] The brain was the black box[18] par excellence. Furthermore, it is telling that schizophrenia was the first object of neuroplastic research. The seemingly far-fetched conundrum of Dr. Walter Bishop, how to purposefully alter the functional structure of the brain, was the holy grail of the first era of neuroplasticity. Unlike Kant, these thinkers were drawn to the seemingly impenetrable object of the brain. But unlike the early brain scientists that Kant mocks, who started with the cranial nerves and fibers that make up the brain, the cyberneticists tried to understand and model the brain's function rather than its structure. The early success of this modeling led almost immediately to its application. Rudimentary brains, the homeostats, were put to use regulating machinery, creating temperature-controlled homes, regulating the firing of naval artillery, and being put to use on actual human brains.[19] The goal in almost all cases was designing systems or altering them so that they could "strive to hold back nature's tendency toward disorder by adjusting its parts to various purposive ends."[20]

Imagined in the first generation of cyberneticists was a kind of secret functionalism that could be leveraged against the otherwise entropic tendencies of the cosmos. So a brain, for cyberneticists, was a machine that could receive information, store information, abstract that information, recombine information, and communicate or output new information that might otherwise be called action, all governed by a life principle to persist in completing in these tasks. The earliest of these works, W. Ross Ashby's 1952 *Design for a Brain*, captures the goal of such research in the first sentence of the text: "How does the brain produce adaptive behavior?"[21] The subsequent works—W. Grey Walter's *The Living Brain* (1953), Pierre de Latil's *La pensee artificielle* (1956), John von Neumann's *The Computer and the Brain* (1958), Stafford Beer's *Decision and Control* (1966) and *Brain of The Firm* (1972), and Gregory Bateson's *Steps to an Ecology of Mind* (1972)—all focus on the same question: what is it that allows a brain, even if not a human brain, to self-steer and adapt in complex ways despite being mechanical at the level of each operation? That is, the basic chemistry of a single neuron is relatively simple. Importantly, in each iteration of this question, every one of these thinkers, like Malabou, begins from the premise that a soul or mind independent of the brain is an insufficient answer.

Why return to the beginning, so to speak? In part, because each of these texts is philosophically sophisticated and challenging in its interplay between the experimental material world and the questions provoked by the various machines and even brain experiments—and in part because much can be learned from cybernetics as a trial run of neuroplasticity. Cybernetics is all the more demanding of Malabou's question because of Ashby's use of his theories to support and perform shock therapy, not in spite of them.

While Ashby's questionable use of electroshock therapy undermined the place of many of these thinkers in philosophical debates and traditions,[22] cybernetics' failure in theory did not follow in practice. Environmental study, artificial intelligence, systems biology, climatology, robotics, complexity theory, anything digital, informatics, techno music, video games: all are explicitly indebted to cybernetics. We live in a cybernetic age even if we do not know it. And if there is a unifying theme in all of these strands of cybernetic thought, it is plasticity, the ability of systems to sustain integrity while changing. To be formed and give form while surviving is not a philosophy to come, as Malabou thinks it, but one at the heart of the technological revolutions of the twentieth century.

In light of this convergence it is worth considering the almost immediate hope and proposal to apply the insights of plasticity, particularly brain plasticity, to human systems.[23] If the brain can be modeled, maybe it can also be hacked, to borrow an anachronism from cybernetics' digital future. Can political systems and the brains that constitute them be steered or completely reengineered to produce a new functionality? Neuropolitics in this iteration is a hope for self-sustaining, systemic, and dynamic homeostasis; that is, control.

This chapter, directly inspired by W. Ross Ashby, examines two neuropoliticians. The first is the political scientist Karl Deutsch, author of *The Nerves of Government: Models of Political Communication and Control*; the second is the founder of the Yale University neuroscience program, José Delgado, whose book is *Physical Control of the Mind: Toward a Psychocivilized Society*. In each of their political programs I see a species-scale revolutionary potential for plasticity and the horror of a designed world. The hope is that in these two early attempts to apply insights of neuroscience, we see the political possibilities in the concept of plasticity.

Deutsch begins his book with a question redolent of Malabou and the cyberneticists: "what is the capacity of this political system for self-transformation with significant preservation of its own identity and continuity?"[24] Deutsch, from the beginning of his exploration of the "essential connection between control and communication," is concerned with Malabou's problem of continuity, the delicate balance between plasticity and a destructive plasticity in which self-transformation obliterates the self that undertook transformation.[25] The stakes of the question for Deutsch are apocalyptic. In 1963, at the time of the book's publication, the dark shadow of the Cuban missile crisis loomed large. As a seasoned international relations theorist Deutsch saw the world as an anarchic system of militarily competing states. That competition creates a security dilemma in which each state is compelled by the danger of anarchy to improve its defensive capability. Tragically, as goes the theory, the indistinguishability of defensive and offensive military capability leaves every other state feeling more threatened by the first state's improvement in military defense. The result is escalating arms races, until crisis and a lack of transparency produce war. As a result the international system, for Deutsch and many others, was a cycle of conflicts and wars created by the opacity of intention and threat. Furthermore, following this view of the international order, as no military innovation has ever been withdrawn, global nuclear war was not a question of *if* but when.[26]

Nerves of Government shows that Deutsch understands the international system and its repetition of the security dilemma as a problem of communication and control. The international system was a defunct brain. Imperfect information and the inability to learn from the past pain of war (i.e., memory) lead to repetition compulsion. Therefore, unless an international system could be designed that overcame what he called the "pathology of power" in favor of plasticity—the ability to learn—war would be dominant until life was no longer dominant. Without a combination of memory and plasticity, Deutsch argues, a "society becomes an automaton, a walking corpse."[27] So beginning with a cybernetic theory of mind, Deutsch attempts to develop various theories of "collective personality," "group mind," and "group learning."[28] Society is, according to Deutsch, a "plural membership of minds," whose autonomy and self-steering is contingent upon the degree of *control* or the "pattern of information flow"[29] rather than the amount of power a state can wield.[30]

In an extreme form of American exceptionalism, Deutsch also equates the US model of democracy with a functional mind and takes the Soviet system as the archetype of a pathological system; the critical difference was the flow of information. For Deutsch, the ability of a system to learn and adapt towards increasingly effective survival was dependent on the flow of information. In a fabulous example of Michel Foucault's repressive hypothesis, Deutsch insists that the truth will in fact set us free.[31]

Unfortunately for Deutsch, he underestimated the warning of his best friend and inspiration, Norbert Wiener, regarding the integrity of information. Wiener argues in *The Human Use of Human Beings*—an apt name for this kind of designed politics—that the value of information is highly dependent upon its integrity, not just the quantity of information or the freedom of its flow.[32] In agreement with Deutsch, Wiener argues that the political system is first and foremost a communication network, with multiple levels of feedback that disseminate and habituate value. However, Wiener sees in the United States not a model for democracy but precisely the opposite. Wiener describes an increasing incentive for corporate and national interests to use bluff and sabotage in the information networks such that what is received and proliferated are the competitive and violently instrumental values of market ideology and state militarism.[33] The national echo chamber is a collective mind adapting, according to Wiener, but it has no transcendent liberal value or telos. Instead, the cybernetic nature of politics and control amplifies the dominant logics we now call neoliberalism.

What is significant for our story is that Deutsch and Wiener are in agreement about the stability of control as a self-organizing and self-amplifying tendency of a complex system of brains. Plasticity is present. However the difference is that Deutsch's naive faith in transparency and his romantic view of existing American values blinds him to the effect of that self-amplifying system. For Wiener what is necessary is the production of new values and techniques to overcome what closely resembles Antonio Gramsci's hegemony or Alexander Galloway and Eugene Thacker's exploit.[34] For all four of these thinkers, tendencies within systems gain dominance even if the distribution of the system is not seemingly hierarchical. Rather than hierarchy or topology generally, what makes an order dominant is precisely the ability to remake the individuals in that system through the various feedbacks of information and plasticity.[35] In Wiener's view ideology is not false consciousness, not because market ideology and state militarism are good or natural, but because there is no true consciousness. Rather, market ideology and state militarism become the native operating system of the United States. According to Wiener there is, as in an Apple computer, no command prompt for individual users in a national system. Therefore those that hack or steer the system determine its outcome. According to Wiener, "a block of human beings to increase their control over the rest of the human race . . . may attempt to control their populations by means not of machines themselves but through political techniques as narrow and indifferent to human possibility as if they had, in fact, been conceived mechanically."[36]

I am not sure Deutsch ever came to agree with Wiener. However, by the second edition of *The Nerves of Government* (1966), Deutsch expresses a deep disappointment that the techniques of cybernetics will not catch up with his hopes for the practical application of control to replace the pathology of power.[37] There is for Deutsch an inexplicable lag in the academy and the political system, a failure to wake up to the functionalism of an adaptation based on the free flow of information and learning.

It is precisely Deutsch's lag that José Delgado responds to in *Physical Control of the Mind*. Also inspired by Ashby's *Design for a Brain*, Delgado lays out a manifesto based in part on his applied research on animals and humans utilizing electrical current to alter brain activity. If it seems we are returning to the fictional world of J. J. Abrams, it is important to remember that Delgado was an MD/PhD in Yale's physiology department faculty and later founded and organized the medical school at the Autonomous University of Madrid in Spain.

The *Physical Control of the Mind* was published in Harper's World Perspectives series, whose mission statement expressed the view that "man is in the process of developing a new consciousness which . . . can eventually lift the human race above and beyond the fear, ignorance, and isolation which beset it today. It is to this nascent consciousness, to this concept of man born out of a universe perceived through a fresh vision of reality, that World Perspectives is dedicated."[38] *Pace* Malabou, it is also worth noting that the series was dedicated to the reunification of the humanities and the sciences in the pursuit of a materialist philosophical thought that could overcome "the false separation of man and nature, of time and space, of freedom and security" in the hope of escaping the "present apocalyptic period."[39] As further evidence to this strange convergence, Delgado's volume in the series was published alongside those of theologian Paul Tillich, psychoanalyst Erich Fromm, Nobel Prize–winning physicist Werner Heisenberg, and Marxist literary theorist Georg Lukacs. I rehearse all of this to make the point that what follows is not marginal or out of hand rejected by many as lunacy. Instead, Delgado was and is considered by many to be a public intellectual and scientific genius who contributed directly to the future of humankind.

Wasting no time, Delgado begins *Physical Control* with a grand and apocalyptic tone consonant with the series mission. In the opening chapter, "Natural Fate versus Human Control," Delgado lays out an argument for overt human intervention into a stalled human evolution in order to save the species from the autogenocide of nuclear war and industrial excess. To set the tableau, Delgado writes: "Manifestations of life depend on a continuous interplay of natural forces. Worms and elephants, mosquitoes and eagles, plankton and whales display a variety of activities . . . which escape human understanding, obeying sets of laws which antedate the appearance of human intelligence."[40]

Although Delgado shows reverence for the complex behavior of the natural world, the appearance of man is a break with evolution thus far. Delgado, close to contemporaries who hope to name our current geological epoch the Anthropocene, argues that humans differentiated themselves from other organisms through their "ecological liberation."[41] By this, Delgado means the use of technics, a built environment that alters not just the chances of a species' survival but of the system in which that species survives.

Like many contemporary systems biologists, Delgado insists upon the epigenetic character of humans. What "liberates" humans is the ability to learn techniques for environmental modification, whether the building of shelter or eradication of disease, and pass that information down through the ages. So an archive of distributed knowledge forms a kind of exogenetic code—hence *epigenetic* legacy—that supplants or changes the determinism of internal genetic traits.[42] Importantly for Delgado, the epigenetic heritage enables what he calls "freedom of choice." However, this freedom is not of the traditional liberal variety; what is important is not freedom at the level of the individual but the species' ability to steer its development with or against genetic possibilities. Thusly, argues Delgado, "our activities are less determined by adaptation to nature than by the ingenuity and foresight of the human mind, which recently has added another dimension to its spectrum of choices—the possibility of investigating its own physical and chemical substratum."[43]

Despite this newfound avenue for control, humanity, according to Delgado, has disproportionately focused upon the development and design of technics rather than alterations to the meat sacks of human being. The result is the accumulation of extraordinary transformative power but in exchange for a "servitude dominated by levers, engines, currency, and computers."[44] Power for Delgado, as for Deutsch, is pathological and regulated by an economy of zero-sum competition that has invested in the destructive technics of "atomic overkill" rather than in human betterment. Therefore responsibility to the species demands a new awareness that can overcome "behavior . . . composed of automatic responses to sensory inputs."[45] The goal of such an awareness would be to counteract the automatism of individual humans and fundamentally alter behavioral patterns. Unlike Deutsch and Wiener, Delgado does not think this is achievable at the level of information transparency and flow or that the creation of new values will be sufficient—although all of this is necessary. Instead, we should "re-examine the universal goals of mankind and pay more attention to the primary objective, which should not be the development of machines, but of man himself" and thus as a species consider intervening physically in the "intercerebral mechanisms."[46]

So in hopes of overcoming the crisis of power and the dead end of politics, Delgado declares the discovery of human plasticity as the next phase of epigenetic evolution.[47] The genetic—or as he reads it, neural—determinism and cultural construction have converged in the discovery and understanding of neuroscience and genetics.[48] What Delgado describes as control is not different in kind or degree from Malabou's concept of plasticity. The difference is in the center of gravity or fulcrum of formation and formability. This difference is not an empirical difference, however. Instead, the weird material and discursive similarity between the two thinkers belies a severe metaphysical difference. For Malabou it is not defensible "to advocate an absolute transparency of the neuronal in the mental."[49] Instead, what she calls "a reasonable materialism . . . would posit that the natural contradicts itself and that thought is the fruit of this contradiction."[50] The wager is that "the brain does not obey itself" because the alea is in reality.[51]

For Delgado it is precisely the opposite. The stability of the substrate of a plastic brain can be brought into harmony with thought and value. In some sense, Delgado represents the specter of Kant. Nature is a kind of mechanistic matter to be brought under the control of the faculties.[52] In the case of Delgado, those faculties can be engineered. Ultimately, though, the difference in concepts of plasticity as process is minimal and may in fact be resolved someday empirically, which could leave Malabou's speculative metaphysics inert. Leaving that aside, it is important to see how much differently Delgado's neurorevolution proceeds from Malabou's precisely because of the bifurcation point between their thinkings' respective commitment to an ordered versus aleatory nature.

Again like Malabou, Delgado sees a promise in neuroplasticity. We are called, as Malabou agrees, by the question "what do we do with our brain?" But Delgado's answer comes from extensive experimentation with brain electrodes rather than as an open-ended philosophical conundrum. Delgado claims to have developed sufficient knowledge of the brain's terrain and function to target aggression instincts that, he argues, are at the heart of human violence. Made famous by dramatic video footage, the Cordoba bull experiment demonstrated Delgado's ability to alter the mood and behavior of complex vertebrate animals.[53] In the experiment, Delgado steps, as a matador, into a bullring with a bull infamous for goring bullfighters. Delgado is armed only with a large remote control. The bull, he explains in the voiceover, has been fitted with an intracranial electrode calibrated to alter its aggression response. Another matador in the ring uses his cape to get the bull's attention; the bull charges. When Delgado engages the electrode, the bull stops

Something Darkly This Way Comes 247

charging and grows increasingly uninterested in the fluttering cape. Delgado then approaches the bull, at which time rather than charge, the bull retreats and cowers in fear.

On the basis of this experimental work Delgado proposes that the perfection of such electrodes represents the possibility of ending the threat of nuclear war and saving humanity from its current fate. Aware that many would find his methods objectionable, Delgado lays out a strong argument for preferring the freedom of the species to the freedom of any one individual. But Delgado is not a communitarian in the sense that he would argue that there are competing collective and individual values the greater good ought to trump. Provocatively, Delgado makes a different argument, one based on the instability and inauthenticity of individual identity. In some sense, Delgado presents us with an affirmative case for Malabou's destructive plasticity.

Like all good technophiles Delgado begins by making the case that altering the human brain is inevitable, as no state regulation will be able to stop the progress of "scientific advance."[54] According to Delgado, the physical control of the mind is, like a knife, neither good nor bad. In a pithy phrase, Delgado states "science should be neutral, but scientists should take sides."[55] By this he means that morality lies in how we put the inevitable technological development to use. His argument begins again to converge with Malabou's when Delgado switches from the tack of inevitability to an argument against the presupposition that there is something lost when minds are altered: "The mind is not a static, inborn entity owned by the individual and self-sufficient but the dynamic organization of sensory perceptions of the external world, correlated and reshaped through the internal and anatomical and functional structure of the brain. Personality is not an intangible and immutable way of reacting but a flexible process in continuous evolution, affected by its medium."[56]

From this, Delgado extrapolates an equivalency between a kind of constructivist position that argues for the cultural and social production of subjectivity and the intentional alteration of neurochemical processes. Similarly, as Malabou rightfully points out, this difference is indeed thin, as discriminating between culture and nature is as arbitrary as it is circular.[57] Furthermore, Malabou writes that in the concept of plasticity, "the entire identity of the individual is in play: her past, her surroundings, her encounters, her activities; in a word, the ability that our brain—that every brain—has to adapt itself, to include modifications, to receive shocks, and to create anew on the basis of this very reception."[58]

Not unlike the minimal difference in argument between Jeremy Bentham's normative account of utilitarianism and Michel Foucault's account of discipline, Delgado and Malabou share a view on the ineluctable absence of either a constitutive inside or outside to the formation of the subject. However, unlike Malabou, Delgado has not left to the imagination how such an insight should be put to use.

Delgado further extends his analogy into the accepted realm of liberal control by comparing physical interventions to the broadly accepted role of education. In a broad appeal to common sense Delgado writes, "culture and education are meant to shape patterns of reaction which are not innate in the human organism; they are meant to impose limits on freedom of choice."[59] Here Delgado aligns his proposal with earlier progressive education advocates, from Immanuel Kant to John Dewey. In an extension of his famous editorial "What is Enlightenment," Kant argues in *Education*, "Man can only become man by education. He is merely what education makes of him, for with education is involved the great secret of the perfection of human nature."[60] Like Delgado, Kant argues that education is necessary because "discipline must be brought early; for when this has not been done, [. . .] undisciplined men are apt to follow every caprice."[61] Despite the differences between Kant's transcendental idealism and Delgado's naive materialism—a difference substantially impacting the technique of intervention—the narrative of paternal development is nearly identical. Malabou's relative silence on technique places her in strange company given her deconstruction of the binary between nature and culture.

Delgado ends his section "Ethical Considerations" with the promise that electrical stimulation can never be total. Instead, electrical stimulation is in a "dynamic equilibrium" with the other forces, "a new factor in the constellation of behavioral determinants."[62] Delgado concludes then that the real threat to human freedom is not brain alteration but remaining "slaves of millenniums of biological history."[63] On the final page of *Physical Control of the Mind*, Delgado implores: "Shape your mind, train your thinking power, and direct your emotions more rationally; liberate your behavior from the ancestral burden of reptiles and monkeys—be a man and use your intelligence to orient the reactions of your mind."[64] One can hear in Delgado's manifesto resonances with those, like Ray Kurzweil and other accelerationists and posthumanists, who drive to take charge of our brains.[65] Although more humble and open-ended, Malabou also implores us to overcome ideological critique and take plasticity as a fact as well as a philosophical provocation; she warns, "so long as we do not grasp the political, economic, social, and cultural implications of the knowledge of cerebral plasticity available today, we cannot do anything with it."[66] I do not think for a moment that Malabou wants to do with our brains what Delgado has in mind. However, what is apparent in both Malabou's call to take the brain seriously and the underlying principles of Deutsch's and Delgado's thinking is that the future of neuroplasticity is politically fraught and no longer science fiction. To put it another way, the challenge of neuroplasticity is necessary but insufficient to formulate a politics or an ethics. Instead, liberal goals of human maturity (Kant) and perpetual peace (Kant again), when armed with techniques of neuroplastic intervention, animate the desire to obliterate the aleatory in favor of a designed order.

THE SOFT MACHINE: THE MUTATION OF CONTROL

> Cut word lines—Cut music lines—Smash the control images—Smash the control machine—Burn the books—Kill the priests—Kill! Kill! Kill! Inexorably as the machine had controlled thought feeling and sensory impressions of the workers, the machine now gave the order to dismantle itself and kill the priests . . .
> —William Burroughs

William Burroughs's essay "The Limits of Control," which inspired both Gilles Deleuze and the later Foucault, is written in direct response to Delgado's proposal of universal mind control.[67] Burroughs, in his signature paranoid style appropriate to the American moment in which he was writing, speculates that techniques of "mind control" have already been deployed in the United States, in particular in the assassination of Robert Kennedy. Burroughs speculates that Sirhan Sirhan was under "posthypnotic suggestion."[68] For Burroughs the brain, at least the physical intervention into the brain, is not ultimately what is threatening. It is language that is the milieu of control: "Suggestions are words. Persuasions are words. Orders are words. No control machine so far devised can operate without words, and any control machine which attempts to do so relying entirely on external force or entirely on physical control of the mind will soon encounter the limits of control."[69] According to Burroughs, control requires "opposition or acquiescence . . . if I establish complete control somehow, by implanting electrodes in the brain then my subject is little more than a tape recorder, a camera, a robot. You don't *control* a tape recorder you *use* it."[70] For Burroughs it is not possible to imagine control without a controller or, at least, the exteriority of control. His subject/object split is misleading and obfuscates a vital distinction between oppositional power, a kind of kinetic microphysics of resistance, and the frictionless character of control.

In this section, I argue that Malabou's conception of neuroplasticity pushes the horizon of control beyond Burroughs's prudish humanism and, further, that plasticity, with its obliteration of an outside to the material seat of consciousness, contributes to a more provocative understanding of control in Deleuze and Foucault.

Instead of entertaining the possibility of total or destructive control, Burroughs extends his sentimental attachment to a residual human nature—an other of control—by elevating resistance to a life principle, not in the sense of what a good life is but as a condition of living at all: "When there is no more opposition, control becomes a meaningless proposition. It is highly questionable whether a human organism could survive complete control. There would be nothing there. No person there. *Life is will!*"

Burroughs's concept of life as resistance is very close to Spinoza's *conatus*, in which a thing is characterized by trajectory, momentum, or force to perdure in its thingness, on its own terms. However, what happens when control is understood in the tune of the steering or homeostasis of cybernetics rather than in opposition? If exteriority—the forming rather than formed—is ephemeral, then what is life or *conatus* opposing? Instead, we would have to consider the possibility that *conatus* can follow control. I see this as the critical insight of destructive plasticity.

Therefore Burroughs is at odds with Delgado and in some sense Malabou, who sees in the interplay of brain and alea "neither an inside or outside world."[71] For Burroughs, control requires a controller and the time and distance to enact control on an object of control.[72] In Burroughs's lingering humanism there is somehow a remainder of the human that exceeds the brain and its ordering functions. So for Burroughs there is a kind of species-wide fail-safe. Following Malabou, exteriority, as well as the distinction between the physical and mental, does not survive the explosive concept of plasticity or its empirical demonstration. So to inject plasticity into the term "control" pushes us to hear Deleuze's Spinozist refrain of "we know not yet what a body can do" in the key of horror rather than hope. We have to consider a body with no essential limit and therefore a concept of control without a humanist horizon. This understanding of control draws on the earlier period of neuroplasticity found amongst the cyberneticists rather than the connection to Burroughs. Among the cyberneticist thinkers and inventors control is architectural or emergent; that is, imminent to a system or machine rather than imposed.[73]

However, pushing Deleuze via Malabou beyond Burroughs does not necessarily land us in the necessity of total control. Instead, it subtracts the human or human essence, as well as interiority and exteriority, from the presence or absence of control. In their study of network behavior, Galloway and Thacker persuasively make the argument that horizontal, even endogenous, network architecture is not necessarily more democratic or less controlled than more hierarchical or externally imposed structures, as has often been advanced by those who celebrate the supposed democracy of the Internet revolution.[74] I might say the same of consciousness and the brain. In fact, this is what marks the transition from disciplinary institutions to control societies. The shift from power or coercion to control: a multivalent, graduated continuum of modulations. In a society of control, interventions occur at the level of populations, whether human or neuronal. What Galloway and Thacker refer to as protocols can alter the arrangement and formation of bodies without anyone being at the wheel (in the anthropocentric sense of the term). A protocol according to Galloway is:

> . . . a set of rules that defines a technical standard. But from a formal perspective, protocol is a type of object. It is a very special kind of object. Protocol is a universal description language for objects. Protocol is a language that regulates flow, directs netspace, codes relationships, and connects life-forms. Protocol does not produce or causally effect objects, but rather is a structuring agent that appears as the result of a set of object dispositions . . . Protocol is always a second-order process; it governs the architecture of the architecture of objects. Protocol is how control exists after distribution achieves hegemony as a formal diagram. It is etiquette for autonomous agents. It is the chivalry of the object.[75]

It is important that an ahuman or inhuman etiquette or chivalry can emerge without having been designed and then become recursive. The neural Darwinist explanation for the embedding of culture in physiology and genetics demonstrates the absurdity of genetic determinism and illustrates the possibility of emergent control in a plastic brain.[76] There has been some controversy about the so-called maternal instincts as an effect in both men and women of a hormone called oxytocin. The mechanistic view that explains humans as a series of brain states is happy to discover such a hormone. However, the existence of oxytocin is insufficient to explain anything other than the existence of a process. For the process to become active in the deep human past, an ecology of inducements and constraints selected individuals with increased social attachment and receptors for hormones that promote a sense of attachment, as well as more complex brain structures for expanded social existence.

However, genes are not rules. They are incipient expressive objects influenced by material and cultural networks—ecology. According to neuroscientists, when humans are born they have some hundreds of trillions of synapses, but only those that are used, that is, activated by experiences, survive. The neurons that remain dormant start to disappear around the age of eight and diminish throughout the course of human life. The synaptic sequence that responds to oxytocin, the so-called parenting hormone, must be used before too long into human maturation, or the individual will not have been primed for the hormone.

Without the responsive synaptic structure, you could fill a person artificially with oxytocin, and it would have no effect. That is to say, there must be a biocultural relationship of care that causes the release of the hormone, fires the synapses, and feeds back into the expression of genes needed to make more oxytocin. All of which again presupposes what can be called a behavioral or cultural characteristic of care.

What emerges is a strong tendency of people to love infants. What makes this process interesting is that there is an ecological history of this hormone and the care of offspring that is not reducible to genetics, physiology, or culture but nonetheless has produced a consistent "etiquette" characterizing hominid behavior since long before *Homo sapiens*. The complex but regularized relationship between all of these agents—DNA, culture, environmental pressures, and brain plasticity—is coordinated by an etiquette or chivalry that while not a law has consistency of interaction necessary to produce a million years or so with few Medeas and Zeuses. It is a protocol; neither solely learned nor hardwired. Control can emerge, assembled as it were, on the fly, but once established, exploits exist for intervention. Hence the ability to tactically steer hormone ecologies, even weaponize them. In the case of oxytocin, the US military has deployed oxytocin in training and high-stress battle situations. As with parent and infant, the artificial levels of oxytocin promote troop bonding. However, in the space of war the artificially induced bonding is not universal; oxytocin is not love. Instead, those hormone-tightened bonds also provoke extreme hostility towards enemies seen to threaten the in-group. Oxytocin fuels militarily useful rage and violence where once it intensified care.[77]

Confronted with *modified* soldiers, the risk is that that protocol, once grafted on to the sociopolitical world, devolves into a kind of brute structuralism, a return to Delgado's dream of total control as an engineered order of the faculties. Protocols are so emergent, so immanent to the system, that resistance, even in its most descriptive sense—the microphysics of power redoubled by the friction or refraction of that power relation by the subject on which power was directed—ceases to have much application. The mobile and plastic nature of the modulation—control protocols within a network architecture—is part of a dynamic equilibrium, a range or average of control with an acceptable and even useful margin of error, that lacks the traction to push back. It is like trying to fight underwater without sand to stand on.[78] So the problem is not the totality of control but the particular organization of a control protocol. The control society, in this reading of Deleuze, optimizes rather than either repress (sovereign/juridical) or manage (specific) bodies. The control system is a difference machine with a refrain or protocol of control, not the rigid state of Burroughs's control system.[79]

The cutting edge of Malabou's destructive plasticity is consonant with this concept of control. Importantly, Malabou's reading of the brain gives control a conceptual reach distinct from concepts such as power and discipline on which Burroughs's oppositional notion of control relies. So if we take Deleuze at his word, that control societies are of a different order than disciplinary societies or carceral logics, we must take leave of Burroughs for an inhuman terra incognito waiting in the virtuality of the human brain and push it farther into the polis, the species, and the planet. Destructive metamorphosis, a plasticity not an elasticity, marks this epoch increasingly known as the Anthropocene. Malabou's distinction between elasticity and plasticity is precisely that metamorphosis is a cascade of transversal changes from which we cannot return. Significantly, at each level of mutation and formation, plasticity may confront us philosophically and practically with the paradox of a subject, even a species, that will not recognizably or self-consciously survive the crisis of philosophy it is called to answer. Destructive plasticity revolts and shudders against the dreams of sovereign steering and control. Rather, the sovereign is the alea, the emergent.[80]

CONCLUSION: AFFIRMING THE HORROR OF MATERIALISM

> This is reality, and we must accept it and adapt to it . . . The concept of individuals as self-sufficient and independent entities is based on false premises.
> —Jose Delgado, *Physical Control of the Mind*

> If those arrangements were to disappear as they appeared . . . without knowing either what its form will be or what it promises . . . then one can certainly wager that man would be erased, like a face drawn in sand at the edge of the sea.
> —Michel Foucault, *The Order of Things*

> Every species can smell its own extinction. The last ones left won't have a pretty time with it. In ten years, maybe less, the human race will just be a bedtime story for their children. A myth, nothing more.
> —"John Trent," character in John Carpenter's *In the Mouth of Madness*

What has to be navigated in the confrontation between Malabou and those that would cash in on plasticity is the tension between "the plasticity of the brain [as] the real image of the world"[81] and "a vision of the brain [as] political"[82] Well-meaning neo-Spinozists of the Deleuzian variety see in the possibility of the brain a hope and the potential for newness. On the latter we can agree without hesitation. However, what Malabou shows us is that the collapse of nature and culture is a beginning, not a sufficient ending. To push this point farther, I am attempting to think the horror of those that would put neuropolitics to use in the existing political order and therefore taking newness to be as capable of destruction as of hope. The fragility of things requires that we take the possibility of destruction seriously.[83] In particular, both Deutsch and Delgado are within the mainstream of liberal thinking and therefore ought not to be seen as outliers in the world of possible tactics of neuropolitics. After all, each focuses on procedural democracy as improved by accountability and the improvement of the populace through the diffusion of norms of open communication and order over conflict and violence.

Importantly, I see in Delgado and Deutsch an easy conquest for what Fred Moten and Stefano Harney call *government prospectors*.[84] Governmentality in search of innovation may in fact find neuropolitical proposals quite reasonable. Certainly the US military already pursues Delgado's agenda albeit in reverse. Soldiers' brains and bodies are continuously altered for performance, including but not limited to the manipulation of memory intensity, sleep needs, depression, and guilt; oxytocin is used to create stronger bonds between troops and a more violent territorial character.[85] These interventions are something quite distinct from the "ideology" of neuroplasticity, of which Malabou makes short shrift.

Techniques of control based on plasticity at the neural, polis, and species level are not discourses that make use of metaphors of networks, of self-organizing and self-healing systems. These techniques are real practices to be put to use in the engineering of an order.[86] Therefore, the *pharmakon* of neural plasticity is not exhausted by the opposition between Malabou's gesture towards a Foucauldian care of the self and a discourse of cognitive capitalism. Instead, the danger is the competitive struggle between attempts to reinvent and innovate the self in the face of the sedimentation of control practices gaining an increasingly global scope. As seen in the work of Edward Bernays, stretching back to the beginning of the twentieth century, the fight to steer the polis of brains is not new. It is merely the case that "manufacturing consent" has escalated from the cottage industry of early advertising firms to full-scale industrialized design.

This is why it is necessary to read plasticity in the context of control. Control here is not a synonym for power or oppression; it is the name we give to an emergent and surviving order often indifferent to those it controls. This is why Malabou insists on "the possibility of destructive plasticity, which refuses the promise, belief, symbolic constitution of all resource to come[.] It is not true that the structure of the promise is undeconstructable. The philosophy to come must explore the space of this collapse of messianic structures."[87] Beyond what is to come, what preceded an order is not always apparent either; *it is possible to lose things*. In this sense, the horror of plasticity and control is not the confrontation with the ineffable but the ineffability of what once was and can never be again. The fragility of things is real; freedom as we currently cultivate it can be broken.[88]

For Burroughs, the limits of control rely on a separation of form and humanity—as if "form could be left hanging like a garment on the chair of being or essence."[89] To move beyond Burroughs toward the bleeding edge of Malabou's and Deleuze's thinking is to accept, even affirm, the virtuality of control; a freedom no longer diminished or infringed upon or even lost but a freedom that never was, the victim of an "annihilating metamorphosis."[90] Such a vestigial appendage of freedom, if it persists at all, may itch from time to time or gnaw at an atrophied consciousness, but it will be relieved by the proverbial butt scratch. This is what Malabou calls "a power of change without redemption," but she also adds a "power without teleology" and "without meaning." What has to be considered when plasticity—formative and destructive—enters into the orbit of control is the possibility of a change with the telos of meaning of an other that cannot be indexed as change by the body or polis changed.

This is the horror of the lobotomy, political plasticity, and the subjective catastrophes of strokes and Alzheimer's disease; it is not the screams of the damned but the blank stare and a mouth hanging open. Horror is the body that need not know that it should scream. The plasticity of control and the accident possess the capability of "forgetting the loss of symbolic reference points."[91] In our current predicament, can we not already observe the body that cannot help but shop; the body of irresistible consent, thoughtless bland calculations; bodies consuming pink slime or worse yet consuming metabolized and sterilized politics lacking almost entirely any relation to the political? Contra Burroughs, there are worse things than death. There is surviving manufactured control. Can we not imagine what Eugene Thacker calls a blasphemous life, a "life that is living but that should not be living" rather than the dignity kill-switch imagined by Burroughs?[92] In this image of the end without ending, "life is weaponized against life itself."[93] In a world without an essential self, without a soul, we are left to ponder that kind of ending.

This is why destructive plasticity is better understood through horror than tragedy. Lesions, decay, dementia, shock therapy, brain manipulation: all demonstrate life's indifference to a particular form of life, not the mourning and melancholia of tragic loss. Tragedy is more about attachment than loss. Horror is the confrontation with a world that does not care or even know what is lost. In Malabou's words the accident or the aleatory compels us to "think a mutation that engages both a form and being, a new form that is literally a form of being."[94] This form of being, in so far as it is one, is characterized by both fragility and perdurance. Such a thought leaves us with little grounding. It is mere life, a life without qualities; what Deleuze calls a life.⁹⁵ This is not reason to flee into the fantasy of a soul or the moralization of intentionalists. The horror of matter is real and cannot be assuaged by persistent argument to the contrary. We live in a world in which decay and catastrophe, not the human subject, are sovereign. That there is no transcendental index for the self that loses its self is without alternative. There is no ideology to attack; it merely is. That so many find this predicament unacceptable changes nothing.

Can we affirm such an inhuman position, or is this all fruitless and cynical nihilism? The affirmation is vital. To confront the unhumanity of the world demonstrates exactly what is at stake in fragility. The brain, the polis, freedom, the world, the earth, are breakable even explosive rather than necessary. It is from the impossible position of extinction or oblivion that providence is eviscerated in favor of the freedom of the aleatory. E. M. Cioran's account of decay is resonant here. Cioran writes, "we cannot elude existence by explanations. We can only endure it, love or hate it, adore or dread it, in that alternation of happiness and horror which expresses the very rhythm of being, its oscillations, its dissonance."⁹⁶ This is the task and the freedom of philosophy at this moment. The violence of destructive plasticity is the true limit of control. Reality, according to Malabou, always contains "a vital hitch, a threatening detour . . . one that is unexpected, unpredictable, dark."⁹⁷ However the radical possibility of otherwise comes at an astronomical cost. This is the lesson of both formative and destructive plasticity at every scale. The thing that changes itself dwells at the precipice of nonbeing.

NOTES

1. Malabou, *What Should We Do*, 58.
2. Kant, *Anthropology*.
3. Kant, *Anthropology*, 5.
4. The account of maturity here bears little resemblance to Kant's description of maturity in *Was Ist Aufklärung?*
5. Kant, *Anthropology*, 15.
6. Kant, *Anthropology*, 34–35.
7. Malabou, *Future of Hegel*.
8. Leys, "Turn to Affect," 434–72. See Rose and Abi-Rached, *Neuro*.

9. For an in-depth discussion of Habermas's resistance to neuropolitics, see Grove, "Must We Persist?"

10. Žižek, "Philips Mental Jacket."

11. Bogost, *Alien Phenomenology*, 48.

12. It is worth considering that the pill popping was the result of the migraine as alea.

13. Habermas, *Future of Human Nature*, 25.

14. Deleuze, "Postscript."

15. Deleuze, "Postscript."

16. Coming to the conclusion of the bankruptcy of ethical theories that attack us with ought was helped a great deal by a conversation with Levi Bryant on his blog *Larval Subjects*. Bryant is always a generous and helpful inspiration and sounding board for ideas. See "Ethics and Politics: What Are You Asking?," *Larval Subjects*, accessed November 6, 2013, http://larvalsubjects.wordpress.com/2012/05/29/ethics-and-politics-what-are-you-asking/.

17. Pickering, *Cybernetic Brain*, 8.

18. For an explanation of the importance of the black box approach to cybernetic experimentation, see Ashby, *Introduction to Cybernetics*, 86–88. For a very provocative critique of black box thinking, see Galloway, "Black Box."

19. For an excellent history and analysis of the formative role of cybernetics in the development of contemporary cognitive science and neuroscience, see Dupuy, *Cognitive Science*.

20. Wiener, *Human Use*, 27.

21. Ashby, *Design for a Brain*, 1.

22. There has been a resurgence in the interest in cybernetics as it becomes more and more evident that thinkers and scientists from Stuart Kaufman to Gilles Deleuze were informed by cybernetics. The significance of cybernetics for the increasing sophistication of artificial intelligence also contributes to this fascination. See Clarke and Hansen. *Emergence and Embodiment*; Pickering, *Cybernetic Brain*.

23. For a history of Stafford Beer's role in Allende's almost cybernetic revolution in Chile, see Medina, *Cybernetic Revolutionaries*.

24. Deutsch, *Nerves of Government*, xiii.

25. Deutsch, *Nerves of Government*, viii.

26. Deutsch, *Nerves of Government*, xiii.

27. Deutsch, *Nerves of Government*, 129.

28. Deutsch, *Nerves of Government*, 134.

29. Deutsch, *Nerves of Government*, 137.

30. Deutsch, *Nerves of Government*, 129.

31. Foucault, *Power/Knowledge*.

32. Wiener, *Human Use*, 131.

33. Wiener, *Human Use*, 161–62.

34. Galloway and Thacker, *Exploit*, 6–7.

35. Gilbert Simondon, the French engineer who was the inspiration for Gilles Deleuze and Félix Guattari, similarly described this process, naming the individuals "logics of individuation." Simondon is trying to capture the formation of something like an individual but through the complex process of identity/difference produced in the systemic orders in which such an event takes place. Simondon, Gilbert. *La individuación*.

36. Wiener, *Human Use*, 181.

37. Deutsch, *Nerves of Government*, ix–x.

38. Delgado, *Physical Control*, 281.

39. Delgado, *Physical Control*, 287.

40. Delgado, *Physical Control*, 3.

41. Delgado, *Physical Control*, 4.

42. Delgado, *Physical Control*, 6.

43. Delgado, *Physical Control*, 7–8.

44. Delgado, *Physical Control*, 8.

45. Delgado, *Physical Control*, 9.

46. Delgado, *Physical Control*, 11.

47. Delgado's vision is creepy but maybe not as insidious as so-called benign imperialists that defend the colonial project as a precondition for global peace. At least in Delgado's case there is wholly absent from the text and argument the racial geographies of superiority and inferiority that underwrite many liberal visions of cosmopolitanism. See Harvey, *Cosmopolitanism*.

48. As fellow travelers in the hope for species control, it is important to note the connection between James Watson and Francis Crick and cybernetics. When Watson and Crick announced their research agenda to discover the language of heredity, they said they hoped to do for genetics what Norbert Wiener had done for cybernetics: to understand the information or code that constituted life, or in their words, show the presence "of cybernetics on the bacterial level." It is then not surprising that in his later life James Watson has embarrassed himself as an advocate of racial eugenics. The search for the genetic code was animated by the desire to steer it. See Conway and Siegelman, *Dark Hero*, 278, and Milmo, "Fury."

49. Malabou, *What Should We Do*, 82.

50. Malabou, *What Should We Do*, 82.

51. Malabou, *What Should We Do*, 79.

52. Simondon instructively distinguishes mechanical versus machinic objects on the basis of the capacity of an object to adapt or ignore its environment. This helps overcome the presumption that all reductions to process are reductionist. Rather, machinic objects have the capacity for creativity and emergent properties despite being made up of parts. Simondon, *Du mode d'existence*.

53. For video footage of the demonstration, see www.youtube.com/watch?v=RLvlZl4WLQQ.

54. Delgado, *Physical Control*, 214. So far Delgado is certainly right. Further the research has been driven primarily by defense-related funding sources. The US military in particular has led the way in brain research with application for brain-machine interfaces and brain-behavior modification. As demonstrated by the exhaustive research of medical ethicist Jonathan Moreno, very little attention has been given to the military-brain nexus by the public or the civilian scientist whose research depends on military financing. See Moreno, *Mind Wars*.

55. Moreno, *Mind Wars*.

56. Delgado, *Physical Control*, 215.

57. Bennett and Connolly. "Contesting Nature/Culture."

58. Malabou, *What Should We Do*, 7.

59. Delgado, *Physical Control*, 215.

60. Kant, *On Education*, 6–7.

61. Kant, *On Education*, 4.

62. Delgado, *Physical Control*, 215.

63. Delgado, *Physical Control*, 233.

64. Delgado, *Physical Control*, 244.

65. Kurzweil, *Singularity Is Near*.

66. Malabou, *What Should We Do*, 82.

67. Burroughs, *Limits of Control*, 38. Deleuze and Guattari took a long road trip across the United States in the summer of 1975. During that trip, in addition to seeing the Grateful Dead, Deleuze and Guattari met with William Burroughs. The meeting, as well as Burroughs's literature more generally, is reflected throughout their collaborative writing. See Demers, "American Excursion."

68. Demers, "American Excursion."

69. Demers, "American Excursion."

70. Burroughs, *Limits of Control*, 39.

71. Malabou, *Ontology of the Accident*, 14.

72. Burroughs, *Limits of Control*, 40.

73. Connolly, *Neuropolitics*, 56–57.

74. Galloway and Thacker, *Exploit*, 6.

75. Galloway, *Protocol*, 74–75.

76. The explanation of neural Darwinism that follows is taken from Daniel Lord Smail's provocative challenge to Stephen Jay Gould's neo-Lamarckian theory of cultural evolution. Smail's attempt is to prevent the "backdoor" Cartesian dualism that often occurs when culture is privileged as something opposed to genetics on the basis that the dissolution of this opposition would result in genetic determinism. See Smail, *Deep History*, 112–15.

77. Wade, "Dark Side." 2011.

78. Kwinter, "Notes," 100–101.

79. Burroughs, *Limits of Control*, 38.

80. Connolly calls this the "wild" element that traverses the multiply layered and intercalated systems of the universe. This wild element is the limit to order or that which cannot be ordered, leaving open the possibility of creativity and the new. See Connolly, *Neuropolitics*, 95.

81. Malabou, *Ontology of the Accident*, 39.

82. Malabou, *Ontology of the Accident*, 52.

83. William Connolly's account in *Neuropolitics* of his father's brain damage shows how we are beholden to our brains for thought. At any moment the contingency of thought, memory, recognitions, and connections, which we desperately wish could transcend the matter of life, can all unravel. The very real confrontation with the limits of organic life makes neuropolitics more than a trend or a new discourse of the human. Instead, neuropolitics is what we all must face in medias res; see Connolly, *Neuropolitics*, preface. On the concept of fragility as the modern predicament, see "First Interlude: Melancholia," in Connolly, *Fragility of Things*.

84. Moten and Harney, "Blackness and Governance," 357.

85. Moreno, *Mind Wars*.

86. Orders go awry in both senses of the word: the command and the underlying organization in which orders take place. Despite the rigor and conditioning of boot camp and the bodily discipline of years of military service, steering soldiers between the purposeful devastation of Fallujah in 2004 and the killing spree of US Army Staff Sergeant Robert Bales in southern Afghanistan is unpredictable at best, despite increasingly sophisticated behavioral and neuroinvasive technics for control. With both Fallujah and Bales, one cannot but wonder how the bodies involved had been altered by go pills for night patrols, oxytocin for morale, antidepressants to fight battle stress, and so on. Furthermore, invasive intracranial intervention into soldiers' brains is no longer speculative. DARPA has begun experiments with mood regulating brain implants to treat veterans suffering from PTSD. The program, armed with a 12 million dollar budget, hopes to have an approved 'cybernetic implant' within five years. If DARPA continues to make progress they will receive an additional 20 million dollars. http://www.defenseone.com/technology/2014/05/D1-Tucker-military-building-brain-chips-treat-ptsd/85360/.

87. Malabou, *Ontology of the Accident*, 88.

88. For an exploration of the relationship between cultivation and the arts of the self required for what I mean by freedom, see Connolly, *Neuropolitics*, 106–8.

89. Malabou, *Ontology of the Accident*, 17.

90. Malabou, *Ontology of the Accident*, 30.

91. Malabou, *Ontology of the Accident*, 18.

92. Thacker, *In the Dust*, 104.
93. Thacker, *In the Dust*, 104.
94. Malabou, *Ontology of the Accident*, 17.
95. Deleuze, *Pure Immanence*.
96. Cioran, *Short History*, 47.
97. Malabou, *Ontology of the Accident*, 7.

CHAPTER **12**

The Touring Machine (Flesh Thought Inside Out)

Fred Moten

1

In a recent review of evolutionary psychologist Robert Kurzban's book *Why Everyone (Else) Is a Hypocrite: Evolution and the Modular Mind*, philosopher and linguist Jerry Fodor takes sharp exception to Kurzban's assertion that our brains, insofar as they are nothing more than a bundle of heuristics capable of performing discrete sets of computational operations, neither imply nor require the organizing principle/principal that we ordinarily call a self. According to Fodor, Kurzban sees no reason for the science of psychology to acknowledge selves. "Well," Fodor retorts, "Here's one in a nutshell: selves are the agents of inference and of behavior; you need executives to account for the rationality of our inferences; you need the rationality of our inferences to account for the coherence of our behavior; and you need the coherence of our behavior to explain the successes of our actions."[1] When Fodor asserts the necessity of the executive, a relation between the knowledge and the care of the self is implied, though what Michel Foucault claims to be the priority of care to knowledge is inverted. In the intensity of his normative philosophical self-regard, Fodor's executive is at least proximate to the one that Foucault, in a brief reading of Seneca's *De Ira*, calls the administrator. For Foucault, however, that nearness also encompasses an unbridgeable distance since knowledge prepares the way for renunciation, which, in the end, cannot abide with care. But insofar as Fodor's critique of Kurzban seems to leave renunciation by the wayside, to consider the representative generality that emerges when Fodor's self, which seeks to "explain the success of [his] actions," and Foucault's self, which prepares "for a certain complete achievement of life," are posed together seems nothing less than an imperative.² At stake in such a pose, in the assumption of the possibility of position, is not only how but also that one looks at oneself, how and that one gives an account of oneself in the end, as an end in a discourse of ends above means. In the meantime, in a temporality of means that might not even be discernible as a moment's absence, the mode of renunciation that derives from philosophical self-absorption is endlessly refused in an ongoing flash of exhaustion and consent. Our flesh of flames burns bright in its submergence. Its (neo-)plastic burr still folds. *I want to study the poetic registration of this immeasurable preface to the world.*

In sketching an outline of the "technologies of the self, which permit individuals to effect by their own means or with the help of others a certain number of operations on their own bodies and souls, thoughts, conduct, and way of being, so as to transform themselves in order to attain a certain state of happiness, purity, wisdom, perfection or immortality," Foucault presumes a clear difference between them and those "technologies of production, which permit us to produce, transform or manipulate things." This is to say that while these technologies "hardly ever function separately," they do operate against the backdrop of a sharp distinction between things and selves, which move within two different technological hemispheres—the technological manipulation of things and signs, which "are used in the study of science and linguistics," and the "technologies of domination and the self," which Foucault concerned himself with in the development of his "history of the organization of knowledge," his historiography of the present.³

Black studies, which does or should consider what Nahum Chandler calls "the problem of the negro as a problem for thought" within and by way of imperatives that are beyond category, is constrained to investigate the integration of these hemispheres and is particularly responsible for forging an understanding regarding the relationship between (the manipulation of) things and (the care of) selves.⁴ This is to say that insofar as the ungovernability of things and signs within and outside or underneath the field that is delineated and enclosed by the manipulative efforts of selves caught up in the exertions of governmentality is or should be our constant study, we have to comport ourselves in and toward the juncture of technological breakthrough and technological breakdown. Black study moves at the horizon of an event where certain instruments, insofar as they can no longer either calculate or be calculated, are bent towards the incalculable. That juncture, that event, doesn't just imply and assume and consider movement; it is itself on the move as a kind of fugitive coalescence of and against more than agential force, more than agential voluntary, as a kind of choir, a kind of *commercium*, whose general refrain—like a buzz or hum underneath self-concern's melodic line—is that it's not your thing, you can't just do what you want to do. Such clamor might best be understood, in its constant improvisational assault on the understanding that was sent to regulate it, as antiadministrative, ante-executive action.

Fodor believes that evolutionary psychologists, like Kurzban, have taken the notion of the modularity of mind—an idea, derived in part from the Chomskyan idea of innate and specific mental device, that states that such a device is evolutionarily developed to have a specific function—too far. Though Fodor is a major contributor to that notion, he believes that too much liberty is taken with and derived from cognitive impenetrability, the condition in which mental mechanisms are understood to be not only distinct but also independent, "encapsulated from beliefs and from one another."[5] And so he takes Kurzban severely to task for attempting to show that such encapsulation predicts, as it were, the absence of the executive. For Kurzban, the fact that we can believe two contradictory beliefs is explained by the fact that the brain contains distinct, discrete modules—bundles of software, as it were—that are devoted to separate operations. It's not the mind or the self that believes contradictory things; it's just two different packages within the brain that do. Contradictory views correspond to different functions, different uses to which the brain is put that correspond, in turn, to different packages of mental processes. As Kurzban puts it,

> this functional approach includes the idea that in the same way computer software that is very flexible consists of a very large number of subroutines, the human mind has a large number of subroutines—modules—designed for particular purposes.
>
> An important consequence of this view is that it makes us think about the "self" in a way that is very different from how people usually understand it. In particular, it makes the very motion of a "self" something of a problem, and perhaps quite a bit less useful than one might think.[6]

Fodor's concern and his critique are derived from his sense that Kurzban's psychological Darwinism—"the theory that some/many/all of the traits that constitute our 'psychological phenotype' are adaptations to problems posed by the environments in which the mind evolved"—can explain negation (the relation or copresence of P and not-P) but not addition (the relation of P and Q).[7] He argues that Kurzban can explain how there can be negation without an executive but not how there can be interpenetrability (interarticulation, interinanimation) without an executive.

> . . . [It is] Kurzban's thesis that we can do without anybody who's in charge. Something has to ensure that, in many, many cases, if you believe P and you believe Q, you also believe P&Q. In traditional intellectualist models, this is part of what executives do. The executive is an inference-making organ; it is structured so that when it finds P is on the list of your beliefs, and Q is on the list of your beliefs, it adds P&Q to the list of your beliefs. Very roughly, it allows for the construction of relatively complex mental states from relatively simple mental states; so it can (maybe) explain how it is possible for a creature with a finite head to have indefinitely many beliefs. On this sort of view, it is not an accident that the belief P is a constituent of the belief P&Q; and it is not an accident that the sentence "John prefers coffee" is a constituent of the sentence "John prefers coffee in the morning." If you have an executive, you can (maybe) make sense of all that. If not, then—so far as anyone knows—you can't. Intellectualism suggests the possibility of a unified treatment of logic, language and thought.[8]

What I've been wondering, by way of the specificity of Fodor's critique of Kurzban but against the grain of what Fodor understands to constitute the ground of that critique and from the perspective of someone who is also interested in certain operations that have been done on bodies and soul, as well as on *Body and Soul*, is whether the self is better understood as something akin to what David Kazanjian calls a "flashpoint" marking a socially generated rebellion against the executive that is manifest in the form of the soloist who can now be thought as sociality's nonfull, nonsimple, anarchic, anarchaic, old-new avatar?[9] The executive function is an exclusionary, regulative function: it says that the issue at hand is about the difference between the negation of P (here called the not-P) and Q. But what is excluded here is a (de)generative, expansive, invaginative, and imaginative totality—given in the undercommon intellectual works and lives of the ones who are constrained to mind their Ps and Qs—that is, neither the negation of P nor Q. More precisely, what is missing is a vast range of extrarational relations for which we cannot, strictly speaking, account; relations, which is to say things, that cannot be accounted for because they cut and augment inference; things like whatever occurs when believing P and believing Q is more or less and/or more and less than P and Q. (In general, the general is more and less, given in new sentences that some might see as unworthy constituents for which we cannot account but which others might see more clearly as instantiations of the invaluable. Worked minds work wonders with 6.2 words, making do with less and more.)[10] At the same time, radical disbelief in cognitive penetrability both within what we refer to as the individual mind and between individual minds does, as Fodor suggests, imply a strict and limiting regulation of mental processes, which is to say of the relation between mind and world, mind and things in the world. While psychological Darwinists might be able to account for contradiction, they cannot account for generative interarticulation, which Fodor speaks of under the rubrics of inference and behavior and Foucault (like Arendt) speaks of under the rubrics of thinking and acting, things which things are said not to be able to do but always in relation to social history insofar as "the way people really think [and act] is not adequately analyzed by the universal categories of logic."[11]

Consider, for instance, by way of Foucault, how the valences of constituency entail both the belief, or the sentence, that is "simpler," more fundamental, and the power to constitute the consent to be governed and represented by a derivative of supposedly greater complexity. This double edge of constituency—a kind of anoriginal potential that is often constrained to submit to what it generates, to what represents or gives accounts (of it), where giving an account is a taking stock of oneself that is inseparable from a taking stock of one's things—returns us to Foucault's concern with self-concern. The constituent is subject to the derivative, the calculation, which is held in and as credit in a kind of freedom from mutuality. The elemental, in its irreducible supplementarity, is given over to a kind of fixed contingency that is called the executive, which, when it is supposed to give an account of what is essential in and as generativity instead gives an account of itself, an account of the self understood as a kind of interplay of slavery and freedom and not as an effect of the generative force of anoriginal fugitivity, an accounting in which that self is misunderstood to be originary.

When the self is understood to be originary, interpenetrability is both warped and lost—warped when the always already given internal difference of "simple" cognitive states or processes is forgotten in a discourse of penetrability that is held in the very idea of the individual mind; lost when interpenetrability between minds is submitted to the notion of the individual mind's originarity rather than its derivation from the social constituency.

There is something like, but both a little bit and a whole lot more than, what Alan Turing described/imagined: an infinite memory capacity with an infinite amount of time whose computational force allows us to chart the limits of what can be computed. This other thing goes over the edge of that limit. It is as if it has been thrown over the side of the vessel, the state-sanctioned ship or self that navigates that limit. The self's or the subject's transcendence has usually been associated with what it is to stand on the edge of the abyss to which it is and has been committed. Transcendence matters to the one who stands there only if it is given in her immanence, her thingliness, her fallenness, her movement in and with submarine sound, in and as the Atlantic underbridge.

Consider that the transition from a philosophy or a natural history to a biology of race accompanies and informs the pseudoscientific emergence of what we now recognize as the science of the brain and that the Kantian revolution in moral, aesthetic, and political theory and the theory of mind are fatefully and fatally coupled with and enabled by the invention of the philosophical concept of race that submits difference to a sovereign power that will have been both refined (in the recovery of a single originary purpose, a monogenetic impetus) and dispersed (wherein that purpose is, as it were, replicated and reproduced as human mental endowment). Do so while keeping in mind that the revolution in theories and techniques of computation (especially the computation of risk and maritime positioning that helped significantly to fuel the transition from mercantilism to [the interplay of the dispersion of sovereignty and the refinement of private accumulation and the conceptualization and regulative exclusion of externalities that we call] capitalism) that began to emerge in the mid-nineteenth century with the work of Charles Babbage and that took more immediately practical and efficient shape in the mid-twentieth century by way of the contributions of Alan Turing, Norbert Wiener, and others coincide roughly with the inception and return of Afro-diasporic revolutionary social movement and the new modes of consciousness (and their globalized dispersal) such movement reflected and helped to shape. The desire to study the black insurgency whose traces remain in and as the dissemination of phonic substance in literature and music is now inseparable from attending to the history of the interplay of calculation, displacement, and abolition. This conjuncture manifests itself in frenzied, troubled, muffled speech over the edge of whatever is supposed to divide sacrament from profanation. Foucault, by way of Philo of Alexandria, recalls "an austere community, devoted to reading, to healing meditation, to individual and collective prayer and to meeting for a spiritual banquet (agape, 'feast')." These common practices, he argues, "stemmed from concern for oneself." Foucault then shows how the movement from self-care to self-knowledge is finally and fully instantiated in techniques of verbalization that are first deployed in the service of ascetic self-renunciation and then, with the advent of the human sciences, are given over to a mode of self-representation that is the necessary accompaniment to what Angela Mitropoulos calls "the proliferation and democratization of sovereignty."[12] The undercommon articulation I want to study, the symposium I want to join, marks the material disbursal of the knowledge and care of flesh, in the flesh, not in the self's or the king's divided body, in and against the terror and privation that attend the long career of self-concern's self-displacement. When drowned speech becomes fire music, embalming burned flesh with a runaway sermon's fragrant sound, an alternative is announced.

2

By way of the din of generative multiplicity, which sounds like a quartet's rhizomatic excess of itself, or like what kids' anarchic sounding does to speech, or like the evolutionary step of loved, invaluable flesh's instantiating interplay of artifice and intelligence, its blessedness inseparable from its woundedness, both new, interinanimate in beatitude, in poverty's radical theoretical attitude: M. NourbeSe Philip's Zong! *(and more generally the black history that is the sea, as Derek Walcott didn't quite say), documents of descent and dissent, experiments in ascension and consent, as an emergence anticipatorily after the fact of the ongoing imposition of a submarine state of emergency that the dispersed sovereign (the executive whose sentences are constrained to administer the brutalities of broken felicity, fractured enjoyment), having commenced merchant, is serially enjoined to declare. What they know of their injury is given in what they know of their blessing.*

There's an unruly interplay of silence and chatter that Ian Baucom's massively illuminating book, assemblage and idiosyncretic archive, Spectres of the Atlantic, replays. There, the Zong's exhausted, inspiriting cargo—132 or 143 persons (documentation of the number always changes as if marking an insistent incalculability) thrown into the sea whose trace was buried in the hold of the official language and documents of the governmental and financial entities that authored their disappearance—enacts its emergence and meta-emergence again. Thinking, but also living, between silence and chatter persists on other registers, in all languages: not only the silencing of things, the silence of an unheard case, of a muffled appeal consigned to lower frequencies, of disruptive wave and terminally colliding particle where no one can observe; and not only that other effect that constantly nascent and dying capitalism and colonialism produces, the ceaseless chatter of administration, regulation and what Baucom calls "phenomenal busy-ness": but also the silence and chatter of song, which thinkers have been known to misrecognize as an unbearable lightness; but also the hard, sweet life of language on "the spectrum," where I am an initiate under the protection of my son. He moves between silence and chatter, where the set pieces that adults usually reserve for the forced participation of kids break down in the face of a constant contact improvisation that you have to be ready for, as Al Green or Danielle Goldman would say. The brilliant surprise of the silly abcs (ba, dc, fe, h . . . sung to the rhythm and melody of the old tune) or the belated christening of a dinosaur (the protocerealbox, his bones discovered in illicit breakfast reading) must be heard to be believed. But those impositions (How old are you? Are you ready for Santa Claus? Are you strong? Show me your muscles! Do you like school?) aren't the only scripts, all of which aren't so easily done without. Every returned I love you is treasure when every incalculable gift was occasioned by an unimaginable loss and when the gift is often harder to accept, or would be, if it weren't for what you had already been given by poems, which Charles Bernstein, thinking about Robin Blaser, calls "the flowers of associational thinking." Lorenzo gives me a fresh bouquet every day as I learn to stop mourning for something I never had.

One of the hard parts of caring for a child with an "Autism Spectrum Disorder" is the problem of where they should go to school. And if you're picky about school to the point of not believing in it even though you love it so much you never want to leave it, if you're so committed to the conservation of the strange and beautiful that your mistrust of the normal is redoubled to a level of intensity that can actually keep up with your desire for your child to have a normal life, then the general necessity of the alternative (school), which may have been a principle you've been trying to live by, now becomes concrete and absolute. It requires you to go back to first grade, at least every Tuesday morning, in order to play and get dirty and paint and make birdbaths and talk about princesses. Lorenzo and I facilitate communication with the other kids for one another out in the woods, where all those flowers grow. On Tuesday afternoon I go to school with the big kids, whose interest in those flowers often goes against the grain of their schooling, where critical and creative attendance upon both silence and chatter is frowned upon in the interest of a whole other kind of preparation. In the afternoon we try to read Zong! This means we get together to decide how to get together to decide how to read it. A collective enterprise is implied here—I don't think anybody can do it by themselves. Philip's memorial bouquet—faded, fading, murmured, submerged, displaced, misspaced, overlaid, is an effect of a range of superimposition exposed as beauty, the amplification of an associational field that evokes the mutual aid that it also requires.

At circle time on Thursday, Lorenzo declared that when he makes smores for Julian (which I wasn't aware that he'd ever done, because I think he's never done it) he makes them with bricks, sticks and snow. He has become an anoriginal king of comedy. When everybody stopped laughing all the other jokes started flying around. Have you ever seen a Bethany eat another Bethany? Have you ever seen a Christopher eat a dishtopher? The circle broke up into a whole bunch of fiery, delectable shapes driven further out by chocolate milk. Orchard Hill School became the river of rivers in North Carolina (centrifugal curriculum, vigor, local abstraction). Then it was time for me to go to real school and time for them to go to the sleds. I wish my class were at the surreal school. That's what I'm trying for. But I have been lecturing my ass off, driven by the Holy Ghost that Philip is giving away. The only way I'm gonna be able to shut up is to go to Chicago. But I hadn't gone yet last week so my poor students had to bear with me, sitting around the table, while I repeated myself again, hoping that it was in a different way and hoping that the difference mattered. Then I said, in desperation, that the thing about this class is that I just want to be in a band, preferably this band, pointing to the speakers, listening to that first modification of the one/s that cause/s Baraka to use atom bomb and switchblade in the same phrase, Miles and them in '60, in Stockholm, with Wynton instead of Red, Jimmy instead of Philly Joe. There's a sped-up deepening of "All Blues" that was only gonna get faster and more lowdown over the next handful of years as the universal machines kept blowing things up. From there we went back to "The Buzzard Song," a Gil Evans installation, arranged horns chasing measure into the room with the moving walls. Abram said, "Well, he's just so cool that he can play his way out of any situation."

In a long set of unmade circles, the conditions and effects of miscommunication are brutal and glorious. They keep going till you stop—to revel in something that breaks you up; to rebel in dread of reverse and whatever brings it because if there were nothing it would be impossible and easier. I'm trying to talk about zones of miscommunication + areas of disaster + their affective ground and atmosphere and terrible beauty. They're the same but really close to one another but unbridgeably far from one another, connected by some inside stories we keep running from, the way people flee a broken park when the island is a shipwreck. The crumbled refuge is a hold and a language lab. Half the school falls away from the other half that escapes. Help in the form of a madman's persistent gunship. The settler's exceptional and invasive mobile fortress. Aggressive, hovering neglect of the instructor. He says the constant variety of distraction makes collaborating impossible and the other story's been buried again, concrete taken for water. The serially disrupted plan should have been disrupted but the disruption is serial—the same, enlarged catastrophe whose sociomusical, sociopoetic anticipation will peek through every once in a while, as suppressed reports of suppression. Somebody has to imagine that, and how we keep dying for the shit we live for. The slave trade's death toll takes another shock today and still we cannot quite engage, always a little turned away and elsewhere, a little alone. At 1:15 we have to see if we want to figure out a way to work through this, which is to say in this. To move in, which is to say through, the obscenity of poetry, of what it is to think about one little boy but removed, upstairs, in the luxurious monastery. The question of how we can read this poem is redoubled now. Now, how can we read this poem? This, too, is what Zong! is about, having claimed the catastrophe. And also: how can we turn the whole world into rubble for what was already held in the catastrophe.

Poetry is rhythm breaking something to say that broke rhythm, an afterlife installation where knowledge takes the form of pauses, a soundscape made of risen questions, a machine made out of what happened when we were together in the open in secret. It miscommunicates catastrophe with unseemly festivity, in an obscenity of objection; it knows not seems, it doesn't know like that, its Julianic showings go past meaning, in social encryption, presuming the form of life whose submergence it represents. But it doesn't represent. It more and less than represents. There's a rough, unsutured transaction that moves against repair to make a scar. The new thing is a scar. It's hard to look at something when you can't look away. In Scenes of Subjection, *Saidiya Hartman says re-dress is "a re-membering of the social body that occurs through the recognition and articulation of devastation, captivity and enslavement . . ." I don't know if redress is obscene; I just know that it's cognate with administration. The social life of poetry strains against a grammar that seeks to defy both decay and generativity in the name of a self-possessed equivalence that, in any case, you know you can't have because you know you can't have a case. Some folks strive for that impossibility, rather than claim the exhaustion they are and have, as if this were either the only world or the real one. Encrypted celebration of the ongoing encryption is an analytic of the surreal world in this one. It's not about cultural identity and it's not about origin; it's the disruptive innovation of one and the voluntary evasion of the other.*

> communism is how you get nasty with enjoyment. good morning is the new catastrophe of our boulevard. so you gave up what you never had and now you're a collection agency. you need a lawyer. at a loss, I say, good morning. he says, good morning. how are you? good. how are you? good. we feel obscenely good about ourselves.[13]

Catastrophe is the absence of the realistic account. Unflinching realism cannot account for such exhaustion. Attempts at such accounting are brazen in their hubris unless whatever such account moves up and down an incalculable scale. The assignment of a specific value to the incalculable is a kind of terror. At the same time, the incalculable is the very instantiation of value. The incalculable is what I think I mean by innovation. You could think about it in relation to Arendt's understanding of natality, but only by way of a suspension of Arendt's brutal exclusions. This is Hartman's encryption. The logic of reparation is vulgar. It's inseparable from representation understood as the thing, which is presumed to have a hole in it, made whole. To make whole, as if one could ever find that completion, as if such completion weren't an absolute brutality, as if the whole were static, as if it were the original, as if it were ever anything other than more and less than itself, as if the simple logic of the synecdoche could ever have been adequate to the mobile assemblage (the Benjaminian constellation where what has been comes together with the now), is an act of violence. It's a heuristic device for attorneys and their literary critical clerks, who have no sense of time. Meanwhile, Jetztsein is the supplement like Selassie is the chapel.

The commitment to repair is how a refusal to represent terror redoubles the logic of representation. The refusal of our ongoing afterlife can only ever replicate a worn-out grammar. The event remains, in the depths. The event-remains are deep and we stand before them, to express them, as their expression. These bits are a mystery, a new machine for the incalculable, which is next, having defied its starting place. I almost remembered this in a dream, where we were just talking, and nothing happened, and then it was over, until just now, with your hands, and light on the breeze's edge. I just can't help feeling that this is what we're supposed to do—to conserve what we are and what we can do by expansion, whose prompt, more often than not, shows up as loss (which shows up, more often than not, as a prompt). More shows up more often than nought if you can stand it.

There's a mutual transformation that occurs when the thing is engaged, a mutual supplement that serrates fantasmatic scenes of repair, that is always manifest as getting through or past or behind it to its essence or its message. What if the message were displaced by the ongoing production of code, which is our social life and what our social life is meant to conserve? What if what we talked about under the rubric of silence were discussed under the rubric of space? Or, in a different register, air? Or water? What is it like to be in the world with some other thing? What does it mean to consider that the relation between the reader, the poem, and history is spatial, a special relation, a north Atlantic entreaty, a plea, an exhortation in the form of a world embrace in resistance to enclosure? To speak the space-time of articulation as futurity, as projection? There's a mutual transportation that occurs when the poem is engaged, a mutual indirection that turns the way back round, this beckoning descent onto the gallery floor or fire or flor or banquet or bouquet.

The logic of reparation is grounded on notions of originary wholeness, on the one hand, and abstract/general equivalence, on the other. Baucom thinks this in relation to credit and imagination but I wonder if it's not really bound up with a strange kind of empiricism. What's the relation between the logic of reparation and the logic of representation? And what does that relation have to do with telling the truth, or the story, or the whole truth, or the whole story, with truth telling as a way of making whole? The normative arc of becoming (a subject, a citizen) is part of this logic. What if there were a radical politics of innovation whose condition of possibility is memory, which remains untranslated, whose resistance, in turn, makes innovation possible? Not to resuscitate! No resurrection. Make it new, like they used to say, so that indexicality is an effect, a technique, so that the recording is part of an experimental impulse. The archive is an assemblage. The assemblage is an image of disaster. But I just want you to enjoy yourself and I want you to believe that. This is an enthusiasm. This is the new thing and a lot of what it's about is just trying to figure out how to say something. How to read. Not (or not only) how to offer a reading, or even an interpretation, but a performance of a text, in the face of its unintelligibility, as if one were forced/privileged to access some other world where representation and unrepresentability were beside the point, so that the response to the terrors and chances of history were not about calculation, not bound to replicate, even in a blunted and ethically responsible way, the horrors of speculation, where new materialities of imagination were already on the other side of the logic of equivalence.

Fragmentation is also about more, an initiation of the work's interior social life, a rending of that interiority by the outside that materializes it. The logic of the supplement is instantiated with every blur, every gliss, every melismatic torque, every twist of the drone, every turn of held syllable. I want to attend to the necessary polyphony. I don't want to represent anything and I don't want to repair anything but I do want to be here more, in another way. I think, in the end, Zong! works this way but even if it doesn't work this way I want it to work this way. I want to work it this way, in coded memory, as the history of no repair, as the ongoing event of more and less than representing. Zong! is about what hasn't happened yet. It is a bridge, which is to say a witness, to the ecstatic and general before. It moves in the irreducible, multiply lined relation between document and speculation, where the laws of time and history, of physics and biochemistry, are suspended, remade, in transubstantiation. The ones who have been rendered speechless are given to and by a speaker, in code, whose message, finally, is that there is speech, that there will have been speech, that radical enunciation (announcement, prophecy, preface, introduction) is being offered in its irreducible animateriality. No mercantile citizenship, no transcendental subject, no neurotypical self matters as much as this: the refusal of administration by those who are destined for a life of being thrown, thrown out, thrown over, overlooked for their enthusiasms, which they keep having to learn to look for and honor in having been thrown, which keep coming to them, which they keep on coming upon, always up ahead, again and again from way back, as out recording, submerged encoding, faded script that can't be faded, joining the sound of the ones who have (been) sounded, under an absolute duress of water, flesh that keeps speaking to us here and now, in contratechnical, counterstrophic, macrophonic amplification of the incalculable.

When we immerse ourselves in Zong!, throw ourselves into its terrible analytic of flesh, its beautiful analyric of being-thrown, we are the touring machine, dedicated to the thinking of the incalculable, suspended in the break of computation, held on the other side in always being sent, saturated in what Édouard Glissant calls our "consent not to be a single being," still in movement, *in the quartet's enthusiastic madness, out of which Trane's glissando emerges to introduce us, once again, to our multiplicity. Which reminds me of a little girl named Mykah, noted for her refusal of administration, her resistance to calculation, her tendency to get in over her head. She keeps caringly, carefully, not taking care of herself with others all the time, is so exorbitantly common that she keeps folks worried about her executive and her administrator, who seem too often to go on tour. One day, standing in front of a hollow place in a tree almost big enough for them to enter, Mykah said to my boy: "Come on, Lorenzo, let's take a walk into the future."*

3

In "Will Sovereignty Ever Be Deconstructed?," Catherine Malabou notes that political philosophy is still organized by or erected around the problem of sovereignty. But what if the theory of politics understands and properly calculates its object? What if political philosophy is and can be nothing other than the theory of sovereignty? Malabou's concern with the fate of sovereignty stems from her sense of the incompleteness of what she calls its "biopolitical deconstruction," wherein the citizen emerges as something on the order of a general equivalent (an abstract and empty signifier that Malabou aligns with symbolic life). With sovereignty's diffusion, the citizen, given in restricted, state-sanctioned protocols of dissemination and delivery, (re)constituted in a right to life that emerges with the regulation of life, takes insubstantial fade as its proper form. Malabou traces the movement of such appearance from natural history to biology, noting its correspondence with the transition from political subject to living subject that might be said to have been initiated in biology's catalogic disenchantment, when the collection of natural facts is accompanied by a deficit of purposiveness that Kant believes to be predicated on the absence of a teleological principle. Kant moves to cut the reduction of *bios* to fact, instrument, immanence—to regulate its fecundity and rupture its finitude—by inventing such a principle and when he engages in such conceptual production it might be said that he is already involved in something like the deconstruction of biopolitical deconstruction, thereby allowing what Malabou now desires—a kind of mutual touch of *bios* and *ta politika* that the biopolitical turns out to interdict and that, in any case, the political is meant to avoid with more or less deadly antisocial revulsion. Kant's anticipation of Malabou is interesting given the particular tools he invents and deploys in the name of that deconstruction. The philosophical conception of race that Robert Bernasconi attributes to Kant would contain and rationalize the differential, (de)generative force, the finitude and fecundity, of *bios*, which now, in the wake of Kant's invention, is inseparable from blackness, which has been pressed into the double duty of signifying life *and* death in the light and echo of their morbid interinanimation. The history of this invention, which we still act out and inhabit, gives pause as we consider Malabou's appeal to the epigenetic and the phenotypical, even if all I can do now is mention in passing an ongoing attempt to think that relation by way of phenomenology's ambivalent appeal to genesis, which is given in and as materiality, thingliness, flesh. What's at stake is that resistance to instrumentalization is driven by a kind of panic in the face of generativity and destruction, of an irregular play of life and death that might be something like what Malabou has been elaborating under the rubric of "plasticity" and might be said to correspond to something Kant spurns and craves under the rubric of "the imagination in its lawless freedom." The transcendental subject, the sovereign, dispersed in and as the new citizen with a right to life, returns in the interest of a certain security, in and as a certain (faculty of the) understanding, in a way that might allow us ultimately to recognize what I think it is that animates Malabou's essay, *the notion that there is nothing other than biological resistance to biopower*. She allows and requires us to ask, what if the *bios* is nothing other than mutual instrumentalization and, even, indebtedness within a massive field of means without end/s? Then, "biological determination" is a conceptual mistake. What we would speak of, instead, constantly and paradoxically, is the necessary and indetermination that the biological performs within the general structure of the interplay of fecundity and finitude; we would attune ourselves to an already given disruptive augmentation of *bios*, articulated in and as its deconstruction, its animation and solicitation by an abolitionist drive; we would engage in the interminable invention of an aleatory principle, improvising through the opposition of immanence and transcendence, addressing ourselves to the angel of dust with the material variability, the anapercussive breath, of N who sits (walks, leaps) in, here, for, and as the incalculable.[14]

Malabou's work requires and allows us again to consider the relationship between sovereignty and law. If it's possible to detach law from the state, as Robert Cover suggests, then it might also be possible to detach law from the sovereign, each in the interest of inviting new worlds.[15]

Malabou differs from those philosophers who see the biological as a field of instrumentality that must be regulated. They fear the play of life and death, which is characterized as the "state of nature," that Hobbes famously anthropomorphizes as "the time men live without a common power to keep them all in awe, [when] they are in that condition which is called war; and such a war as is of every man against every man," delimiting life as "solitary, poor, nasty, brutish, and short."[16] What's just as crucial as the articulation of an assumed need for common power to keep men in awe is the rhetorical maneuver that submits biological anarchy to statist terminology, a kind of transcendental clue that allows one to consider that nature is nothing other than resistance to the sovereignty that it brings online, whether the common power that keeps *bios* in awe is the proper, enclosive, regulatory husbandry of an invading army or the moral law within. Insofar as Kant appeals to natural history he tries to deconstruct biopolitical deconstruction, insofar as he remains committed to sovereignty in the dispersed, democratized form of the free and self-regulated world citizen, he remains committed to a biopolitical deconstruction that insofar as it works, finally, to protect the political from the biological, engages in sovereignty's serial reconfiguration. The idea of a natural (or universal) history, which would organize the prolific, destructive informality of the biological, given as the continual giving and taking rather than the absence of form, reifies and recollects the dispersed sovereign. Malabou puts it this way and as a general formulation: "It is then striking to notice that the critique or deconstruction of sovereignty is structured as the very entity it tends to critique or deconstruct. By distinguishing two lives and two bodies, contemporary philosophers reaffirm the theory of sovereignty, that is, the split between the symbolic and the biological."[17]

How is symbolic life delineated? By way of Foucault and also by way of Eric Santner's updating of Ernst Kantorowicz, Malabou implies that the distinction between the symbolic and the biological (given first in the king's two bodies and then dispersed throughout the citizenry) corresponds to the distinction between the body and (divested, devalued [insofar as it has been assigned and reduced to an exchange value], supposedly deanimated) flesh. She accesses Agamben's assertion that the bare life of divested flesh is somehow incorporated into every body, as a kind of essence, that dwells in the biological body. Mere flesh is within, as well as outside, the symbolic economy. Necessarily degraded essence, flesh is within, at the core of, the body, as its reduction to the deadliness of merely living. Flesh is unaccommodated, which implies the impossibility of something like an analytic of flesh that might pierce the distinction between the biological and the symbolic, between two bodies and two modes of life, by thinking the flesh as invaluable, as the continual disruption of the very idea of (symbolic) value, which moves by way of the reduction of substance. This is to say that the reduction to substance (body to flesh) is inseparable from the reduction of substance. Saussure speaks, for instance, of the reduction of phonic substance as a fundamental maneuver for the formation of a universal science of language; Derrida and Lacan endorse this reduction in their different ways; Guattari, on the other hand, asserts that this materiality is irreducible, and Malabou refines and extends that assertion, challenging the ascription of nonvalue to the one whose value is only in the arbitrariness of exchange or signification. I want to link the rematerializing energy of Malabou's notion of plasticity to the actuality of an analytic of the fugitive's, the noncitizen's, flesh that is predicated not on the flesh's nonvalue but on its being invaluable. That analytic is given to us twice in 1987, in the work of Toni Morrison and Hortense Spillers. In Morrison's *Beloved*, is Baby Suggs's fugitive sermon to the fugitives who embody the disruption of the distinction between things and persons, her injunction to them to love the flesh that they are, the flesh that is unloved and unvalued, a reinvestment, or does she preach the impossibility of flesh's divestment, which then further implies something like a radical displacement of the symbolic and its supposed force? Now we touch on a certain problematic of resurrection and transubstantiation that comes into quite specific analytic relief in experience of, which is always also to say over, the edge where being valued in exchange and having no value outside exchange converge. In the age of the biopolitical deconstruction of sovereignty, such experience is racialized and gendered. Perhaps Malabou's resounding of Derrida's insight that "the dignity of life can only subsist beyond the present living being" comes fully into its own by way of the analytic of invaluable flesh that is given in the exhaustive "consent not to be a single being" that Édouard Glissant locates in the emergence from the brutal im/possibilities of the middle passage. This is something that Spillers more fully elaborates in her distinction "between 'body' and 'flesh' . . . between captive and liberated subject-positions. In that sense, before the 'body' there is the 'flesh,' that zero degree of social conceptualization that does not escape concealment under the brush of discourse, or the reflexes of iconography. . . . If we think of the 'flesh' as a primary narrative, then we mean its seared, divided, ripped-apartness, riveted to the ship's hole, fallen, or 'escaped' overboard. . . . This materialized scene of unprotected female flesh—of female flesh 'ungendered'—offers a praxis and a theory, a text for living and for dying, and a method for reading both through their diverse mediations."[18] Bare life is (degraded) essence, sacred and sacrificeable. But flesh and bare life are not the same. If, as Malabou suggests, "the space which separates bare life from the biological body can only be the space of the symbolic," then flesh is the biological, in its finitude and fecundity, that is before the body. The biological is the essence of the symbolic (its impetus, its initiation) just as flesh is the essence of the body. Essence is, here, as Malabou suggests, neither and both inside and outside. It has no place, it is insofar as it is displacement. Flesh is the irreducible materiality of *différance*, "the non-full, non-simple structured and differentiating origin of differences."[19] This is what is given in and as Baby Suggs's festival of things.

Perhaps Malabou would say, by way of Lévi-Strauss that the flesh, as Spillers theorizes it, is a floating signifier, possessing a "value zero," a symbolic value; that it is the very engine of the symbolic, the very instantiation of valuation. And Spillers would agree except for the fact that it also constitutes the most radical endangerment of the system of value, of the symbolic, of the discursive. What happens, then, if the traditional placement of flesh within the king's two bodies is displaced by the flesh-in-displacement that initiates what Spillers calls her "American grammar"? What if we follow Spillers in claiming the monstrosity of "mere" flesh? This is another way of thinking about Malabou's assertion of the brain's plasticity. If Malabou wants to put an end to the split between the two bodies, it is by lingering in/with the flesh, the merely biological, for a while. She lingers with the analytic that it makes possible, as if there were something already there, in the persistence of its difference from rather than in its reintegration with the discursive body, in and as the very exhaustion and exhaustibility of the flesh. There is something in the flesh, in its disintegration from and of the body, its personality, and its place. There is something to be thought from the flesh's givenness in displacement, the violence it does to positionality that instantiates positional violence. Sovereignty may very well be located or instantiated in the split between the two bodies, but this still requires us to consider that sovereignty, which can never be separated from the (symbolic) body, is detachable from the (biological) flesh, which would justify some interest in the fleshliness, the thingliness, of the noncitizen. Flesh renders the difference and distance between the king's two bodies inoperative and inarticulate. The merger and dispersion of those bodies is biopolitics. In this sense, the merger of *bios* and *ta politika* is inseparable from and is manifest as the political rejection of the biological, which is given in the regulative conferral of the right to life. This is why, as Gayatri Chakravorty Spivak has suggested, the first right must be the right to refuse, not to have, rights, even if it is exercised as the refusal of what has been refused, which is in the end the monstrous emergence that occurs where right, power, life, and death converge.

Malabou wants something like a rehabilitation of the biological that will have been accomplished by way of a liberation of "continental philosophy from the rigid separation it has always maintained between the biological, hence the material, and the symbolic, that is, the nonmaterial or the transcendental."[20] And it is at this point that the brain appears as reinvested, symbolical, transcendental, *plastic* flesh. But in this regard, isn't the deconstruction of biopolitical deconstruction still a sovereign operation? Isn't the brain, in a way that flesh precisely exhausts, where the sovereign now resides? Will it be anything other than the occasion for the plasticization of sovereignty, with all the attendant hierarchization left intact? Maybe the trouble we have with the king's head, its indefatigable resistance to all our would-be decapitative weaponry, is that it has a brain in it. Maybe we can appose the transcendental brain with the flesh's dislocative immanence. Malabou says, "We are the authors of our own brains."[21] But who are "we"? How can "we" resist a tendency to isolate the brain from the rest of "our" (phenotypical/genotypical) flesh so that authorship doesn't reify an old administrative or executive function that is nothing other than a new version of sovereignty? How can we prevent the body's inspirited materiality (the brain) leaving the flesh behind? Or a plasticization of sovereignty, which is also a placement of sovereignty, a reconfiguration or opening of sovereignty's place, leaving behind what flesh-in-displacement allows us to think, a new analytic of sociality, a new analytic of thingliness-in-festivity?

Consider the music that Baby Suggs evokes—its disruption of the opposition of score and performance, writing and reading; consider its disruption of the executive function. Recall the intrication of nature and history in the philosophical invention of race, in the philosophical deployment of the phenotypical difference that, in the century after Kant introduces it, very quickly gets enacted through a certain racial and gender discourse of the brain. The history of the racialized, gendered philosophical interplay of phenotype and genotype, nature and culture (history), is a familiar horror. It's not enough to say that we can separate this from a given racial and gender discourse; it's the fact that racial and gender discourses emerge from it. I invoke Spillers and Morrison because the theory of flesh preserves what Foucault once called "the thought of the outside."[22] It's not just the historical fact of biological determinism's exclusions with which we still have to contend; it's that there is no organization that I can imagine wanting to be a part of that wouldn't be open to the outside's propelling, transformative, antesovereign force. Isn't the work of sovereignty given precisely in an essentially prophylactic protocol, where self-transformation and self-organization are now mobilized in the work of self-protection? Is there a danger of the brain becoming a kind of epigenetic wall? If there is, such a danger—given in the potential solipsism that autonomy and autopoesis might be said to carry—is revealed to us by Malabou's analysis, which brings us to the point of being able to express a desire for the informal, which is to say that which informs, that which gives and takes form. The informal will have also been given or will have been seen to have been instantiated in every undercommon ruptural social generativity that goes over the edge. Over the edge of the ship. Overboard. Thrown. Fallen. Inescaped. The touring machine is a diving bell, an instrument for sounding that becomes, at the end of exhaustion, ascent, accent, a certain songlike, singsong quality, a sing sing sing kinda quality, a fugitive sing sing kinda thing, an instrument whose forced movement in thinking the unregulated, the un-self-possessed, its rubbed, performed, informal interiority, is flesh thought inside out.

NOTES

1. Fodor, "Fire the Press Secretary," 24.
2. Fodor, "Fire the Press Secretary," 25; Foucault, "Technologies of the Self"; Martin, Gutman, and Hutton, *Technologies of the Self*, 31.
3. Foucault, "Technologies of the Self," 18.
4. See Chandler, "Of Exorbitance," 345–410.
5. Fodor, "Fire the Press Secretary," 24.
6. Kurzban, *Everyone (Else)*, 22.
7. Fodor, "Fire the Press Secretary," 24.
8. Fodor, "Fire the Press Secretary," 25.

9. See Kazanjian, *Colonizing Trick*, 27. Kazanjian writes, "in the strictest sense the term refers to the process of igniting a liquid, of turning a liquid into flame. Here, I interpret such a process less as a breaking out of chaos than as a material transformation with powerful effects. 'Flashpoint' in this sense refers to the process by which someone or something emerges or bursts into action or being, not out of nothing but transformed from one form to another; and, it refers to the powerful effects of that emergence or transformation." In its concern with the conjunction of form and explosiveness, Kazanjian takes a theoretical path that can be said to parallel that of Catharine Malabou, about whom more later.

10. I'm thinking a very specific interpenetration, which is, I think, only disguised as an impenetrability. The first permutation/permeation emerges in part of an epigraph for Greenberg, *Devil Has Slippery Shoes*, xv: "'Course CDGM's good,' said a large lady from Lauderdale County. "'Cept the things about it that's bad. There's a lotta good folks come here to help us. 'Course, there's a lot just come to cause a fuss too. And the federal government's finally recognized us down here—'course sometimes that ain't so good, 'cause for every smile it gives us, it gives us a kick too. Well, at least it's got us colored peoples workin' for oursel's. 'Cept the ones that won't. One thing, though, it's great for the kids. On'y thing, it's kinda hard on 'em when they get to real school and it ain't like our school. God's helpin' us, ain't no doubt. It's just that the Devil keeps skippin' in and outa things so's we won't get spoilt. He really keeps you guessin'! Each thing, you gotta study it to see if it's God in the disguise of difficulty, or the Devil in the disguise of somebody good. This whole thing really keep us workin' our mind." The second comes into relief in Chomsky, "What We Know": "A significant insight of the first cognitive revolution was that properties of the world that are informally called mental may involve unbounded capacities of a finite organ, the 'infinite use of finite means,' in Wilhelm von Humboldt's phrase. In a rather similar vein, Hume had recognized that our moral judgments are unbounded in scope, and must be founded on general principles that are part of our nature though they are beyond our 'original instincts.' That observation poses Huarte's problem in a different domain, where we might find part of the thin thread that links the search for cognitive and moral universals. By mid-20th century, it had become possible to face such problems in more substantive ways than before. By then, there was a clear understanding, from the study of recursive functions, of finite generative systems with unbounded scope—which could be readily adapted to the reframing and investigation of some of the traditional questions that had necessarily been left obscure—though only some, it is important to stress. Humboldt referred to the infinite use of language, quite a different matter from the unbounded scope of the finite means that characterize language, where a finite set of elements yields a potentially infinite array of discrete expressions:

discrete, because there are six-word sentences and seven-word sentences, but no 6.2-word sentences; infinite because there is no longest sentence (append "I think that" to the start of any sentence). Another influential factor in the renewal of the cognitive revolution was the work of ethologists, then just coming to be more widely known, with their concern for 'the innate working hypotheses present in subhuman organisms' (Nikolaas Tinbergen) and the 'human a priori' (Konrad Lorenz), which should have much the same character. That framework too could be adapted to the study of human cognitive organs (for example, the language faculty) and their genetically determined nature, which constructs experience and guides the general path of development, as in other aspects of growth of organisms, including the human visual, circulatory, and digestive systems, among others."

11. Martin, "Truth, Power, Self," 10.
12. Mitropoulos, "Oikopolitics," 68.
13. Moten, "Block Chapel," 250–60.
14. See Mackey, *Broken Bottle*.
15. See Cover, "*Nomos* and Narrative," 4–68.
16. Hobbes, *Leviathan*, 84.
17. Malabou, ch. 1, 39.
18. Spillers, "Mama's Baby," 67–68.
19. Derrida, "Différance," 11.
20. Malabou, ch. 1, 40.
21. Malabou, ch. 1, 43.
22. See Foucault, "Maurice Blanchot," in Foucault and Blanchot, *Maurice Blanchot*, 54.

CHAPTER **13**

Interview with Catherine Malabou

QUESTION 1

BRENNA BHANDAR and JONATHAN GOLDBERG-HILLER: What is the role of the philosopher today? In chapter 1, you argue that the philosopher must deconstruct biopolitical deconstruction in an effort to expose and uncover its ideological character. In several of your writings, you have framed a major contribution to this ideological distortion as a neoliberal capitalist one. One implication seems to be that the task of philosophy will end with the critique of capitalism and a renewed appreciation of the unruliness of the biological species-being. Yet Marx, to whom you often allude, also examined the historical sedimentation of capitalist appropriation that limited the choices confronting those who resisted capitalist relations, and he famously argued that the task of philosophy had ended. Why has it been necessary to keep philosophy alive after Marx? In what ways should we understand the philosophical relationship of biological unruliness, in which your own materialism is invested, to historical constraint that preoccupied Marx's ideas of materialism?

In a related vein, Alberto Toscano's paper suggests that there may be some loss in posing questions of metaphysics and capitalism to Heidegger (as you do in *The Heidegger Change*) but not also to Hegel (we note that capitalism is never referenced in *The Future of Hegel*). Is there a particular reason today why a Marxist critique of materialism, which in Marx's day was directed towards much of the Hegelian philosophical enterprise, should not add to our understanding of plasticity and biological materialism?

CATHERINE MALABOU: My relationship with Marx is not unconditional. I do not think that the Marxist critique can be, by its own strength, a sufficient instrument for the subversion of capitalist ideology. When I say "by its own strength," I mean this critique is not, nor any longer, philosophically independent. It has to be coupled with the Heideggerian critique of ontology (*Destruktion*) and with deconstruction. Reciprocally, *Destruktion* and deconstruction have to be confronted with Marxism.

All the readings I developed in *The Heidegger Change* affirm that it is not possible to act as if the destruction of metaphysics—and later its deconstruction—had no connection with what Marx calls the history of capitalism, or historical materialism. There is an undeniable solidarity between the reduction of the metaphysical tradition initiated by Heidegger and that of capital undertaken by Marx. In both cases, it is a question of bringing up to date a double fetishization, that of Being and that of money. Being as it is always being confused with being in the history of metaphysics, and money as it is always thought of as the origin of value. There is, of course, a coincidence between capitalism and ontology. Coincidence at the same time between critique of capital and destruction of traditional ontology.

In *The Heidegger Change*, I tried to show that the relationship between Being and being in the way Heidegger thinks them should be read as exchange relations. Within the tradition of metaphysics, it is the exchange as "value for" (*gelten*) that dominates all the figures of the takeover of Being by being, all the logics of ontic substitution. The economy of this exchange is very close to capitalism. However, that which Heidegger calls the "other thinking," which comes after metaphysics, is another type of exchange, irreducible in the former and consequently in capitalism. The other exchange is called "favor" (*Gunst*) and is not unrelated to Communism. Under the rules of this new exchange, Being and being continue to circulate within one another but without violence, without domination, without any of the two overlooking, in the manner of a fetish, the game of their circulation. I therefore proposed a materialist reading of Heidegger, for which I borrowed Marx's method. A reading that builds on the concepts of change (*Wandel*), transformation (*Wandlung*) and metamorphosis (*Verwandlung*). Let me quote here a passage from the conclusion of the book that expresses very clearly the need for not an ontological but an *economic* interpretation of Heidegger:

> *Ereignis*, it should be recalled, is *the appropriating event that suspends the proper* while in the same move rendering thought susceptible to a break with the logic of appropriation conceived as servitude. But

this rupture does not lead thought to transcend the economic or exit the sphere of exchange and substitution. The announcement of the other (ex)change has nothing to do with the aneconomic coming of god knows what nonpromising promise or nongiving gift. A proximity between Heidegger and Marx indeed exists, and it doubtlessly lies in the possibility of the ontological and the economic coinciding within the definition of exchange, of exchange and mutability, of the metamorphosable and displaceable character of value, and of the impossibility of transgressing all this plasticity.[1]

In contrast and vice versa, I submit that the Marxist corpus cannot and must not escape deconstructive vigilance today. Heidegger has revealed what remains unperceived in the materialism of Marx that inscribes itself, as no other philosophical doctrine, in the history of Being and mobilizes without analyzing concepts such as production, structure, property and ownership, man, value, and essence. Concepts that, uncriticized, continue to stifle thought in the thick smoke of idealism. Following Heidegger, Derrida has brilliantly shown, in *Specters of Marx*, that Marxism situates itself in a messianic horizon (even if this is, for him, a question of "messianicity without messianism") of difference and *différance*. This is a horizon that is not, stricto sensu, that of history. We must then question one of the most sensitive points of Marxism—and of its failure—namely, the nature and value of his promise, of his announcement, of that which signifies the coming of Communism. More than Communism, in fact; it is perhaps its mode of coming which, in Marx, remains problematic.

To sum up in a word, therefore, no deconstruction without materialism but no Marxism without deconstruction. Those who do not see the point of a cross between Marx and Heidegger or between Marx and Derrida or among Marx, Heidegger, and Derrida still confuse, in my critical opinion, political thinking and dogmatism in their belief that philosophy is an obstacle to this same critique. It is true, as you say yourself, that Marx has developed the dialectic that simultaneously unites and separates philosophy and ideology. But he never said that the philosophical critique of philosophy should be canceled or overtaken. I think the Marxist corpus can only gain in strength and effectiveness when it is filtered through the destruction of ontology.

Althusser I think would have agreed, as he described authentic materialism in one of his later texts as "materialism of the encounter," a materialism opposed to rationalist, teleological materialism. The materialism of the encounter, he wrote, "is opposed, as a wholly different mode of thought, to the various materialisms on record, including that widely ascribed to Marx, Engels and Lenin, which, like every other materialism in the rationalist tradition, is a materialism of necessity and teleology, that is to say, a transformed, disguised form of idealism."[2] Teleological materialism has unfortunately suppressed the aleatory materialism of contingency, a materialism without a goal for which the model remains the atomic rain of Epicurus. Marx is obviously no stranger to this sort of materialism (he did his thesis, let's not forget, on classical atomism), yet he masked it with the other materialism: the dialectic subservient to *teleological* necessity. It is therefore important to liberate the materialism of Marx from the materialism of Marx! Let's freely talk about what is secretly brewing beneath the framework of the system, this thought which says that it is the "deviation," not the goal, which is originary! Even Heidegger sees himself summoned to the aid of this repressed materialism! Althusser writes, "We can start with a surprising comparison: between Epicurus and Heidegger."[3] A beginning can escape to itself, be secretly doubled by another beginning, which Heidegger calls an origin. Althusser then admits that the bourgeoisie may have had another origin than the one Marx has assigned to it! For Marx, bourgeoisie "is produced as an antagonistic class by the decay of the dominant feudal class." Althusser continues, "Here we find the schema of dialectical production again, a contrary producing its contrary. We also find the dialectical thesis of negation, a contrary naturally being required, by virtue of a conceptual necessity, to replace its contrary and become dominant in its turn. But what if this was not how things happened? What if the bourgeoisie, far from being the contrary product of the feudal class, was its culmination and, as it were, acme, its highest form and, so to speak, crowning perfection?"[4]

Obviously, it is what I have called the *mode of coming*[5] of the result that it is necessary to interrogate in Marx, which, in the first place, is philosophically possible only in the staging of a confrontation between different types of thinking and concurrent ontologies.

What matters to me in my reference to Althusser is not the content of his thesis, namely that, ultimately, "there is no satisfactory theory of the bourgeoisie in Marx."[6] What is essential for me here is to see that Althusser refers to a non-Marxist paradigm to question Marx. Althusser confronts Marx with Heidegger but also, in the same text, with Machiavelli and Spinoza. In a way of speaking, it is important, indeed vital, to *pluralize Marxism*. One could choose to see in this statement a relativization of the importance of Marxism. Or one can have here the opposite: a means to reengage current events, to replay our fate, and to affirm its inescapable character. It is obviously to the second option that I subscribe.

What is philosophy for, for me today, you ask? The deconstruction of all axiomatic evidence whatsoever. That of Marxism, that of deconstruction itself. For this, the two movements must work together, one against the other and with each other.

QUESTION 2

BB and JG-H: Your recent philosophical work has emphasized the scientific revolution surrounding our understanding of biological regulation, tracing the significance of the decline of understanding DNA as a reproductive code and the rise of epigenetics, a model that you understand to integrate the biological and the symbolic through metabolic cellular processes of interpretation of genetic information. You have suggested that this symbolism is its political significance, an argument you have also made regarding neuroplasticity. This implies that some aspects of scientific modeling are ideological. Are all? We recall that Max Weber famously argued that all science was swept up in the commitment to progress (an idea resonating with capitalist and imperialist ideologies) and that he argued that the fate and meaning of scientific discovery was to "ask to be surpassed and outdated." How robust must discovery and modeling be before science challenges philosophical thinking? In what ways is science interested in and equipped to deal with its own ideological models? Were scientists to rethink the explanatory power of epigenetics one day, what might that tell us about plasticity?

CM: This question gives me the opportunity once more to invert these perspectives and return to the necessity of a Marxist critique of destruction and of the deconstruction of metaphysics. It is from this point of view that we must tackle the relationship between philosophy and science. I note that, from these perspectives, it is impossible and meaningless to speak *in general*. I am not, moreover, an epistemologist and have therefore no comprehensive theory of these relations. So I will respond by taking the specific example of my thinking about biopolitics and about the discrepancy between this concept and categories used in some contemporary biological fields, such as epigenetics, that permits us to intervene through philosophical discourse.

That a resistance to what is today called "biopower"—the monitoring, regulation, exploitation, and instrumentalization of the living organism (*du vivant*) can emerge from possibilities inscribed in the structure of the living organism itself and not from philosophical concepts that skate on the surface of this structure without ever grasping it; that there may be a *biological* resistance to biopolitics; that the *bio-* might be seen as a complex and contradictory instance, opposed to itself and pointing to, on the one hand, the ideological vehicle of modern sovereignty, and on the other hand, that which applies its brakes: *this* seems never to have been considered by contemporary philosophers.

By "structure of the living organism," we must understand both the internal organization of the living organism and, through its biology, the categories that describe it or bring it to light. We will designate a single word, the "biological," for these two inseparable dimensions, that of biological life and that of biological science. Contemporary philosophical thoughts about life, which precisely articulate the biological, systematically subordinate the former to the latter and thus do not accord the biological any autonomy. Affirming the existence of a political counteroffensive inscribed within the biological itself proposes, therefore, to renew philosophical analysis.

The process of integrating the politicization of life and the biologization of politics, initiated by Foucault, takes place without tension because the biological is deprived of a right to reply and seems to fill the mold without force (*pouvoir*). Everything happens as if biology prepares itself from its birth, in the eighteenth century, for its political investiture while lending to power some of its categories. It seems there cannot exist *bio*political resistance to bio*politics*.

Such thinking clearly leaves on the side of the road that which, in the biological, turns itself against technobiopolitics. Anything that relates to traits or training of bodies or to the control of behavior or to management of health or control of reproduction. It is a question of the reservoir of possibilities recorded in the living organism itself. A dimension that reveals the revolutionary discoveries of molecular and cellular biology today. These findings, which remain largely ignored by philosophers, are precisely likely to renew the political question. As evidenced by the progress of epigenetics.

I do not deny that the meaning of biological categories remains highly ambiguous and ideologically suspect nor that biology is, in an essential manner, a fierce ally of biopolitics. The instrumentalization of the living organism is a fact: genetic manipulation, cloning, transgenic agriculture—the list is long. But I want to ensure that there is, within biological research itself—and I mean by "research" as well experimental practice, the conceptual and theoretical dimension that is inseparable from it—the elaboration of a strategy of resistance to biopolitics itself! It is thus necessary to philosophically elaborate this dialectical relationship of biology to itself. You are right to emphasize that biology, like other "technosciences" today, is engaged in a logic of progress and frantic discovery and that epigenesis certainly has value, in part, as the theoretical gadget of the moment. But one cannot deny that our ways of thinking and living find themselves transformed in depth by the discovery of the importance of epigenetic factors in the formation of the living organism. Regenerative medicine, therapeutic cloning, gene therapy, ecology, brain development . . . Gradually, all these questions change our perceptions of the body, of genetic determinism, of the environment. The race to discovery is not, therefore, the only engine of science, and this includes the heart of global capitalism, where science is one of the most significant agents and normative instruments.

In other words, sovereignty and biopower are, of course, inseparable from the production of biological values today. But I want to ensure that the latter is not reduced to it. Usually, the philosophical critique of biopower returns to the opposite to show that nothing in biology allows for a resistance to sovereignty. Such resistance can result only from a conflict between what I call symbolic life and biological life. Philosophers generally agree that it is necessary to have a *different* concept of life than that of biological life in order to think about an aspect of the living organism that biology could not capture. Call this dimension that of meaning, of existence, of history, of all that is assumed to come from purely "cultural" practices.

I try to show in the book that I am presently writing that the *body* (Foucault), the *animal* (Derrida), and *bare life* (Agamben) in the end expel the biological supposed to be at their heart and yet still remain expressions of a body, an animal, or a symbolic fragility—dematerialized and disembodied and thus idealized. Not deconstructed in any case.

My intention is not to develop a univocal "critique" of these three thought-objects, which clearly offer a concept of life other than that which is developed in the tradition of spiritualist philosophy, for example, or phenomenology. Contemporary issues of the formation of the body, the difference between sex and gender, the generations and parenthood, the ethical issues raised by advances in biotechnology, reflections on the precariousness and fragility of life, on the animal, the environment—all these must obviously reflect on biopolitics and exposure of life to sacrifice.

However, as I endeavor to show, the "meaning" of life remains, within these reflections, compartmentalized by differences and boundaries. The wall remains that separates life from itself: biological life is still, in one way or another, always derived and once more relegated under symbolic life. This cut has not been overcome, and philosophers today, inheritors of critical thought, of poststructuralism and of deconstruction, continue to develop a unilateral approach to biology without interest in radically new definitions of the living organism apparent since the turn of the 1990s. The dialogue between philosophy and biology has not yet occurred.

It should be noted that biologists do not any longer make this discussion possible. None of them has yet seen fit to respond to philosophers by situating in a precise manner the discoveries and advances in the life sciences in the political debate opened by the double angle of attack of biopower and technoscience. It seems hard to believe that biologists know neither Foucault nor Derrida nor Heidegger, for example, nor have never encountered the word *biopolitics*. Surprisingly, biology does not try to resist its status as political-ideological instrument of sovereign power that is reserved for it by contemporary philosophy. Attached to the two poles of ethics (endless debates about reproductive technologies and the status of the embryo) and evolutionism (various responses to the ideological challenge of Darwinism), scientists fail to reflect on how the science of living organisms could and should now worry itself about the identification between biological determination and political normalization of life. The ethical shield surrounding biological discourse today is not sufficient to define the space of a theoretical disobedience to accusations of complicity between life sciences, sovereignty, capitalism, and the technological manipulation of life.

It is therefore necessary to lay the foundations of dialogue, to ask of contemporary biology "permission," to borrow a phrase from Canguilhem, to identify its "fundamental philosophical concepts."[7] But what is a biological concept? It is a question, as explained further by Canguilhem, of a notion on the way to becoming "a universal and obligatory mode of apprehending the experience and existence of living beings" and that constitutes itself thus as "a universal and obligatory mode of apprehending the experience and existence of living beings."[8]

Aware of the risk run by any philosopher who "tr[ies] his hand at biological philosophy" of "compromising the biologists he uses or cites" and thereby achieving the position of a "fanciful" biology,[9] I try to bring out these categories, which, starting from the experience of the living organism, become the fundamental modes of thought while transforming philosophy itself.

QUESTION 3

BB and JG-H: Since *The Future of Hegel*, you have stressed the significance of subjectivity for the concept of plasticity, making the grasping subject a key element of your notion of plastic reading. You wrote in that book, "the concept of plastic reading accords a determinative and decisive role to the subjectivity of the reader, the reader having become the author of the enunciation. The reader rewrites what he or she reads. Yet it is incumbent on no one but the reader to present, in return, the movement which, paradoxically enough, led to the collapse of the 'knowing I,' hence to individuality itself." In *Plasticity at the Dusk of Writing* and again in *Changing Difference* you demonstrate the significance of autobiography, particularly an intellectual autobiography, to our understanding of how reading gives life to the concept of plasticity and your own sense of subjectivity. In *The New Wounded*, you draw more upon experience, noting at the outset of the book the significance of your grandmother's struggle with Alzheimer's disease as a provocation for developing the concept of cerebrality. Many of the pieces in this collection have addressed the particular experiences of violence and of race for assessing the radical politics that plasticity heralds. What is the role of experience in philosophy? In what ways can experience be a provocateur to understanding plasticity? Specifically, do you see the experience of your family living in Algeria and moving back to France when you were young making a particular contribution to your later philosophical work? Does this colonial experience have an explicit or implicit influence on your insights into plasticity?

CM: Among the colonizing ex-powers, France is one of those that will have taken longest to reflect on its past. Postcolonial studies have met with success there only recently, and the French often deny the colonial trauma. As Benjamin Stora, the greatest living historian of the Algerian War, writes:

> France is sick with its colonial past. Having shunted it to the margins of its history for far too long, marginalizing it in universities and school textbooks, it has returned like a boomerang into public debate. Like a family secret that blows up, one evening, at the dinner table, the colonial question has reemerged with the February 2005 law that sought to sanction the "positive role" of French colonization. A year later President Jacques Chirac had to backtrack and disavow his parliamentary majority. This retreat was very revealing: France is still not reconciled when it comes to decolonization to the loss of French Algeria.[10]

In France we are witnessing the very beginning of real research on this memory, which remains, according to Stora, "at war." In fact, French postcolonial investigations remain for the most part undistributed and untranslated (I think that Stora himself remains unknown in the anglophone world). One has the impression that nothing new has been written since Fanon, which is not true, but it all still remains concealed. Few French people know what the Algerian War was, which is to say *also* a civil war among the Algerians themselves (the conflict between the FLN and Messali Hadj's MNA). We could even speak of a double civil war, since the binary confrontation is doubled by a war within the communities themselves.

In other words, few people know that there is no Algerian War but Algerian *wars* (let us also note that the expression "Algerian War" was officially adopted in France only on October 18, 1999). Memories, inheritances. Neither single nor united. Nor is there a united front on the French side. Pierre Nora has recently included, by way of a preface to the new edition of his book *Les français d'Algérie*, the letter that Jacques Derrida, at the time a student, had sent to him upon publication.[11] An admirable letter, in which Derrida gently reproaches Nora for having an excessively uniform vision of *the* Algerian French. Here, too, they are many! A long labor, carefully untying the knots, has been started by Stora and other young historians, but there is a way to go. Endless disputes bar free access to the archives. We are dealing with a real black spot in the country's history. A foreclosure.

I think it's important to mention this before answering your question, to underline that no "repatriated" from Algeria—for that is what I am!—finds it easy to place her own history in the more global context which serves as its background. My own family was totally silent, during my whole childhood and to the present day, on the complexity of the memories and conflicts that "French Algeria" represents. I lived, through my mother, the myth of the lost paradise. Something extremely painful but also extremely univocal. For a long time, I myself didn't try to find out more.

So you can imagine from this point of view just how shaken up I was by my meeting with Derrida! It's as if someone in me was waiting to meet at last an "other" *pied-noir*, different than the familiar faces, introducing me to an entirely other dimension of things, something that was later confirmed by my readings of Edward Said in particular.

This encounter was also decisive to the extent that Derrida taught me that it is impossible to separate biography, or rather autobiography, and theory. Recall this passage from "Otobiographies: The Teaching of Nietzsche and the Politics of the Proper Name": "We no longer consider the biography of a 'philosopher' as a corpus of empirical accidents that leaves both a name and a signature outside a system which would itself be offered up to an immanent philosophical reading—the only kind of reading held to be philosophically legitimate.... Neither 'immanent' readings of philosophical systems (whether such readings be structural or not) nor external, empirical-genetic readings have ever in themselves questioned the *dynamis* of that borderline between the "work" and the "life," the system and the subject of the system."[12] Now it is precisely this frontier that Derrida incessantly explored.

This is in effect why I think, to return to your question, that "personal" experience plays a key role in any philosophical undertaking, even if this role is never easy to define.

What I can say, about my personal experience of Algeria, is that it is very strange not to have a country of birth, to live with the idea that one's country of birth was in some sense confiscated. I don't even know where my maternal grandmother is buried. There is nothing there anymore. It's funny. It's a little as if one didn't exist. This means a very great sadness, a very, very great sadness, something that never heals, the idea of a solitude that is difficult to measure. But it also gives you a great strength, like an eternal desire to laugh.

QUESTION 4

BB and JG-H: Frantz Fanon argued that the lived and embodied experiences of colonialism and race impeded the universalizing moment promised by Hegel's *Phenomenology*. Building on this critique, Fred Moten, in his piece in this collection, uses a concept of flesh to indicate the excesses of blackness—its insurgent, incalculable, and ungovernable dimensions—and he suggests that, like your own work, flesh is invaluable, a challenge to the critics of sovereignty (Foucault, Agamben, and others) who ascribe "non-value to the one whose value is only in the arbitrariness of exchange or signification." Yet, Moten points out, in contemporary efforts to deconstruct sovereignty through the theory of biopolitics, the flesh remains racialized and gendered. This is quite evident in the science of the brain, which has long been plagued by white supremacist notions. He therefore questions whether "the deconstruction of biopolitical deconstruction [is] still a sovereign operation? Isn't the brain, in a way that flesh precisely exhausts, where the sovereign now resides? Will it be anything other than the occasion for the plasticization of sovereignty, with all the attendant hierarchization left intact?" If philosophical discourses have historically bred racial and gender discourses, as Moten suggests, how do you assure yourself that the task of deconstructing the deconstruction of biopolitics doesn't repeat this odious history with its dangerous politics?

CM: I have great admiration for the work of Fred Moten. I am entirely convinced by his analysis of the risk of a constant rebirth of sovereignty. Including on the basis of its own deconstruction. A sovereignty that inscribes, in the bodies and flesh of its subjects, new subordinations, new colonizations whose effects are constantly displaced but never truly suppressed. In this sense, I am very conscious that the very modest deconstruction of the concept of biopolitics that I have undertaken is not sufficient to counter the risk of a return of sovereignty that may be borne by contemporary biological categories, including the ones that seem to threaten the sovereignty of the code, of the program, and of determinism in general. It is also true that the brain, the organ of command par excellence, can be considered the sovereign of the body—its cybernetics, if you will, since cybernetics is etymologically the art of government.

How could one not see, as I already noted in *What Should We Do with Our Brain?*, that the plasticity of the brain has today become the model for the new spirit of capitalism? It may be supple, malleable, even decentered, but neural government is still government! How could one not see that this plasticity is recuperated at all levels to affix new labels and fashion new categories? Schizo brains, criminal brains, female brains, and male brains . . . Neurobiology today is undeniably the new discourse of power.

Against this, I am obviously powerless. Nevertheless, I think that to propose an analysis of this new domination can at least allow us to produce a form of consciousness of this situation. I call this paradoxical consciousness "the consciousness of the brain." I believe that it is important today to be able to draw out everything that is implied by this formula.

NOTES

1. Malabou, *Heidegger Change*, 276–77.
2. Althusser, "Underground Current," 167, 168.
3. Althusser, "Underground Current," 168.
4. Althusser, "Underground Current," 201.
5. Malabou, *Heidegger Change*, 136. This is Skafish's translation of *mode d'advenue*.
6. Althusser, "Underground Current," 202.
7. Canguilhem, *Knowledge of Life*, 59.
8. Canguilhem, *Knowledge of Life*, 98.
9. Canguilhem, *Knowledge of Life*, 59.
10. Stora and Leclère, *La guerre des mémoires*, 7.
11. Nora, *Les français d'Algérie*.
12. Derrida, "Otobiographies," 5.

Adorno, Theodor W. *Negative Dialectics*. Trans. E. B. Ashton. New York: Continuum, 1973.
Agamben, Giorgio. *Homo Sacer: Sovereign Power and Bare Life*. Stanford, CA: Stanford University Press, 1998.
Agamben, Giorgio. *The Open: Man and Animal*. Stanford, CA: Stanford University Press, 2004.
Agamben, Giorgio. *The Signature of All Things: On Method*. Trans. Luca D'Isanto with Kevin Attell. New York: Zone Books, 2009.
Agamben, Giorgio. *State of Exception*. Chicago: University of Chicago Press, 2005.
Alexander, James McKinney. *Mission Life in Hawaii: Memoir of Rev. William P. Alexander*. Oakland, CA: Pacific Press, 1888.
Allewaert, Monique. *Ariel's Ecology: Plantations, Personhood, and Colonialism in the American Tropics*. Minneapolis: University of Minnesota Press, 2013.
Althusser, Louis. "Appendix: On Jacques Monod." In *Philosophy and the Spontaneous Philosophy of the Scientists: And Other Essays*, 145–66. London: Verso, 1990.
Althusser, Louis. "The Underground Current of the Materialism of the Encounter." In *Philosophy of the Encounter: Later Writings, 1978–87*, edited by François Matheron and Olivier Corpet, 163–207. London: Verso, 2006.
Anghie, Antony. *Imperialism, Sovereignty and the Making of International Law*. 1st ed. Cambridge: Cambridge University Press, 2007.
Apess, William. *On Our Own Ground: The Complete Writings of William Apess, a Pequot*. Amherst: University of Massachusetts Press, 1992.
Aron, Raymond. *Introduction à la philosophie de l'histoire: Essai sur les limites de l'objectivité historique, complétée par des textes récents*. Paris: Gallimard, 1981.
Ashby, W. Ross. *Design for a Brain*. 2nd ed. London: Chapman and Hall, 1960.
Ashby, W. Ross. *Introduction to Cybernetics*. London: Chapman and Hall, 1956.
Atlan, Henri. "Biological Medicine and the Survival of the Person." *Science in Context* 8, no. 1 (1995): 265–77.

Bakhtin, Mikhail M. "Author and Hero in Aesthetic Activity." In *Art and Answerability: Early Essays by M. M. Bakhtin*, 4–256. Austin: University of Texas Press, 1990.

Bakhtin, Mikhail M. "The *Bildungsroman* and Its Significance in the History of Realism (toward a Historical Typology of the Novel)." In *Speech Genres and Other Late Essays*, translated by Vern McGee, 10–59. Austin: University of Texas Press, 1999.

Bakhtin, Mikhail M. "Epic and Novel." In *The Dialogic Imagination: Four Essays*, translated by Michael Holquist and Caryl Emerson, 3–40. Austin: University of Texas Press, 1981.

Balbus, Isaac. "Commodity Form and Legal Form: An Essay on the 'Relative Autonomy' of the Law." *Law and Society Review* 11 (1977): 571.

Baldwin, J. Mark. "A New Factor in Evolution." *American Naturalist* (1896): 536–53.

Balibar, Étienne, and Immanuel Wallerstein. *Race, Nation, Class: Ambiguous Identities*. London: Verso, 1992.

Bannerji, Himani. *Thinking Through: Essays on Feminism, Marxism and Anti-Racism*. Toronto: Women's Press, 1995.

Barad, Karen. "Quantum Entanglements and Hauntological Relations of Inheritance: Dis/continuities, SpaceTime Enfoldings, and Justice-to-Come." *Derrida Today* 3, no. 2 (2010): 240–68.

Barker, Joanne. *Native Acts: Law, Recognition, and Cultural Authenticity*. Durham, NC: Duke University Press, 2011.

Barthes, Roland. *Mythologies*. New York: Hill and Wang, 1972.

Bauman, Zygmunt. "Reconnaissance Wars of the Planetary Frontierland." *Theory, Culture and Society* 19, no. 4 (2002): 81–90.

Bauman, Zygmunt. *Society under Siege*. Hoboken, NJ: Wiley, 2013.

BBC Food Blog. "Why Not Eat Insects?" Accessed February 24, 2014. www.bbc.co.uk/blogs/food/2011/03/why-not-eat-insects.shtml.

Benjamin, Walter. "On the Concept of History." In *Walter Benjamin: Selected Writings*, vol. 4, *1938–1940*, edited by Michael W. Jennings, translated by Edmund Jephcott. Cambridge, MA: Harvard University Press, 2003.

Benjamin, Walter W. "Two Poems by Friedrich Holderlin." In *Walter Benjamin: Selected Writings: 1913–1926*, vol. 1, trans. Stanley Corngold. Cambridge, MA: Harvard University Press, 1996.

Benjamin, Walter, and Peter Demetz. *Reflections: Essays, Aphorisms, Autobiographical Writing*. New York: Schocken, 1986.

Bennett, Jane. *Vibrant Matter: A Political Ecology of Things*. Durham, NC: Duke University Press, 2009.

Bennett, Jane, and William E. Connolly. "Contesting Nature/Culture: The Creative Character of Thinking." *Journal of Nietzsche Studies* 24, no. 1 (2002): 148–63.

Benyus, Janine M. *Biomimicry: Innovation Inspired by Nature*. New York: HarperCollins, 2009.

Bergson, Henri. *Creative Evolution*. Mineola, NY: Dover, 1998.

Beurton, Peter J., Raphael Falk, and Hans-Jörg Rheinberger. *The Concept of the Gene in Development and Evolution: Historical and Epistemological Perspectives*. Cambridge: Cambridge University Press, 2000.

Bhabha, Homi K. "Culture's In-Between." In *Questions of Cultural Identity*, edited by Stuart Hall and Paul du Gay, 53–60. Thousand Oaks, CA: Sage, 1996.

Bhandar, Brenna. "Plasticity and Post-Colonial Recognition: 'Owning, Knowing and Being.'" *Law and Critique* 22, no. 3 (2011): 227–49.

Bhandar, Brenna. "Resisting the Reproduction of the Proper Subject of Rights: Recognition, Property Rights, and the Movement towards Post-Colonialism in Canada." London: University of London, 2007.

Bhandar, Brenna. "Strategies of Legal Rupture: The Politics of Judgment." *Windsor Yearbook of Access to Justice* 30, no. 2 (2012): 59–78.

Bignall, Simone. "Potential Postcoloniality: Sacred Life, Profanation and the Coming Community." In *Agamben and Colonialism*, edited by Marcelo Svirsky and Simone Bignall, 261–84. Edinburgh: Edinburgh University Press, 2012.

Bird, Isabella Lucy. *The Hawaiian Archipelago: Six Months among the Palm Groves, Coral Reefs, and Volcanoes of the Sandwich Islands*. London: John Murray, 1875.

Black, C. F. *The Land Is the Source of the Law: A Dialogic Encounter with Indigenous Jurisprudence*. Abingdon, UK: Routledge-Cavendish, 2010.

Bogost, Ian. *Alien Phenomenology; or, What It's Like to Be a Thing*. Minneapolis: University of Minnesota Press, 2012.

Boltanski, Luc, and Eve Chiapello. *The New Spirit of Capitalism*. Trans. Gregory C. Elliott. London: Verso, 2007.

Borrows, John. "Frozen Rights in Canada: Constitutional Interpretation and the Trickster." *American Indian Law Review* 22, no. 1 (1997): 37–64.

Borrows, John. *Recovering Canada: The Resurgence of Indigenous Law*. Toronto: University of Toronto Press, 2002.

Bouabdellah, Zoulikha. "Set Me Free from My Chains." Accessed February 24, 2014. www.docstoc.com/docs/75806900%20/.

Bouabdellah, Zoulikha, and Jérôme Sans. *Soft Transgression: Zoulikha Bouabdellah*. Paris: BANK, 2010.

Bourdieu, Pierre, and Jean-Claude Passeron. *The Inheritors: French Students and Their Relation to Culture*. Chicago: University of Chicago Press, 1979.

Braun, Bruce. "Biopolitics and the Molecularization of Life." *Cultural Geographies* 14, no. 1 (2007): 6–28.

Brilman, M. C. "Georges Canguilhem: Norms and Knowledge in the Life Sciences." PhD diss., London School of Economics, 2009.

Brown, Richard Harvey, and Beth Davis-Brown. "The Making of Memory: The Politics of Archives, Libraries and Museums in the Construction of National Consciousness." *History of the Human Sciences* 11, no. 4 (1998): 17–32.

Bryant, Levi R. *The Democracy of Objects*. Ann Arbor: Open Humanities Press, 2011. Accessed June 30, 2014. http://quod.lib.umich.edu/o/ohp/9750134.0001.001/.

Bryant, Levi R. "Ethics and Politics: What Are You Asking?" *Larval Subjects*. Accessed November 6, 2013. http://larvalsubjects.wordpress.com/2012/05/29/ethics-and-politics-what-are-you-asking/.

Burroughs, William S. "The Limits of Control." *Semiotexte* 3, no. 2 (1978): 38.

Butler, Judith. *Gender Trouble: Feminism and the Subversion of Identity*. New York: Routledge, 1990.

Butler, Judith. *Giving an Account of Oneself*. New York: Fordham University Press, 2005.

Butler, Judith. *The Psychic Life of Power: Theories in Subjection*. Stanford, CA: Stanford University Press, 1997.

Butler, Judith. *Undoing Gender*. New York: Routledge, 2004.

Butler, Judith, and Catherine Malabou. *Sois mon corps: Une lecture contemporaine de la domination et de la servitude chez Hegel*. Paris: Bayard Centurion, 2010.

Butler, Judith, and Gayatri Chakravorty Spivak. *Who Sings the Nation-State? Language, Politics, Belonging*. London: Seagull, 2007.

Bynum, Caroline Walker. *Metamorphosis and Identity*. New York: Zone Books, 2005.

Byrd, Jodi A. *Transit of Empire: Indigenous Critiques of Colonialism*. Minneapolis: University of Minnesota Press, 2011.

Canguilhem, Georges. *Knowledge of Life*. Edited by Paola Marrati and Todd Meyers. New York: Fordham University Press, 2008.

Canguilhem, Georges. *Le Normal et le pathologique*, 79. PUF, Quadrige, Paris, 2006.

Canguilhem, Georges. *A Vital Rationalist: Selected Writings from Georges Canguilhem*. New York: Zone Books, 1994.

Canguilhem, Georges. "Le vivant et son milieu." In *La connaissance de la vie*, 2nd ed., 129–54. Paris: Presses Universitaires de France, 1998.

Carey, Nessa. *The Epigenetics Revolution: How Modern Biology Is Rewriting Our Understanding of Genetics, Disease, and Inheritance*. New York: Columbia University Press, 2012.

Casarino, Cesare. "Philopoesis: A Theoretico-Methodological Manifesto." *Boundary 2* 29, no. 1 (2002): 65–96.

Césaire, Aimé. *Discourse on Colonialism*. Translated by Joan Pinkham. New York: Monthly Review Press, 2001.

Chakrabarty, Dipesh. *Provincializing Europe: Postcolonial Thought and Historical Difference*. Princeton, NJ: Princeton University Press, 2008.

Charlot, John. *The Kamapuaʻa Literature: The Classical Traditions of the Hawaiian Pig God as a Body of Literature*. Laie, HI: Institute for Polynesian Studies, Brigham Young University / Hawaii Campus, 1993.

Cheah, Pheng. "Biopower and the New International Division of Labor." In *Can the Subaltern Speak? Reflections on the History of an Idea*, edited by Rosalind C. Morris, 179–212. New York: Columbia University Press, 2010.

Chen, Mel Y. *Animacies: Biopolitics, Racial Mattering, and Queer Affect*. Durham, NC: Duke University Press, 2012.

Chomsky, Noam. "What We Know: On the Universals of Language and Rights." *Boston Review* 30 (2005): 3–4.

Cioran, E. M. *A Short History of Decay*. New York: Arcade, 1998. Accessed June 29, 2014.

Clarke, Bruce, and Mark B. N. Hansen, eds. *Emergence and Embodiment: New Essays on Second-Order Systems Theory*. Durham, NC: Duke University Press, 2009.

Connolly, William E. *The Fragility of Things: Self-Organizing Processes, Neoliberal Fantasies, and Democratic Activism*. Durham, NC: Duke University Press, 2013.

Connolly, William E. *Neuropolitics: Thinking, Culture, Speed*. Minneapolis: University of Minnesota Press, 2002.

Conway, Flo, and Jim Siegelman. *Dark Hero of the Information Age: In Search of Norbert Wiener, the Father of Cybernetics*. New York: Basic Books, 2005.

Coole, Diana, and Samantha Frost. *New Materialisms: Ontology, Agency, and Politics*. Durham, NC: Duke University Press, 2010.

Cooper, Davina. *Sexing the City: Lesbian and Gay Politics within the Activist State*. London: Rivers Oram Press, 1994.

Coulthard, Glen S. "Subjects of Empire: Indigenous Peoples and the 'Politics of Recognition' in Canada." *Contemporary Political Theory* 6, no. 4 (2007): 437–60.

Cover, Robert M. "*Nomos* and Narrative." *Harvard Law Review* 97 (1983): 4–68.

Crenshaw, Kimberlé. "Demarginalizing the Intersection of Race and Sex: A Black Feminist Critique of Antidiscrimination Doctrine, Feminist Theory and Antiracist Politics." *University of Chicago Legal Forum* (1989): 139–67.

Dahlbom, Bo. "Mind Is Artificial." In *Dennett and His Critics: Demystifying Mind*, ed. Bo Dahlbom. Oxford: Basil Blackwell, 1998.

Dao, James. "More Military Dogs Show Signs of Combat Stress." *New York Times*, US section, December 1, 2011. Accessed December 4, 2011. www.nytimes.com/2011/12/02/us/more-military-dogs-show-signs-of-combat-stress.html.

Darian-Smith, Eve, and Peter Fitzpatrick. *Laws of the Postcolonial: Law, Meaning, and Violence*. Ann Arbor: University of Michigan Press, 1999.

Darwin, Charles. *On the Origin of Species by Means of Natural Selection; or, The Preservation of Favoured Races in the Struggle for Life*. 2nd ed. London: John Murray, 1860.

da Silva, Denise Ferreira. *Toward a Global Idea of Race*. Minneapolis: University of Minnesota Press, 2007.

Davies, Margaret. "Queer Property, Queer Persons: Self-Ownership and Beyond." *Social and Legal Studies* 8, no. 3 (1999): 327–52.

Deleuze, Gilles. *Cinema 2: The Time-Image*. London: Continuum, 2005.

Deleuze, Gilles. *Difference and Repetition*. New York: Columbia University Press, 1994.

Deleuze, Gilles. "How Do We Recognize Structuralism?" In *Desert Islands and Other Texts (1953–1974)*, translated by Mike Taormina, 170–92. Cambridge, MA: MIT Press, 2003.

Deleuze, Gilles. *Logic of Sense*. London: Continuum, 2005.

Deleuze, Gilles. *Nietzsche and Philosophy*. New York: Columbia University Press, 1983.

Deleuze, Gilles. "Postscript on Control Societies." In Gilles Deleuze, *Negotiations, 1972–1990*, 177–82. New York: Columbia University Press, 1995.

Deleuze, Gilles. *Pure Immanence: Essays on a Life*. 2nd ed. New York: Zone, 2005.

Deleuze, Gilles. *Spinoza: Practical Philosophy*. San Francisco: City Lights, 1988.

Deleuze, Gilles, and Félix Guattari. *Milles plateaux*. Paris: Minuit, 1980.

Deleuze, Gilles, and Félix Guattari. *What Is Philosophy?* New ed. New York: Columbia University Press, 1996.

Delgado, José Manuel Rodríguez. *Physical Control of the Mind: Toward a Psychocivilized Society*. New York: Harper and Row, 1971. Accessed June 29, 2014. http://books.google.com/books?id=0EwyQgAACAAJ, 281.

De Luca, Michael. *In the Mouth of Madness*. Dir. John Carpenter. Transcript of the screenplay. Accessed February 25, 2014. www.script-o-rama.com/movie_scripts/i/in-the-mouth-of-madness-script.html.

Demers, Jason. "An American Excursion: Deleuze and Guattari from New York to Chicago." *Theory and Event* 14, no. 1 (2011).

Den Ouden, Amy E., and Jean M. O'Brien. *Recognition, Sovereignty Struggles, and Indigenous Rights in the United States*. Chapel Hill: University of North Carolina Press, 2013.

Derrida, Jacques. *Acts of Religion*. London: Routledge, 2001.

Derrida, Jacques. *Aporias: Dying—Awaiting (One Another at) the "Limits of Truth" (Mourir—s'attendre aux "limites de la vérité")*. Stanford, CA: Stanford University Press, 1993.

Derrida, Jacques. *Archive Fever: A Freudian Impression*. Chicago: University of Chicago Press, 1998.

Derrida, Jacques. *The Beast and the Sovereign*. Vol. 1. Chicago: University of Chicago Press, 2011.

Derrida, Jacques. *The Death Penalty*. Chicago: University of Chicago Press, 2013.
Derrida, Jacques. "Différance." In Jacques Derrida, *Margins of Philosophy*, translated by Alan Bass, 1–28. Chicago: University of Chicago Press, 1982.
Derrida, Jacques. "The Ends of Man." In Jacques Derrida, *Margins of Philosophy*, trans. Alan Bass, 109–36. Chicago: University of Chicago Press, 1982.
Derrida, Jacques. "Form and Meaning: A Note on the Phenomenology of Language." In Jacques Derrida, *Margins of Philosophy*, translated by Alan Bass, 155–73. Chicago: University of Chicago Press, 1982.
Derrida, Jacques. "From Restricted to General Economy: A Hegelianism without Reserve." In Jacques Derrida, *Writing and Difference*, translated by Alan Bass, 251–77. London: Routledge and Kegan Paul, 1978.
Derrida, Jacques. *Glas*. Paris: Éditions Galilée, 1974.
Derrida, Jacques. *Glas*. Lincoln: University of Nebraska Press, 1986.
Derrida, Jacques. *Learning to Live Finally: The Last Interview*. Ed. J. Birnbaum. Brooklyn, NY: Melville House, 2007.
Derrida, Jacques. "Manquements du droit à la justice (mais que manque-t-il donc aux 'sans-papiers'?)." In Jacques Derrida, Marc Guillaume, and Jean Pierre Vincent, *Marx en Jeu*. Paris: Descartes, 1997.
Derrida, Jacques. "Marx and Sons." In *Ghostly Demarcations: On Jacques Derrida's "Specters of Marx,"* edited by Michael Sprinker, 213–69. London: Verso, 1999.
Derrida, Jacques. "Marx, c'est quelqu'un." In Jacques Derrida, Marc Guillaume, and Jean Pierre Vincent, *Marx en Jeu*. Paris: Descartes, 1997, 9–28.
Derrida, Jacques. *Negotiations: Interventions and Interviews, 1971–2001*. Stanford, CA: Stanford University Press, 2002.
Derrida, Jacques. "Otobiographies: The Teaching of Nietzsche and the Politics of the Proper Name." In *The Ear of the Other*, edited by Christie McDonald, translated by Peggy Kamuf. New York: Schocken, 1985.
Derrida, Jacques. *Paper Machine*. Stanford, CA: Stanford University Press, 2005.
Derrida, Jacques. "Paper or Me." In Jacques Derrida, *Paper Machine*, 41–65. Stanford, CA: Stanford University Press, 2005.
Derrida, Jacques. *Points . . . : Interviews, 1974–1994*. Stanford, CA: Stanford University Press, 1995.
Derrida, Jacques. *Specters of Marx: State of the Debt, the Work of Mourning and the New International*. New York: Routledge, 1994.
Derrida, Jacques. *Il tempo degli addii*. Milan: Mimesis, 2006.
Derrida, Jacques. "Le temps des adieux." *Revue philosophique de la France et de l'étranger* 123, no. 1 (1998): 3–47.
Derrida, Jacques. "A Time for Farewells: Heidegger (Read by) Hegel (Read by) Malabou." Preface to Catherine Malabou, *The Future of Hegel: Plasticity, Temporality, and Dialectic*, translated by Joseph D. Cohen, vii–xlvii. New York: Routledge, 2005.

Derrida, Jacques. "To Unsense the Subjectile." In Jacques Derrida and Paule Thévenin, *The Secret Art of Antonin Artaud*, translated by Paule Thévenin, 59–148. Cambridge, MA: MIT Press, 1998.

Derrida, Jacques, and Keith Reader. "Paper or Myself, You Know . . ." *Paragraph* 21, no. 1 (March 1998): 1.

Derrida, Jacques, and Paule Thévenin. *The Secret Art of Antonin Artaud*. Cambridge, MA: MIT Press, 1998.

Derrida, Jacques, Geoffrey Bennington, Marc Crépon, and Thomas Dutoit. *La peine de mort: Séminaire*, vol. 1. Paris: Éditions Galilée, 2012.

Derrida, Jacques, Marc Guillaume, and Jean Pierre Vincent. *Marx en Jeu*. Paris: Descartes, 1997.

Descola, Philippe. *Beyond Nature and Culture*. Translated by Janet Lloyd. Chicago: University of Chicago Press, 2013.

Deutsch, Karl Wolfgang. *The Nerves of Government: Models of Political Communication and Control, with a New Introduction*. Vol. 90729. Glencoe, IL: Free Press, 1975

Dore, Florence. "Law's Literature, Law's Body: The Aversion to Linguistic Ambiguity in Law and Literature." *Law, Culture and the Humanities* 2, no. 1 (2006): 17–28.

Dosse, François. *History of Structuralism*. Vol. 1: *The Rising Sign: 1945–1966*. Minneapolis: University of Minnesota Press, 1997.

Dupuy, Jean-Pierre. *On the Origins of Cognitive Science*. Cambridge, MA: MIT Press, 2009.

"Dutchman Urges World to Eat Bugs." *BBC*, Europe, January 18, 2011. Accessed October 1, 2011. www.bbc.co.uk/news/world-europe-12216355.

Emmanuelli, Xavier, and Catherine Malabou. *La grande exclusion: L'urgence sociale, symptôme et thérapeutique*. Paris: Bayard Centurion, 2009.

Énard, Mathias. *Zone*. Translated by Charlotte Mandell. Rochester, NY: Open Letter, 2010.

Esmeir, Samera. *Juridical Humanity: A Colonial History*. Stanford, CA: Stanford University Press, 2012.

Esposito, Roberto. *Bios: Biopolitics and Philosophy*. Vol. 4. Minneapolis: University of Minnesota Press, 2008.

Evans, David. *Sexual Citizenship: The Material Construction of Sexualities*. London: Routledge, 1993.

Evans, Dylan. *An Introductory Dictionary of Lacanian Psychoanalysis*. New York: Routledge, 1996.

Everson, Brian. "Introduction." In Mathias Énard, *Zone*, translated by Charlotte Mandell, vii–xi. Rochester, NY: Open Letter, 2010.

Fanon, Frantz. *Black Skin, White Masks*. New York: Grove Press, 1967. Reprint, London: Pluto, 2008.

Fanon, Frantz. *The Wretched of the Earth*. Translated by Richard Philcox. New York: Grove Press, 2004.

Feinman, Jay, and Peter Gabel. "Contract Law as Ideology." In *The Politics of Law: A Progressive Critique*, edited by David Kairys, 373. Rev. ed. New York: Pantheon, 1990.

Felman, Shoshana. "Beyond Oedipus: The Specimen Story of Psychoanalysis." *MLN* 98, no. 5 (December 1, 1983): 1021–53.

Fenves, Peter. *The Messianic Reduction: Walter Benjamin and the Shape of Time*. Stanford, CA: Stanford University Press, 2011.

Fine, Ben. "Development as Zombieconomics in the Age of Neoliberalism." *Third World Quarterly* 30, no. 5 (2009): 885–904.

Fine, Ben, and Dimitris Milonakis. *From Economics Imperialism to Freakonomics: The Shifting Boundaries between Economics and Other Social Sciences*. New York: Routledge, 2009.

Fine, Robert, Richard Kinsey, John Lea, and Jock Young, eds. *Capitalism and the Rule of Law: From Deviancy Theory to Marxism*. London: Hutchinson, 1979.

Fitzpatrick, Peter. *Modernism and the Grounds of Law*. Cambridge Studies in Law and Society. Cambridge: Cambridge University Press, 2001.

Fitzpatrick, Peter. *The Mythology of Modern Law*. London: Routledge, 1992.

Fodor, Jerry. "Fire the Press Secretary." *London Review of Books*, April 28, 2011, 24–25.

Foucault, Michel. *The Archaeology of Knowledge*. New York: Pantheon, 1972.

Foucault, Michel. *The Birth of Biopolitics: Lectures at the Collège de France, 1978–79*. Houndmills, UK: Palgrave Macmillan, 2008.

Foucault, Michel. "The Confession of the Flesh." In Michel Foucault, *Power/Knowledge: Selected Writings and Other Interviews 1972–1977*, 194–228. New York: Pantheon, 1980.

Foucault, Michel. *L'herméneutique du sujet: Cours au Collège de France (1981–1982)*. Édition établie sous la direction de François Ewald et Alessandro Fontana, par Frédéric Gross (Coll. Hautes Études). Paris: Seuil/Gallimard, 2001.

Foucault, Michel. *The History of Sexuality: An Introduction*. New York: Vintage, 1990.

Foucault, Michel. *The Order of Things: An Archaeology of the Human Sciences*. London: Routledge, 2002.

Foucault, Michel. *Power/Knowledge: Selected Writings and Other Interviews 1972–1977*. New York: Pantheon, 1980.

Foucault, Michel. *Security, Territory, Population: Lectures at the Collège de France, 1977–78*. Houndmills, UK: Palgrave Macmillan, 2007.

Foucault, Michel. *"Society Must Be Defended": Lectures at the Collège de France, 1975–76*. 1st ed. New York: Saint Martin's Press, 2003.

Foucault, Michel. *Le souci de soi*. Vol. 3 of *Histoire de la sexualité*. Paris: Gallimard, 1984.
Foucault, Michel. "Les techniques de soi." In Michel Foucault, *Dits et écrits*, vol. 4, 783–813. Paris: Gallimard, 1988.
Foucault, Michel. *Technologies of the Self: A Seminar with Michel Foucault*. Amherst: University of Massachusetts Press, 1988.
Foucault, Michel. "Truth and Power." In *Power/Knowledge: Selected Writings and Other Interviews 1972–1977*, 109–33. New York: Pantheon, 1980.
Foucault, Michel, and Maurice Blanchot. *Maurice Blanchot: The Thought from Outside*. Translated by Brian Massumi and Jeffrey Mehlman. New York: Zone Books, 1987.
Franke, Katherine M. "The Domesticated Liberty of Lawrence v. Texas." *Columbia Law Review* 104 (2004): 1399–426.
Franklin, Sarah. *Dolly Mixtures: The Remaking of Genealogy*. Durham, NC: Duke University Press, 2007.
Freud, Sigmund. "Beyond the Pleasure Principle." In *The Standard Edition of the Complete Psychological Works of Sigmund Freud*, edited by James Strachey, vol. 18. London: Verso, 2001.
Freud, Sigmund. "Inhibitions, Symptoms and Anxiety." In *The Standard Edition of the Complete Psychological Works of Sigmund Freud*, edited by James Strachey, vol. 20. London: Verso, 2001.
Freud, Sigmund. *Three Contributions to the Theory of Sex*. Translated by A. A. Brill. Reprint, Eastford, CT: Martino Fine Books, 2011.
Friday, Chris. *Lelooska: The Life of a Northwest Coast Artist*. Seattle: University of Washington Press, 2003.
Galloway, Alexander. "Black Box, Black Bloc." In *Communization and Its Discontents: Contestation, Critique, and Contemporary Struggles*, edited by Benjamin Noys, 237–52. New York: Minor Compositions, 2012.
Galloway, Alexander R. "Catherine Malabou, or The Commerce in Being." French Theory Today pamphlet series. Accessed June 22, 2012. http://cultureandcommunication.org/galloway/FTT/.
Galloway, Alexander R. "The Poverty of Philosophy: Realism and Post-Fordism." *Critical Inquiry* 39, no. 2 (January 1, 2013): 347–66.
Galloway, Alexander R. *Protocol: How Control Exists after Decentralization*, 74–75. Cambridge, MA: MIT Press, 2004.
Galloway, Alexander R., and Eugene Thacker. *The Exploit: A Theory of Networks*. Minneapolis: University of Minnesota Press, 2007.
Gasché, Rodolphe. *The Idea of Form: Rethinking Kant's Aesthetics*. Stanford, CA: Stanford University Press, 2003.
Glimcher, Paul W. *Foundations of Neuroeconomic Analysis*. 1st ed. New York: Oxford University Press, 2010.

Goldberg-Hiller, Jonathan. *The Limits to Union: Same-Sex Marriage and the Politics of Civil Rights*. Ann Arbor: University of Michigan Press, 2004.

Goldberg-Hiller, Jonathan. "Reconciliation and Plasticity in a Postcolonial Hawai'i." *Law, Culture and the Humanities*, June 30, 2011.

Goldberg-Hiller, Jonathan, and Noenoe Silva. "Sharks and Pigs: Animating Hawaiian Sovereignty against the Anthropological Machine." *South Atlantic Quarterly* 110, no. 2 (2011): 429–46.

Goldschmit, Marc. "Cosmopolitique du marrane absolu." *Sens-Public* (2007). Accessed July 21, 2014. http://sens-public.org/spip.php?article469.

Goodrich, Peter. *Law in the Courts of Love: Literature and Other Minor Jurisprudences*. London: Routledge, 1996.

Goodyear-Kaopua, N. "Kuleana Lahui: Collective Responsibility for Hawaiian Nationhood in Activists' Praxis." *Affinities: A Journal of Radical Theory, Culture, and Action* 5, no. 1 (2011).

Gorman, James. "The Snails of War, and Other Robotics Experiments." *New York Times*, Science, March 20, 2012. Accessed March 20, 2012. www.nytimes.com/2012/03/21/science/the-snails-of-war-and-other-robotics-experiments.html.

Gould, Stephen Jay. "An Evolutionary Perspective on Strengths, Fallacies, and Confusions in the Concept of Native Plants." *Nature and Ideology: Natural Garden Design in the Twentieth Century* 18 (1997): 11–19.

Gould, Stephen Jay. *The Mismeasure of Man*. New York: Norton, 1996.

Gould, Stephen Jay. *Ontogeny and Phylogeny*. Cambridge, MA: Belknap Press / Harvard University Press, 1977.

Greenberg, Polly. *The Devil Has Slippery Shoes: A Biased Biography of the Child Development Group of Mississippi*. London: Macmillan, 1969.

Groh, Claudia, and Ian A. Meinertzhagen. "Brain Plasticity in Diptera and Hymenoptera." *Frontiers in Bioscience (scholar edition)* 2 (2010): 268–88.

Grove, Jairus Victor. "Must We Persist to Continue? William Connolly's Critical Responsiveness beyond the Limits of the Human Species." In *Democracy and Pluralism: The Political Thought of William E. Connolly*, edited by William E. Connolly and Alan Finlayson. London: Routledge, 2010.

Habermas, Jürgen. *The Future of Human Nature*. Trans. Hella Beister and William Rehg. Cambridge: Polity Press, 2003.

Haeckel, Ernst Heinrich Philipp August. *The Evolution of Man: A Popular Exposition of the Principal Points of Human Ontogeny and Phylogeny*. New York: D. Appleton, 1903.

Halberstam, J. "What's That Smell? Queer Temporalities and Subcultural Lives." *International Journal of Cultural Studies* 6, no. 3 (2003): 313–33.

Haldar, Piyel. *Law, Orientalism and Postcolonialism: The Jurisdiction of the Lotus-Eaters*. 1st ed. Abingdon, UK: Routledge-Cavendish, 2008.

Hall, Brian K. "Organic Selection: Proximate Environmental Effects on the Evolution of Morphology and Behaviour." *Biology and Philosophy* 16, no. 2 (2001): 215–37.

Hamacher, Werner. "Guilt History: Benjamin's Sketch 'Capitalism as Religion.'" Translated by Kirk Wetters. *Diacritics* 32, no. 3 (2005): 81–106.

Haraway, Donna. "Encounters with Companion Species: Entangling Dogs, Baboons, Philosophers, and Biologists." *Configurations* 14, no. 1 (2006): 97–114.

Haraway, Donna. *Simian, Cyborgs, and Women: The Reinvention of Nature*. New York: Routledge, 1991.

Haraway, Donna. *When Species Meet*. Minneapolis: University of Minnesota Press, 2008.

Harris, Verne. *Archives and Justice: A South African Perspective*. Chicago: Society of American Archivists, 2007.

Harvey, David. *Cosmopolitanism and the Geographies of Freedom*. New York: Columbia University Press, 2009.

Hawaii v. Office of Hawaiian Affairs. 129 S. Ct. 1436 (2009).

Hegel, Georg Wilhelm Friedrich. *Elements of the Philosophy of Right*. Edited by Allen W. Wood, Translated by Hugh Barr Nisbet. Cambridge: Cambridge University Press, 1991.

Heidegger, Martin. "Letter on Humanism." In *Basic Writings: Revised and Expanded*, 213–66. New York: HarperCollins, 1993.

Heidegger, Martin. *Nietzsche*. Vols. 1 and 2. Translated by David Farrell Krell. San Francisco: Harper, 1991.

Heidegger, Martin. "Why Poets?" In Martin Heidegger, *Off the Beaten Track*, 200–41. Cambridge: Cambridge University Press, 2002.

Helmreich, Stefan. "How Scientists Think—about 'Natives,' for Example: A Problem of Taxonomy among Biologists of Alien Species in Hawaii." *Journal of the Royal Anthropological Institute* 11, no. 1 (2005): 107–28.

Hennessy, Rosemary. *Profit and Pleasure: Sexual Identities in Late Capitalism*. New York: Routledge, 2000.

Herman, Didi. *The Antigay Agenda: Orthodox Vision and the Christian Right*. Chicago: University of Chicago Press, 1997.

Hobbes, Thomas. *Leviathan*. Edited by J. C. A. Gaskin. Oxford: Oxford University Press, 1996.

Holliday, Robin. "The Inheritance of Epigenetic Defects." *Science* 238, no. 4824 (1987): 163–70.

Horn, Tammy. *Bees in America: How the Honey Bee Shaped a Nation*. Lexington: University Press of Kentucky, 2005.

Hunter, Tera. "Putting an Antebellum Myth to Rest." *New York Times*, August 2, 2011.

Hussain, Nasser. "Beyond Norm and Exception: Guantánamo." *Critical Inquiry* 33, no. 4 (2007): 734–53.

Irigaray, Luce. *The Forgetting of Air in Martin Heidegger*. Austin: University of Texas Press, 1999.
Jablonka, Eva, and Marion J. Lamb. *Evolution in Four Dimensions: Genetic, Epigenetic, Behavioral, and Symbolic Variation in the History of Life*. Cambridge, MA: MIT Press, 2005.
Jacob, François. *The Logic of Life: A History of Heredity*. New York: Pantheon, 1973.
Jameson, Fredric. "Imaginary and Symbolic in Lacan: Marxism, Psychoanalytic Criticism, and the Problem of the Subject." *Yale French Studies*, nos. 55–56 (January 1, 1977): 338–95.
Jameson, Fredric. *Valences of the Dialectic*. London: Verso, 2010.
Johnston, Adrian. "The Weakness of Nature: Hegel, Freud, Lacan, and Negativity Materialized." In *Hegel and the Infinite: Religion, Politics, and Dialectic*, ed. Slavoj Žižek, Clayton Crockett, and Creston Davis, 159–80. New York: Columbia University Press, 2011.
Kafka, Franz. *The Metamorphosis, In the Penal Colony, and Other Stories*. Translated by Willa Muir and Edwin Muir. New York: Schocken, 1995.
Kameʻeleihiwa, Lilikalā, trans. *He Moʻolelo Kaʻao O Kamapuaʻa* (A Legendary Tradition of Kamapuaʻa, the Hawaiian Pig-God). Annotated Translation of a Hawaiian Epic, from *Ka Leo O Ka Lāhui*, June 22, 1891–July 23, 1891. Honolulu: Bishop Museum Press, 1996.
Kant, Immanuel. *Anthropology from a Pragmatic Point of View*. Trans. and ed. Robert B. Louden. New York: Cambridge University Press, 2006.
Kant, Immanuel. *The Critique of Judgement*. Oxford: Clarendon Press, 1952.
Kant, Immanuel. *Critique of Pure Reason*. New York: Saint Martin's Press, 1929.
Kant, Immanuel. *On Education*. Mineola, NY: Dover, 2012. Accessed June 29, 2014.
Kant, Immanuel. *Was ist Aufklärung? Ausgewählte kleine Schriften*, vol. 512. Hamburg: Meiner Verlag, 1999.
Kantorowicz, Ernst Hartwig. *The King's Two Bodies: A Study in Mediaeval Political Theology*. Princeton, NJ: Princeton University Press, 1957.
Kauanui, J. Kēhaulani. *Hawaiian Blood: Colonialism and the Politics of Sovereignty and Indigeneity*. Durham, NC: Duke University Press, 2008.
Kay, Lily E. *Who Wrote the Book of Life? A History of the Genetic Code*. Stanford, CA: Stanford University Press, 2000.
Kazanjian, David. *The Colonizing Trick: National Culture and Imperial Citizenship in Early America*. Minneapolis: University of Minnesota Press, 2004.
Keahiolalo-Karasuda, RaeDeen. "The Colonial Carceral and Prison Politics in Hawaiʻi." PhD diss., University of Hawaiʻi at Mānoa, 2008.
Keller, Evelyn Fox. *The Century of the Gene*. Cambridge, MA: Harvard University Press. 2002.

Kincaid, Jamaica. "The Little Revenge from the Periphery." *Transition*, no. 73 (1997): 68–73.

Kittler, Friedrich. *Gramophone, Film, Typewriter*. Translated by Geoffrey Winthrop-Young and Michael Wutz. 1st ed. Stanford, CA: Stanford University Press, 1999.

Kittler, Friedrich. "Towards an Ontology of Media." *Theory, Culture and Society* 26, nos. 2–3 (2009): 23–31.

Klopotek, Brian. *Recognition Odysseys: Indigeneity, Race, and Federal Tribal Recognition Policy in Three Louisiana Indian Communities*. Durham, NC: Duke University Press, 2011.

Kosek, Jake. "Ecologies of Empire: On the New Uses of the Honeybee." *Cultural Anthropology* 25, no. 4 (2010): 650–78.

Kurzban, Robert. *Why Everyone (Else) Is a Hypocrite: Evolution and the Modular Mind*. Princeton, NJ: Princeton University Press, 2011.

Kurzweil, Ray. *The Singularity Is Near: When Humans Transcend Biology*. New York: Penguin, 2005.

Kwinter, Sanford. "Notes on the Third Ecology." In *Ecological Urbanism*, edited by Mohsen Mostafavi and Gareth Doherty, 94–105. Zurich, Switzerland: Lars Muller, 2010.

Lacan, Jacques. *The Other Side of Psychoanalysis*. Vol. 17. New York: Norton, 2007.

Lacan, Jacques, and Dennis Porter. *The Ethics of Psychoanalysis, 1959–1960*. New York: Norton, 1997.

Lane, Robert C., and Saralea E. Chazan. "Symbols of Terror: The Witch/Vampire, the Spider, and the Shark." *Psychoanalytic Psychology* 6, no. 3 (1989): 325–41.

Lawrence, Charles, III. "The Id, the Ego, and Equal Protection: Reckoning with Unconscious Racism." *Stanford Law Review* 39 (1987): 317.

Lecourt, Dominique. "Georges Canguilhem on the Question of the Individual." *Economy and Society* 27, no. 2–3 (1998): 217–24.

Levander, Caroline. *Cradle of Liberty: Race, the Child, and National Belonging from Thomas Jefferson to W. E. B. DuBois*. Durham, NC: Duke University Press, 2006.

Lévi-Strauss, Claude. "Anthropology: Its Achievements and Future." *Current Anthropology* 7, no. 2 (April 1, 1966): 124–27.

Lévi-Strauss, Claude. "Introduction a l'oeuvre de Marcel Mauss." In Marcel Mauss, *Sociologie et Anthropologie*. Paris: Presses Universitaires de France, 1966, 9–52.

Lévi-Strauss, Claude. *Introduction to the Work of Marcel Mauss*. London: Routledge and Kegan Paul, 1987.

Lévi-Strauss, Claude. *The Savage Mind*. Chicago: University of Chicago Press, 1966.

Lévi-Strauss, Claude. *The Way of the Masks*. Seattle: University of Washington Press, 1988.

Leys, Ruth. "The Turn to Affect: A Critique." *Critical Inquiry* 37, no. 3 (March 2011): 434–72.

Lindqvist, Sven, and Joan Tate. *Exterminate the Brutes*. London: Granta, 1996.

Livingston, J., and J. K. Puar. "Interspecies." *Social Text* 29, no. 1, 106 (Spring 2011): 3.

Lockwood, Jeffrey A. *Six-Legged Soldiers: Using Insects as Weapons of War*. Oxford: Oxford University Press, 2008.

Loizidou, Elena. *Judith Butler: Ethics, Law, Politics*. Abingdon, UK: Routledge-Cavendish, 2007.

Lorimer, Jamie. "Nonhuman Charisma." *Environment and Planning D* 25, no. 5 (2007): 911.

Luhmann, Niklas. "On the Cognitive Program of Constructivism and a Reality That Remains Unknown," in *Theories of Distinction: Redescribing the Descriptions of Modernity*, ed. William Rasch. Stanford, CA: Stanford University Press, 2002.

Luhmann, Niklas. *The Reality of the Mass Media*. Trans. Kathleen Cross. Stanford, CA: Stanford University Press, 2000.

Luhmann, Niklas. *Social Systems*. Stanford, CA: Stanford University Press, 1995.

Luhmann, Niklas. *Theories of Distinction: Redescribing the Descriptions of Modernity*. Ed. William Rasch. Stanford, CA: Stanford University Press, 2002.

Lyotard, Jean-François. *Discourse, Figure*. Translated by Antony Hudek and Mary Lydon. Minneapolis: University of Minnesota Press, 2010.

Mackey, Nathaniel. *From a Broken Bottle Traces of Perfume Still Emanate*. New York: New Directions, 2010.

Mahoney, Daniel J. *The Liberal Political Science of Raymond Aron: A Critical Introduction*. New York: Rowman and Littlefield, 1992.

Malabou, Catherine. "Catherine Malabou—What Is a Psychic Event? Freud and Contemporary Neurology on Trauma/Backdoor Broadcasting Company." Accessed February 23, 2014. http://backdoorbroadcasting.net/2010/10/catherine-malabou-what-is-a-psychic-event-freud-and-contemporary-neurology-on-trauma/.

Malabou, Catherine. *Le change Heidegger: Du fantastique en philosophie*. Paris: Léo Scheer, 2004.

Malabou, Catherine. *Changer de différence: Le féminin et la question philosophique*. Galilée, 2009.

Malabou, Catherine. *Changing Difference*. Hoboken, NJ: Wiley, 2011.

Malabou, Catherine. *Counterpath: Traveling with Jacques Derrida*. Cultural Memory in the Present. Stanford, CA: Stanford University Press, 2004.

Malabou, Catherine. "The Eternal Return and the Phantom of Difference." *Parrhesia* 10 (2010): 21–29.

Malabou, Catherine. "An Eye at the Edge of Discourse." *Communication Theory* 17, no. 1 (2007): 16–25.

Malabou, Catherine. "Following Generation." Translated by S. Porzak. *Qui Parle: Critical Humanities and Social Sciences* 20, no. 2 (2012): 19–33.

Malabou, Catherine. *The Future of Hegel: Plasticity, Temporality and Dialectic.* New York: Routledge, 2005.

Malabou, Catherine. *The Heidegger Change: On the Fantastic in Philosophy.* Trans. Peter Skafish. Albany: SUNY Press, 2011.

Malabou, Catherine. "History and the Process of Mourning in Hegel and Freud." *Radical Philosophy* 106 (Mar.–Apr. 2001): 15–20.

Malabou, Catherine. "How Is Subjectivity Undergoing Deconstruction Today? Philosophy, Auto-Hetero-Affection, and Neurobiological Emotion." *Qui Parle: Critical Humanities and Social Sciences* 17 (2009): 111–22.

Malabou, Catherine. *Jacques Derrida: La contre-allée.* Paris: Quinzaine littéraire, 1999.

Malabou, Catherine. *The New Wounded: From Neurosis to Brain Damage.* New York: Fordham University Press, 2012.

Malabou, Catherine. *Les nouveaux blessés: De Freud à la neurologie, penser les traumatismes contemporains.* Paris: Bayard, 2007.

Malabou, Catherine. *Ontology of the Accident: An Essay on Destructive Plasticity.* Translated by Carolyn Shread. Cambridge: Polity Press, 2012.

Malabou, Catherine. *Plasticité.* Paris: Léo Scheer, 2000.

Malabou, Catherine. "Plasticity and Elasticity in Freud's *Beyond the Pleasure Principle*." *Diacritics* 37, no. 4 (2007): 78–86.

Malabou, Catherine. *Plasticity at the Dusk of Writing: Dialectic, Destruction, Deconstruction.* New York: Columbia University Press, 2010.

Malabou, Catherine. *Que faire de notre cerveau?* 2nd ed. Montrouge: Bayard, 2011.

Malabou, Catherine. "Les régénérés: Cellules souches, thérapie génique, clonage." *Critique* 62, nos. 709–710 (2006): 529–40.

Malabou, Catherine. *What Should We Do with Our Brain?* 1st ed. New York: Fordham University Press, 2008. Accessed June 28, 2014.

Malabou, Catherine. "Who's Afraid of Hegelian Wolves?" In *Deleuze: A Critical Reader*, 114–38, edited by Paul Patton. Oxford: Basil Blackwell, 1996.

Malabou, C., and J. Butler. "You Be My Body for Me: Body, Shape, and Plasticity in Hegel's *Phenomenology of Spirit*." In *A Companion to Hegel*, ed. Stephen Houlgate and Michael Bauer. New York: Wiley-Blackwell, 2011, 611–40.

Malabou, C., and Jacques Derrida. *La contre-allée.* Paris: Quinzaine Littéraire, 1999.

Mamdani, M. *When Victims Become Killers: Colonialism, Nativism, and the Genocide in Rwanda.* Princeton, NJ: Princeton University Press, 2002.

Marder, Michael. *Plant-Thinking: A Philosophy of Vegetal Life.* New York: Columbia University Press, 2013.

Markell, Patchen. *Bound by Recognition*. Princeton, NJ: Princeton University Press, 2003.
Martin, Luther H., Huck Gutman, and Patrick H. Hutton, eds. *Technologies of the Self: A Seminar with Michel Foucault*. Amherst: University Press of Massachusetts, 1988.
Martin, Rux. "Truth, Power, Self: An Interview with Michel Foucault, October 25, 1982." In *Technologies of the Self: A Seminar with Michel Foucault*, ed. Luther H. Martin, Huck Gutman, and Patrick H. Hutton, 10. Amherst: University of Massachusetts Press, 1988.
Martinon, Jean-Paul. *On Futurity: Malabou, Nancy and Derrida*. Houndmills, UK: Palgrave Macmillan, 2007.
Marx, Karl. *Capital*. Vol. 1: *A Critique of Political Economy*. Harmondsworth, UK: Penguin Classics, 1992.
Marx, Karl. *The Communist Manifesto*. Chicago: Regnery, 1954.
Marx, Karl. "Concerning Feuerbach." In *Early Writings [of] Karl Marx*, 421–23. Harmondsworth, UK: Penguin, 1975.
Marx, Karl. *Critique of Hegel's "Philosophy of Right."* Ed. Joseph O'Malley. Cambridge: Cambridge University Press, 1977.
Marx, Karl. *Early Writings*. New York: McGraw-Hill, 1964.
Marx, Karl. *The Eighteenth Brumaire of Louis Bonaparte*. New York: International, 1963.
Marx, Karl. *Grundrisse: Foundations of the Critique of Political Economy*. Harmondsworth, UK: Penguin Classics, 1993.
Marx, Karl, and Friedrich Engels. "Economic and Philosophic Manuscripts of 1844." In *The Marx-Engels Reader*, ed. Robert C. Tucker. New York: Norton, 1972.
Marx, Karl, and Friedrich Engels. *Karl Marx, Frederick Engels: Collected Works*, vol. 5. New York: International, 1975.
Masri, Mazen. "Love Suspended: Demography, Comparative Law and Palestinian Couples in the Israeli Supreme Court." *Social and Legal Studies* 22, no. 3 (2013): 309–34.
Massumi, B. "National Enterprise Emergency Steps toward an Ecology of Powers." *Theory, Culture and Society* 26, no. 6 (2009): 153–85.
Matsuda, Mari J. *Where Is Your Body? and Other Essays on Race, Gender, and the Law*. Boston: Beacon Press, 1996.
Maturana, Humberto, and Jorge Mpodozis. *De l'origine des espèces par voie de la dérive naturelle*. Lyon: Presses Universitaires de Lyon, 1999.
Maturana, Humberto, and Jorge Mpodozis. "El origen de las especies por medio de la deriva natural." *Revista Chilena de Historia Natural* 73, no. 2 (2000): 261–310.
Maturana, Humberto R., and Francisco J. Varela. *Autopoiesis and Cognition: The Realization of the Living*. Dordrecht: Reidel, 1980.

Maturana, Humberto R., and Francisco J. Varela. *The Tree of Knowledge: The Biological Roots of Human Understanding.* Boston: New Science Library / Shambhala, 1987.

Mavhunga, C. C. "Vermin Beings: On Pestiferous Animals and Human Game." *Social Text* 29, no. 1, 106 (April 2011): 151–76.

Mawani, Renisa. *Colonial Proximities: Crossracial Encounters and Juridical Truths in British Columbia, 1871–1921.* Vancouver: University of British Columbia Press, 2009.

Mbembe, A. "Necropolitics." *Public Culture* 15, no. 1 (2003): 11.

Mbembe, Joseph-Achille. *On the Postcolony.* Berkeley: University of California Press, 2001.

McCann, Michael. *Rights at Work: Pay Equity Reform and the Politics of Legal Mobilization.* Chicago: University of Chicago Press, 1994.

Medina, Eden. *Cybernetic Revolutionaries.* Cambridge, MA: MIT Press, 2011.

Merry, Sally Engle. *Colonizing Hawai'i: The Cultural Power of Law.* Princeton, NJ: Princeton University Press, 2000.

Milmo, Cahal. "Fury at DNA Pioneer's Theory: Africans Are Less Intelligent than Westerners." *The Independent.* Accessed February 25, 2014. www.independent.co.uk/news/science/fury-at-dna-pioneers-theory-africans-are-less-intelligent-than-westerners-394898.html.

Milner, Neal, and Jonathan Goldberg-Hiller. "Feeble Echoes of the Heart: A Postcolonial Legal Struggle in Hawai'i." *Law, Culture and the Humanities* 4, no. 2 (2008): 224–47.

Mirowski, Philip. *Science-Mart: The Privatization of American Science.* Cambridge, MA: Harvard University Press, 2011.

Mitchell, Timothy. *Rule of Experts: Egypt, Techno-Politics, Modernity.* Berkeley: University of California Press, 2005.

Mitchell v. Minister of National Revenue. 1 S.C.R. (Canada) 911 (2001).

Mitropoulos, Angela. "Oikopolitics, and Storms." *Global South* 3, no. 1 (2009): 66–82.

Moczek, Armin P. "Phenotypic Plasticity and Diversity in Insects." *Philosophical Transactions of the Royal Society B: Biological Sciences* 365, no. 1540 (2010): 593–603.

Moeller, Hans-Georg. *Luhmann Explained: From Souls to Systems.* Chicago: Open Court, 2006.

Montag, Warren. *Althusser and His Contemporaries: Philosophy's Perpetual War.* Durham, NC: Duke University Press, 2013.

Moreno, Jonathan D. *Brain Research and National Defense.* New York: Dana Press, 2006.

Moreno, Jonathan D. *Mind Wars: Brain Science and the Military in the Twenty-First Century.* New York: Bellevue Literary Press, 2012.

Moreton-Robinson, Aileen. "I Still Call Australia Home: Indigenous Belonging and Place in a White Postcolonizing Society." In *Uprootings/Regroundings: Questions of Home and Migration*, edited by Sara Ahmed, 23–40. 1st ed. New York: Berg, 2003.

Moretti, Franco. *Atlas of the European Novel: 1800–1900*. London: Verso, 1999.

Moten, Fred. Excerpt is from "Block Chapel." *Hambone* 20 (Fall 2012): 250–60.

Moten, Fred, and Stefano Harney. "Blackness and Governance." In *Beyond Biopolitics: Essays on the Governance of Life and Death*, edited by Patricia Ticineto Clough and Craig Willse, 351–62. Durham, NC: Duke University Press, 2011, 351–62.

Nancy, Jean-Luc. "Introduction." In *Who Comes after the Subject?*, ed. Eduardo Cadava, Peter Connor, and Jean-Luc Nancy, 1–8. London: Routledge, 1991.

Negri, Antonio. "The Specter's Smile." In *Ghostly Demarcations: On Jacques Derrida's "Specters of Marx,"* edited by Michael Sprinker. London: Verso, 1999.

Nietzsche, Friedrich. *On the Genealogy of Morals and Ecce Homo*. Translated by Walter Kaufmann. New York: Vintage, 1989; Random House, 2010.

Nietzsche, Friedrich. *Thus Spoke Zarathustra: A Book for All and None*. Translated by Adrian del Caro. Cambridge: Cambridge University Press, 2006.

Niewöhner, Jörg. "Epigenetics: Embedded Bodies and the Molecularisation of Biography and Milieu." *BioSocieties* 6, no. 3 (2011): 279–98.

Nora, Pierre. *Les français d'Algérie*. Paris: Christian Bourgois, 2012.

Noys, Benjamin. *The Persistence of the Negative: A Critique of Contemporary Continental Theory*. Edinburgh: Edinburgh University Press, 2010.

Nylin, S., and K. Gotthard. "Plasticity in Life-History Traits." *Annual Review of Entomology* 43, no. 1 (1998): 63–83.

Oaknin, Marc-Alain. *The Burnt Book: Reading the Talmud*. Trans. Llewellyn Brown. Princeton, NJ: Princeton University Press, 1986.

O'Connell, Barry. "Introduction." In William Apess, *On Our Own Ground: The Complete Writings of William Apess, a Pequot*, xiii–lxxxi. Amherst: University of Massachusetts Press, 1992.

Ong, Aihwa. *Neoliberalism as Exception: Mutations in Citizenship and Sovereignty*. Durham, NC: Duke University Press, 2006.

O'Sullivan, Simon. *Art Encounters Deleuze and Guattari: Thought beyond Representation*. Houndmills, UK: Palgrave Macmillan, 2006.

Palmater, Pamela Doris. *Beyond Blood: Rethinking Indigenous Identity*. Saskatoon: Purich, 2011.

Panagia, Davide. *The Political Life of Sensation*. Durham, NC: Duke University Press, 2009.

Pandian, A. "Pastoral Power in the Postcolony: On the Biopolitics of the Criminal Animal in South India." *Cultural Anthropology* 23, no. 1 (2008): 85–117.

Papadopoulos, Dimitris. "The Imaginary of Plasticity: Neural Embodiment, Epigenetics and Ecomorphs." *Sociological Review* 59, no. 3 (2011): 432–56.

Pashukanis, Evgeni i Bronislavovich. *Law and Marxism: A General Theory.* Translated by C. J. Arthur. London: Ink Links, 1978.

Pickering, Andrew. *The Cybernetic Brain: Sketches of Another Future.* Chicago: University of Chicago Press, 2010.

Pisters, Patricia. "Plasticity and the Neuro-Image." Accessed February 24, 2014. www.patriciapisters.com/blog/events/79-plasticity-and-the-neuro-image.

Pitts-Taylor, Victoria. "The Plastic Brain: Neoliberalism and the Neuronal Self." *Health* 14, no. 6 (November 1, 2010): 635–52.

Povinelli, Elizabeth A. *The Cunning of Recognition: Indigenous Alterities and the Making of Australian Multiculturalism.* Durham, NC: Duke University Press, 2002.

Povinelli, Elizabeth A. *Economies of Abandonment: Social Belonging and Endurance in Late Liberalism.* Durham, NC: Duke University Press, 2011.

Pratt, Mary Louise. *Imperial Eyes: Travel Writing and Transculturation.* London; New York: Routledge, 1992.

Proctor, Hannah. "Neuronal Ideologies: Catherine Malabou in Light of A. R. Luria." *Dandelion* 2, no. 1 (2011).

Purcell, Edward A., Jr. *The Crisis of Democratic Theory: Scientific Naturalism and the Problem of Value.* Lexington: University Press of Kentucky, 1973.

Rabinow, Paul, and Nikolas Rose. "Biopower Today." *BioSocieties* 1, no. 2 (2006): 195.

Race: The Floating Signifier. Film. Dir. Sut Jhally. Northampton, MA: Media Education Foundation, 1997. Not released in video form.

Raffles, Hugh. *Insectopedia.* New York: Random House, 2010.

Rancière, Jacques. "Afterword / The Method of Equality: An Answer to Some Questions." In *Jacques Rancière: History, Politics, Aesthetics*, edited by Gabriel Rockhill and Philip Watts, 273–88. Durham, NC: Duke University Press, 2009.

Rancière, Jacques. *Disagreement: Politics and Philosophy.* Minneapolis: University of Minnesota Press, 1999.

Rand, Sebastian. "Organism, Normativity, Plasticity: Canguilhem, Kant, Malabou." *Continental Philosophy Review* 44, no. 4 (October 29, 2011): 341–57.

Razack, Sherene H. "Gendered Racial Violence and Spatialized Justice: The Murder of Pamela George." *Canadian Journal of Law and Society* 15 (2000): 91.

Razack, Sherene H. "Making Canada White: Law and the Policing of Bodies of Colour in the 1990s." *Canadian Journal of Law and Society* 14 (1999): 159.

Rheinberger, Hans-Jorg. *Toward a History of Epistemic Things: Synthesizing Proteins in the Test Tube (Writing Science).* Stanford, CA: Stanford University Press, 1997.

Rice v. Cayetano. 528 U.S. 495 (2000).

Ricoeur, Paul. *Time and Narrative.* Vol. 3. Chicago: University of Chicago Press, 2003.

Rifkin, Mark. "Indigenizing Agamben: Rethinking Sovereignty in Light of the 'Peculiar' Status of Native Peoples." *Cultural Critique* 73 (2009): 88–124.

Rilke, Rainer Maria. *Rilke's Book of Hours: Love Poems to God.* Harmondsworth, UK: Penguin, 2005.

Ritte, Walter, and Bill Freese. "Haloa." *Seedling,* October 2006, 11–14.

Robinson, Gene E., and Fred C. Dyer. "Plasticity of Spatial Memory in Honey Bees: Reorientation following Colony Fission." *Animal Behaviour* 46, no. 2 (1993): 311–20.

Ronell, Avital. *The Test Drive.* Chicago: University of Illinois Press, 2005.

Rose, Nikolas. "The Politics of Life Itself." *Theory, Culture and Society* 18, no. 6 (2001): 1–30.

Rose, Nikolas. *The Politics of Life Itself: Biomedicine, Power, and Subjectivity in the Twenty-First Century.* Princeton, NJ: Princeton University Press, 2006.

Rose, Nikolas S., and Joelle M. Abi-Rached. *Neuro: The New Brain Sciences and the Management of the Mind.* Princeton, NJ: Princeton University Press, 2013.

Ross, Luana. *Inventing the Savage: The Social Construction of Native American Criminality.* Austin: University of Texas Press, 1998.

Saghafi, Kas. "Derrida, Blanchot, and 'Living Death.'" *Derrida Seminar Translation Project,* 2010. Accessed February 24, 2014. http://derridaseminars.org/workshops.html.

Said, Edward W. "The Totalitarianism of Mind: Review of Claude Lévi-Strauss, *The Savage Mind.*" *Kenyon Review* 29, no. 2 (1967): 256–68.

Santner, Eric. *The Royal Remains: The People's Two Bodies and the Endgames of Sovereignty.* Chicago: University of Chicago Press, 2011.

Sartre, Jean-Paul. *Existentialism Is a Humanism.* New Haven, CT: Yale University Press, 2007.

Sassen, Saskia. *The De-facto Transnationalizing of Immigration Policy.* Jean Monnet Chair Papers, 35. Robert Schuman Centre at the European University Institute, Florence, 1996.

Schlais, Gregory K. "The Patenting of Sacred Biological Resources—the Taro Patent Controversy in Hawai'i: A Soft Law Proposal." *University of Hawai'i Law Review* 29 (2007): 581.

Schürmann, Reiner. *Heidegger on Being and Acting: From Principles to Anarchy.* Studies in Phenomenology and Existential Philosophy. Bloomington: Indiana University Press, 1987.

Schwartz, Jeffrey M., and Sharon Begley. *The Mind and the Brain: Neuroplasticity and the Power of Mental Force.* New York: HarperCollins, 2003.

Shapiro, Michael J. *Deforming American Political Thought: Ethnicity, Facticity, and Genre.* Lexington: University Press of Kentucky, 2006.

Shapiro, Michael J. "Slow Looking: The Ethics and Politics of Aesthetics." *Millennium—Journal of International Studies* 37, no. 1 (2008): 181–97.

Shapiro, Michael J. *The Time of the City: Politics, Philosophy and Genre*. London: Taylor and Francis, 2010.

Shaw, Ronald, Ian Graham, and Majed Akhter. "The Unbearable Humanness of Drone Warfare in FATA, Pakistan." *Antipode* 44, no. 4 (2012): 1490–509.

Sherman, Daniel J. *French Primitivism and the Ends of Empire, 1945–1975*. Chicago: University of Chicago Press, 2011.

Shukin, Nicole. *Animal Capital: Rendering Life in Biopolitical Times*. Minneapolis: University of Minnesota Press, 2009.

Simondon, Gilbert. *Du mode d'existence des objets techniques*. Translated by John Hart and Yves Deforge. Paris: Aubier, 2001.

Simondon, Gilbert. *La individuación a la luz de las nociones de forma y de información*. Buenos Aires: Ediciones la Cebra y Editorial Cactus, 2009.

Smail, Daniel Lord. *On Deep History and the Brain*. Berkeley: University of California Press, 2008.

Sohn-Rethel, Alfred. *Intellectual and Manual Labour: A Critique of Epistemology*. Atlantic Highlands, NJ: Humanities Press, 1978.

Spillers, Hortense J. "Mama's Baby, Papa's Maybe: An American Grammar Book." *Diacritics* (1987): 65–81.

Sprinker, Michael, ed. *Ghostly Demarcations: On Jacques Derrida's "Specters of Marx."* London: Verso, 1999.

Stoler, Ann Laura. *Race and the Education of Desire: Foucault's History of Sexuality and the Colonial Order of Things*. Durham, NC: Duke University Press, 1995.

Stora, Benjamin, and Thierry Leclère. *La guerre des mémoires: La France face à son passé colonial*. La Tour d'Aigues: Aube, 2007.

Strohman, Richard C. "Epigenesis and Complexity: The Coming Kuhnian Revolution in Biology." *Nature Biotechnology* 15 (1997): 194–200.

Stychin, Carl. *Law's Desire: Sexuality and the Limits of Justice*. London: Routledge, 1995.

Subramaniam, Banu. "The Aliens Have Landed! Reflections on the Rhetoric of Biological Invasions." *Meridians: Feminism, Race, Transnationalism* 2, no. 1 (2001): 26–40.

Sunder Rajan, Kaushik. *Biocapital: The Constitution of Postgenomic Life*. Durham, NC: Duke University Press, 2006.

Taylor, Charles. *Multiculturalism and "The Politics of Recognition": An Essay*. Ed. Amy Gutmann. Princeton, NJ: Princeton University Press, 1992.

Thacker, Eugene. *After Life*. Chicago: University of Chicago Press, 2010.

Thacker, Eugene. *In the Dust of This Planet*. Alresford, UK: Zero Books, 2011.

Thacker, Eugene. "The Shadows of Atheology Epidemics, Power and Life after Foucault." *Theory, Culture and Society* 26, no. 6 (2009): 134–52.

Thompson, E. P. *Whigs and Hunters: The Origin of the Black Act*. London: Allen Lane, 1975.
Trigger, David S. "Indigeneity, Ferality, and What 'Belongs' in the Australian Bush: Aboriginal Responses to 'Introduced' Animals and Plants in a Settler-Descendant Society." *Journal of the Royal Anthropological Institute* 14, no. 3 (2008): 628–46.
Tsirkas, Stratēs. *Drifting Cities*. New York: Knopf, 1974.
Tucker, Mark, and Duke Ellington. "Interview in Los Angeles: On *Jump for Joy*, Opera and Dissonance." In *The Duke Ellington Reader*, ed. Mark Tucker, 148–151. Oxford: Oxford University Press, 1993.
Uexküll, Jakob von. *Niegeschaute Welten: Die Umwelten meiner Freunde. Ein Erinnerungsbuch*. Berlin: S. Fischer, 1936.
"Unemployed Negativity: January 2011." Accessed February 24, 2014. www.unemployednegativity.com/2011_01_01_archive.html.
US Army. *Eyes of the Army: U.S. Army Roadmap for Unmanned Aircraft Systems—2010–2035*. Fort Rucker, AL: UAS Center of Excellence, 2010, 205. Accessed June 21, 2014. www.rucker.army.mil/usaace/uas/US%20Army%20 UAS%20RoadMap%202010%202035.pdf.
Vahanian, Noelle. "A Conversation with Catherine Malabou." *Journal for Cultural and Religious Theory* 9, no. 1 (2008): 1–13.
Waddington, Conrad H. "Epigenetics and Evolution." In *Evolution*, ed. R. Brown and J. F. Danieli, 186–199. Cambridge: Cambridge University Press, 1953.
Waddington, Conrad H. "The Epigenotype." *Endeavour* 1 (1942): 18–20.
Waddington, Conrad H. *An Introduction to Modern Genetics*. New York: Macmillan, 1939.
Wade, Nicholas. "The Dark Side of Oxytocin, the Hormone of Love: Ethnocentrism." *New York Times*, Science, January 10, 2011. Accessed November 7, 2013. www.nytimes.com/2011/01/11/science/11hormone.html.
Waldby, Catherine. *The Visible Human Project: Informatic Bodies and Posthuman Medicine*. 1st ed. New York: Routledge, 2000.
Walker, David. *Appeal*. New York: Hill and Wang, 1965.
Warner, Michael. *The Trouble with Normal: Sex, Politics and the Ethics of Queer Life*. New York: Free Press, 1999.
Watson, Sean. "The Neurobiology of Sorcery: Deleuze and Guattari's Brain." *Body and Society* 4, no. 4 (1998): 23–45.
Weber, Samuel. *Return to Freud: Jacques Lacan's Dislocation of Psychoanalysis*. Cambridge: Cambridge University Press, 1991.
Weizman, Eyal. *Hollow Land: Israel's Architecture of Occupation*. London: Verso, 2007.
Wenner, Adrian M. "Sound Production during the Waggle Dance of the Honey Bee." *Animal Behaviour* 10, no. 1 (1962): 79–95.

Wenner, Adrian M., and Dennis L. Johnson. "Simple Conditioning in Honey Bees." *Animal Behaviour* 14, no. 1 (1966): 149–55.

"What Is Epigenetics?" Accessed January 3, 2012. www.epigenetics.ch/citations.htm11.html.

White, Garry. "UN Food Advisor Says Let Them Eat Insects." *Telegraph.co.uk*, Commodities, 17, 43. Accessed July 21, 2014. ww.telegraph.co.uk/finance/commodities/8486704/UN-food-advisor-says-let-them-eat-insects.html.

White, H. V. *The Content of the Form: Narrative Discourse and Historical Representation.* Baltimore: Johns Hopkins University Press, 1990.

White, Morton G. "The Revolt against Formalism in American Social Thought of the Twentieth Century." *Journal of the History of Ideas* 8, no. 2 (April 1, 1947): 131–52.

Wiener, Norbert. *The Human Use of Human Beings: Cybernetics and Society.* New York: Da Capo Press, 1988.

Wilson, Edward O. *Nature Revealed: Selected Writings, 1949–2006.* Baltimore: Johns Hopkins University Press, 2006.

Winston, Mark L. *The Biology of the Honey Bee.* Cambridge, MA: Harvard University Press, 1987.

Winthrop-Young, Geoffrey. "Silicon Sociology; or, Two Kings on Hegel's Throne? Kittler, Luhmann, and the Posthuman Merger of German Media Theory." *Yale Journal of Criticism* 13, no. 2 (2000): 391–420.

Wolfe, Patrick. "Settler Colonialism and the Elimination of the Native." *Journal of Genocide Research* 8, no. 4 (2006): 387–409.

Wolfe, Patrick. *Settler Colonialism and the Transformation of Anthropology: The Politics and Poetics of an Ethnographic Event.* London: Continuum, 1999.

Žižek, Slavoj. "Bring Me My Philips Mental Jacket." *London Review of Books*, May 22, 2003. Accessed June 29, 2014. www.lrb.co.uk/v25/n10/slavoj-zizek/bring-me-my-philips-mental-jacket.

Žižek, Slavoj. *Living in the End Times.* London: Verso, 2011.

Žižek, Slavoj. *The Parallax View.* Cambridge, MA: MIT Press, 2006.

CONTRIBUTORS

BRENNA BHANDAR is Senior Lecturer in Equity and Trusts, School of Law, SOAS, University of London. She has published widely on theories of recognition, indigenous rights, property law, and settler colonialism. She is coeditor of a forthcoming special issue of *Feminist Legal Studies* entitled "Reflections on Dispossession."

JONATHAN GOLDBERG-HILLER is Professor of Political Science at the University of Hawai'i, where he teaches sociolegal theory. He is the author of *The Limits to Union: Same-Sex Marriage and the Politics of Civil Rights* (University of Michigan Press, 2004) and has published widely on sexual and indigenous rights. He is the former coeditor of *Law and Society Review*.

SILVANA CAROTENUTO is an associate professor at the University of Naples L'Orientale, Italy, where she has been the director of the Centre for Postcolonial Studies and teaches contemporary English literature. She has translated Hélène Cixous's *Three Steps on the Ladder of Writing* (Columbia University Press, 2000) into Italian. She is author of *Cleopatra's Language: Deconstructive Translations and Survivals* (Marietti, 2009) and many articles on postcolonial poetry, contemporary visual art, deconstruction, and *écriture feminine*.

JAIRUS VICTOR GROVE is Director of the University of Hawai'i Center for Futures Studies. His research focuses on the ecology and future of global warfare—in particular, the ways war continues to expand, bringing an ever-greater collection of participants and technologies into the gravitational pull of violent conflict.

CATHERINE KELLOGG is Associate Professor in the Department of Political Science, University of Alberta. She is the author of *Law's Trace: From Hegel to Derrida* (Routledge / Glasshouse Press, 2010). Her research engages in a conversation with contemporary thinkers on questions of democracy, justice, and sovereignty. She has published widely in the fields of political and legal theory, philosophy, and human rights.

CATHERINE MALABOU is Professor of Modern European Philosophy at the University of Kingston, London, and Professor at the European Graduate School, Leuk-Stadt, Switzerland. She is the author of twelve books, many translated into English, including *The Heidegger Change* (SUNY Press, 2011), *Changing Difference* (Wiley, 2011), *The New Wounded* (Fordham University Press, 2012), *Ontology of the Accident* (Polity Press, 2012), and *Self and Emotional Life* (Columbia University Press, 2013).

RENISA MAWANI is Associate Professor in the Department of Sociology, University of British Columbia Founding Chair of the Law and Society Minor Program at the University of British Columbia (2009/10). She is a sociolegal historian who works on the conjoined histories of Asian migration and settler colonialism. She is the author of *Colonial Proximities* (University of British Columbia Press, 2009).

FRED MOTEN is Professor of English at the University of California, Riverside. He is the author of *In the Break* (University of Minnesota Press), *Hughson's Tavern* (Leon Works), *B. Jenkins* (Duke University Press), *The Feel Trio* (Letter Machine Editions) and coauthor, with Stefano Harney, of *The Undercommons* (Minor Compositions/Autonomedia). His current projects include two critical texts, *consent not to be a single being* (forthcoming from Duke University Press) and *Animechanical Flesh*, which extend his study of black art and social life, and a new collection of poems, *The Little Edges*.

ALAIN POTTAGE is Professor of Law at the London School of Economics. His work focuses on historical and theoretical aspects of intellectual property law. His most recent book, written with Brad Sherman, is *Figures of Invention* (Oxford University Press, 2010). He is also editor, with Martha Mundy, of *Law, Anthropology and the Constitution of the Social* (Cambridge University Press, 2004). He has published widely in the fields of legal theory, property law, critical social theory, and law and anthropology.

ALBERTO TOSCANO is Reader in Critical Theory at the Department of Sociology, Goldsmiths, University of London. He is the author of *Fanaticism* (2010; translated into Korean, Chinese, French, Turkish, Spanish) and of the forthcoming *Cartographies of the Absolute* (2014), with Jeff Kinkle. He edits the

Italian list for Seagull Books (Calcutta), for which he has recently produced editions of Luigi Pintor, Franco Fortini (with a newly subtitled version of Straub-Huillet's *Fortini-Cani*), and Furio Jesi. He is also an editor of the journal *Historical Materialism*.

MICHAEL J. SHAPIRO is a Professor of Political Science at the University of Hawai'i at Mānoa. Among his publications are *The Time of the City* (Routledge, 2010) and *Studies in Trans-Disciplinary Method* (Routledge, 2012). His latest publication is *War Crimes* (Polity Press, 2014).

INDEX

Abrams, J. J., 233, 245
Abstraction, 12, 84, 93–98, 100–101, 107, 144
Adorno, Theodor, 93, 96
Agamben, Giorgio, 22, 28, 36, 41, 172, 181–82, 222, 298, 301; and bare life 23, 38–39, 280, 293; and biology, 38; and state of exception, 222; and symbolic, 40
Aletheia, 81, 82, 84, 90
Alexander, William P., 222, 301
Alterity, 4, 18, 27, 97, 103, 108, 136–38
Althusser, Louis, 13, 28, 47–58, 105–6, 218–19; 289–90, 301
Animal, 37–39, 62, 64, 65, 67, 77–78, 160–65, 177–80, 182, 198, 222–24, 226, 228, 231, 236, 244, 247, 293–94; and animalization, 172, 181–82, 222–23
Apess, William, 204, 301
Apollinaire, Guillaume, 6, 199
Archive, 16, 145, 189, 196, 198–203, 205–6, 246, 272, 276, 296; as open, 201; as plastic, 16, 202, 205
Arendt, Hannah, 269, 275
Aron, Raymond, 32, 301
Ashby, W. Ross, 241, 242, 244, 301
Aurelius, Marcus, 83
Autoaffection, 113, 118

Autoplasticity, 24, 76, 77, 80, 81, 86, 87
Autopoiesis, 24, 75, 77, 85–87

Babbage, Charles, 270
Bakhtin, Mikhail M., 16, 192–94, 195, 197, 301–2; and genre as plasticity, 193
Barthes, Roland, 159–62, 302
Bataille, George, 45, 152
Bateson, Gregory, 241
Baucom, Ian, 272, 276
Beer, Stafford, 241
Being, 97, 288–89
Bentham, Jeremy, 249
Benyus, Janine, 70
Bergson, Henri, 8, 162, 164–66, 177–80, 182, 302
Bernays, Edward, 256
Bernstein, Charles, 272
Biology, 3, 4, 6, 8, 10, 12, 38, 111, 292–94; and access to, 222; and autopoiesis, 24, 77; and accident, 129; and bare life, 39, 41, 282; as biological concept, 294; as biological life, 293; and biopolitics, 37–38, 171, 283, 293–94; and Canguilhem, 78; and capitalism, 104; and colonialism, 222; and control, 42; and determinism, 4, 45, 284, 294; and diversity, 227; and environment,

Biology (*continued*)
24, 80, 86; and essence, 14–15; and flesh, 282; and history, 25, 37–38, 44, 160, 162; and identity, 14, 43; as ideology, 8, 293; and law, 23, 38, 222; and Luhmann, 76; and malleability, 15; and metamorphosis, 210; and materialism, 9, 287; and plasticity, 7, 9, 40, 43, 53, 75, 77, 164, 212; and politics, 171, 185, 292; and philosophy, 45, 270, 294–95; and racism, 218–19, 270; and repetition, 70; and resistance, 40, 44, 104, 279–80, 292–93; and sacrifice, 23; and self, 15, 25; and sovereignty, 38, 39, 42, 86, 278, 280, 293–94, 298; and symbolic, 23–25, 28, 39–40, 42–43, 45, 85, 212, 222, 225–26, 228–29, 280–82, 291, 294; and systems, 241, 246

Biopolitics, 25, 28, 36–39, 160, 167, 171–74, 179, 181, 185, 186, 212, 222–25, 229, 231, 283, 291–94, 298; and colonialism, 222–25, 229

Biopower, 23, 25, 28, 37–39, 86, 90, 171, 172, 184, 185, 226, 279, 292, 293, 294

Black studies, 27, 266

Black, Christine, 228, 303

Blaser, Robin, 272

Blood, 23, 42, 70, 86, 225; as quantum, 219, 225

Body, the, 14, 36, 127, 142, 175, 257, 293; and Bouabdellah, 149; and biopolitics, 36, 38–39, 294; and Derrida, 143; divided between symbolic and biological, 25, 40, 42, 280–82; and feminism, 111; and flesh, 280, 282–83; and Freud, 114, 120; and Hegel, 22, 219–21; as imaginary unity (Lacan), 19, 122, 127; and sacrifice, 294; and sovereignty, 298

Boltanski, Luc, 9, 13, 103, 105
Bouabdellah, Zoulikha, 16, 136, 145–51, 303
Bourdieu, Pierre, 55, 303
Brain, 7–15, 18, 26, 27, 40, 43, 70–71, 103, 104, 105, 107, 111–14, 117, 118, 130, 164, 177, 233–7, 240–55, 265, 267, 270, 283–84, 293, 299; and capitalism, 103–6, 112; and consciousness, 193, 252; and cybernetics, 240–43, 259, 298; and Kant, 235–36, 240, 270; and materialism, 112, 113, 129, 235–36, 240, 283; and mind, 8, 11, 103, 235–36, 241; and plasticity, 12, 104, 140, 164, 183, 186, 193, 236, 242, 244, 247, 253, 255, 258, 282, 283, 298; and psychoanalysis, 112, 116, 118; and race, 283–84, 298; and science, 27, 40, 70, 193, 236, 244, 270, 298; and sovereignty, 18, 27, 169, 247, 283, 298, 299; and symbolism, 28, 103, 140, 151, 235, 237, 240, 255, 283, 299; and trauma or damage, 7, 19, 112, 115, 117, 118, 128, 130, 238, 240, 262

Bryant, Levi, 211
Burroughs, William, 250–52, 254, 257, 261, 304
Butler, Judith, 22, 133, 141, 218, 220–21, 304
Butor, Michel, 199
Bynum, Caroline, 3, 29, 304

Canguilhem, Georges, 52, 78–80, 89, 294, 304
Capitalism, 1, 2, 4, 8–10, 13, 50, 57, 93, 93–94, 100–101, 106, 111–12, 129, 152, 160, 169–70, 177, 184, 197, 256, 270, 272, 287–88, 293–94; as global, 104, 160, 169–70, 172, 177, 197, 293; and Heidegger, 100–101;

and plasticity, 10, 13, 93, 103–4;
as neoliberal, 1, 2, 8, 10, 13, 20, 93,
244, 287
Carpenter, John, 255
Carroll, Lewis, 41
Casarino, Cesare, 191–92, 304
Cerebrality, 19, 114, 116, 117, 118, 129,
131, 295
Chandler, Nahum, 266
Chiapello, Eve, 9, 13, 103, 105
Child, the, 20, 28, 117, 125, 236, 272;
and colonialism, 210, 219; as childhood, 28, 297; and Freud, 121–22;
and Kant, 236; as technique of
reading, 28, 210; and temporality,
219
Chirac, Jacques, 296
Chronotope, 194
Clone, 140, 227
Closure, 7–8, 10, 15, 18, 20, 22, 25,
66, 82, 135, 140, 160, 161, 167, 220,
276, 296
Colonialism, 3, 21, 174, 210–13, 272,
298; and law, 21, 212–13
Commodities, 4, 9, 30, 94–95, 99,
101, 106, 108, 197, 216
Communism, 102, 275, 288, 289
Connolly, William, 235, 262, 302, 305
Conrad, Joseph, 199, 200
Control, 14, 26, 36–37, 42, 85, 104–5,
142, 174, 204, 211, 214, 227, 234,
239, 242, 246, 251–52, 254, 257;
and animals, 162, 170; of bodies,
262, 292; and communication,
242–43; and consciousness, 236;
cybernetics as the study of, 103;
and Deleuze, 239; and ethics, 248;
in ecological science, 227–28; as
machine, 250, 254; of the mind,
248, 250; and neuropolitics, 242,
244, 249; and plasticity, 239, 247,
252, 253, 254, 256, 257; and protocol, 252, 254; and psychoanalysis,
237; of the self, 112, 234, 238; and
self-organization, 244; "societies of
control," 239, 252, 254; and sovereignty, 255; as virtual, 257
Cover, Robert, 279
Crick, Francis, 260
Cynicism, 42, 85, 103, 198

Damasio, Antonio, 113, 128
Darwin, Charles, 28, 48–53, 59,
165, 305
Darwinism, 53, 294; as Malthusian,
51; as neural, 261; as psychological,
267; as social, 10, 28, 51
Dasein, 6, 62–63, 66, 71
Declaration of Independence, 203–4
Deconstruction, 9, 13, 16, 20, 24, 27,
36, 37, 39–40, 45, 65, 86, 133–36,
142, 146, 151–52, 154, 192, 209,
211–12, 220, 249, 278, 287–89, 291,
294; of the human, 62–63; of sovereignty, 24, 39, 45, 86, 280, 298,
279–81, 283, 298
Deleuze, Gilles, 1, 7, 8, 13, 29, 31,
38, 41–42, 46, 48, 56, 60, 89, 109,
140, 153, 190–91, 203, 206–7, 239,
250–52, 254, 257–61, 263, 306;
and bodies, 38; and ethics, 203;
and genres, 191; and life, 258; and
societies of control, 239, 251, 254,
257; and subject, 13; and symbolic,
41, 42
Delgado, José, 242, 244–51, 254,
255–56, 260, 306
Derrida, Jacques, 1, 3, 6, 16, 17, 20,
22–23, 27, 28–30, 32, 36, 38–41,
45–48, 59, 61–66, 68, 70–72, 133–35,
141, 143–45, 151–57, 192, 196, 202,
207, 281, 286, 289, 293–94, 296–97,
299, 306–8; and Algeria, 296; and
the animal, 39, 293; and biology,

Index   331

Derrida, Jacques (*continued*)
  38, 294; and biopolitics, 36; and biography, 297; and human, 62–66, 69; and life, 39, 281; and new materialism, 48; and mourning, 134; and Nietzsche, 66, 68, 140; and ontology, 27; and plasticity, 17, 135, 141, 151, 152; and sovereignty, 28, 36, 38; and supplement, 41; and symbolic, 40; and time, 6, 135, 143, 153, 202; and voir venir, 135, 140, 151
Deutsch, Karl, 242–44, 246, 250, 255–56, 308
Dewey, John, 249
Dialectics, 3, 8, 10–13, 16, 21–22, 40, 44–45, 49, 63–64, 91–93, 95–97, 101–5, 107, 133–34, 137–38, 142, 146–47, 153, 194, 209, 218–21, 289–90, 293
Différance, 282, 289
Dispositif, 16, 22, 26, 74, 161, 171, 176, 180, 189–91, 201–3, 206, 226
DNA, 43, 44, 74, 76–78, 87, 105, 227, 253, 291
Drift, 77, 155–56, 196

Elasticity, 4, 18, 107, 112, 238, 254
Ellington, Duke, 205
Emergence, 105–6, 108, 271, 272, 283; and Bergson, 164, 166; of biology, 38; of biopolitics, 38; of biopower, 37, 171; of the body, 220; of difference, 56, 155; of epigenetics, 24; and Glissant, 281; and Kazanjian, 285; of law, 21; of life, 164, 166; of modernity, 36; of new materialism, 50; novel of (Bakhtin), 193; of the philosopher, 139; of plasticity, 140, 141; of production network, 105; of singularities, 54; of the subject, 22, 127, 220; of social abstraction, 94, 98; of the world, 194

Énard, Mathias, 15, 189–203
Engels, Friedrich, 32, 47, 57, 58, 290
Entomology, 161, 166–68, 182
Environment, 24–25, 43, 52, 76–81, 82, 84, 86–89, 121, 165–66, 173–76, 229, 245–46, 260, 268, 293–94
Epic form, 195
Epicurus, 48, 290
Epigenesis, 73, 75, 77–78, 87, 293
Epigenetics, 43, 44, 73, 76, 78, 291–92
Esmeir, Samera, 223, 308
Esposito, Robert, 171–72, 185, 308
Eternal return, 140
Ethopoiesis, 24–25, 81–87. *See also* Technologies of the self
Event, the, 31, 82–84, 114, 120, 190. *See also* Psychic event

Fanon, Frantz, 175, 213, 218–19, 222, 230, 296, 298, 308
Flesh, 27, 39, 40, 266, 271, 277, 279, 280–84, 298; and bare life, 282; of difference, 27
Flexibility, 2, 4, 8, 15, 18, 19, 91, 101, 103, 106–7, 112, 152, 177, 186, 239, 248, 267
Floating signifier, 41–42, 86, 211–12, 230, 282
Fodor, Jerry, 265, 267–69, 309
Fold in discourse, 18, 19, 33, 87, 235, 266; in neuronal materialism, 26
Form, 1, 2, 3–8, 12, 17–21, 23, 29, 35, 37, 43, 48, 49–58, 80, 83, 89, 91, 94, 97, 100, 102- 103, 105, 107, 108, 111, 116, 119, 128–29 133, 135, 137, 139, 141, 146, 152, 160–61, 164, 167–68, 177, 182, 192–96, 199, 203, 209, 212, 214, 221–22, 226, 236–38, 241, 246, 257, 274; and absolute, 139; and abstraction, 97; and Althusser, 49, 53, 54, 57; and annihilation of, 116, 139, 141, 152,

160, 161, 164, 168; and anticipation, 129, 137; and being, 160, 257; and biology, 43, 50, 51, 74; and biopolitics, 222; and the body, 43, 89, 161, 221; and Canguilhem, 52; and capitalism, 20, 97, 103; and death, 52; and the human, 29; and identity, 167; and Kant, 237; and knowledge, 246; and law, 21, 37, 212, 221, 228; and life, 119, 161, 177, 182, 274; and Luhmann, 80; and Machiavelli, 53; and materialism, 48, 97; and money, 94, 98, 102; and the novel, 16, 195, 199, 203; and Nietzsche, 56; and plasticity, 4, 9, 17–19, 26, 27, 49, 91, 107, 108, 111, 116, 133, 135, 139, 141, 146, 160, 161, 177, 194, 236, 238, 241; and power, 23, 36; and recognition, 21, 214; and society, 91, 94; and sovereignty, 35, 226; and subjectivity, 128, 195, 196, 214; and value, 95, 100; and writing, 21

Foucault, Michel, 1, 16, 20, 22, 24–25, 28, 35, 36, 40, 42, 45–46, 81–86, 88, 90, 160, 171–76, 181, 185–86, 190, 206, 225, 231, 243, 249–51, 255, 259, 265–66, 269–71, 280, 284, 286, 292–94, 298, 309, 310; and biopolitics, biopower, 22–23, 36, 38, 40, 90, 171–74, 181, 185, 225, 292; and care of the self, 256, 265, 269, 271; and control, 251; and discipline, 249; and dispositif, 16, 22, 176, 190; and ethopoeisis, 24, 81–83, 85–86; and future, 84; and sovereignty, 24, 28, 35–36, 85, 171–72, 298; and subject, 42; and symbolic, 42

Freedom, 4, 27, 51, 139, 154, 160, 204, 213, 237, 239–40, 245, 249, 256, 262, 269; as aleatory and contingent, 238, 258; as chimerical, 257; as imagination, 279; and information, 243; as moral, 238; and plasticity, 177; as sexual, 14; as species, 248; as steering, 246; and symbolic structure, 45

Freud, Sigmund, 1, 6–7, 15, 17–20, 111, 113–32, 310; and anxiety, 119, 120, 122; and death drive, 7, 18–19, 114, 124, 126; and libido, 113, 116; and ego, 124; and materiality of the brain, 128; and plasticity, 7, 18, 126; and pleasure principle, 19, 116, 122–28; and psyche, 17; and psychic event, 19, 114, 119–20; and sexuality, 116–18, 124–25; and time, 120, 126; and trauma, 115, 119

Frisch, Karl von, 162
Fromm, Erich, 245

Galloway, Alexander, 12, 153, 244, 252, 259, 310
Genome, 40, 43, 73, 76, 163
Glissant, Édouard, 277, 281
Goldman, Danielle, 272
Gould, Stephen Jay, 261, 311
Governmentality, 256, 266
Gramsci, Antonio, 244
Green, Al, 272

Habermas, Jurgen, 237–39, 259, 311
Habit, 11, 137–38, 142
Haeckel, Ernst, 210, 229, 311
Harney, Stefano, 256, 319, 326
Harris, Verne, 201–2, 312
Hartman, Saidiya, 275
Hegel, Georg, 1, 3, 5–8, 11, 20–21, 45, 55, 59, 62–64, 91–92, 94, 96, 108, 111, 114, 133, 135, 137–41, 144, 152–55, 182, 192, 218–20, 230, 287, 312; and consciousness, 220; and

Hegel, Georg (*continued*)
  plasticity, 21, 22, 135, 220; and recognition, 22, 219; and subject, 22, 63, 64, 220; and time, 5, 137, 138, 140, 220
Heidegger, Martin, 1, 3, 6, 13, 20, 48, 62–69, 72, 88, 90, 92–94, 97–101, 108, 120, 153, 155–56, 192, 287–90, 294, 312; and capitalism, 94, 97, 99–102, 287, 288; and critique of humanism, 65; and Dasein, 62–63; and materialism, 289–90; and money, 98; and originary, 97; and plasticity, 99; and revenge, 67–69; and technical domination, 100
Heisenberg, Werner, 245
Hemingway, Ernest, 199
Heraclitus, 56
Hobbes, Thomas, 35, 48, 280, 312
Homer, 195, 199
Humanism, 62–65, 68, 251
Husserl, Edmund, 62–64
Hyppolite, Jean, 63, 230

Idealism, 10, 47, 49, 106, 249, 289–90
Identity and difference, 52, 135, 139–41, 151
Ideology, 7, 16, 18, 27, 55, 106, 153, 189, 243, 244, 258, 289; and archives, 16; and biology, 294; and biopolitics, 37, 287, 293; and closure, 7; as colonial or imperial, 210; as critique, 103; as excess, 10; and flesh, 27; as market, capitalist, 243–44, 288; as neoliberal, 93; as neural, neuronal, 10, 11, 93, 103, 104, 256; as norm, 14; as practical, 106; and science, 291; and sovereignty, 23, 36, 37, 292; of space, 190; as superstructure, 104–5

Indigeneity, 21, 22, 69, 209–13; and colonialism, 211–12; and philosophy, 211; and plasticity, 218–29; and recognition, 212–17
Irigaray, Luce, 1, 155, 312

Jakobson, Roman, 211
Jameson, Frederick, 3, 10, 29, 31, 92, 103, 107, 313
Johnston, Adrian, 123, 313
Jones, Ernest, 122
Jouissance, 19, 114, 122–27, 129, 149
Joyce, James, 199
Justice, 1, 2, 13–20, 21, 56, 154, 198, 214; as archive, 200–201, 203, 206; dispositif, of 189–91, 199, 201, 203; as ontological, 22, 105; as pedagogy, 197; as repetition, 29, 69

Kafka, Franz, 13, 183, 313
Kant, Immanuel, 73, 96, 235–38, 240, 249–50, 258, 278, 279, 280, 283, 313; and *bios*, 278–79; and epigenesis, 87; and neurophilosophy, 235–36
Kantorowicz, Ernst, 39, 280, 313
Kauanui, Kehaulani, 225, 313
Kazanjian, David, 268, 285, 313
Kennedy, Robert, 250
Kincaid, Jamaica, 204, 313
Kittler, Friedrich, 88, 314
Klein, Melanie, 122
Kurzban, Robert, 265, 267–68, 314
Kurzweil, Ray, 249, 314

Lacan, Jacques, 10, 122, 128–29, 281, 314; and death drive, 114, 124; and materiality of the subject, 19, 127; and jouissance, 123–26, 131; and the real, 31
Latil, Pierre de, 241
Laughter, 68, 134, 152, 219

Law, 1–4, 10, 14, 20–23, 29, 176, 190, 202; and Benjamin, 202, 206; of capitalist development, 57, 101; and colonialism, 21, 212–30, 279, 296; and Derrida (*force of*), 135, 144–45, 154–55; and Freud, 119, 123; as indigenous rights, 21, 212–13, 217, 227; as international, 144, 175; as moral, 280; as natural, 245; and Nietzsche, 68–69; and plasticity, 24, 28; and recognition, 14, 69, 212–22, 228; and revenge, 68–69; of science, 52, 119, 253, 277; and sovereignty, 23, 35–38, 42, 225, 279

Land, 11; and colonialism, 21, 69, 211–17, 224–29; and law, 228–29

Lear, Jonathan, 123

Lenin, Vladimir Ilyich, 47, 290

Lévi-Strauss, Claude, 6, 23, 41, 209–11, 314

Lévinas Emmanuel, 27, 63, 155

Lindqvist, Sven, 200

Luhmann, Niklas, 24–25, 75–76, 85, 315; and autopoiesis, 85–86, 90; and closure, 82; and environment, 80–81

Lukacs, Georg, 245

Machiavelli, Nicolo, 48, 53, 56–57, 291–92

Man-as-species, 160, 172, 174, 176, 179, 181

Marx, Karl, 2, 4, 10–12, 30, 32, 47–48, 54–58, 92–93, 95–97, 101–8, 111–12, 129, 136, 145, 155, 192, 287–90, 317; and metamorphosis, 30; and form, 97

Marxism, 9, 13, 20, 47, 103, 104–5, 152, 219, 220, 287–91

Masks, 22, 36–37, 192, 209–11, 228

Massumi, Brian, 173–75, 235, 317

Materialism, 1, 2, 11, 47–48, 58, 111, 287, 290; as aleatory (*see below* of the encounter); and Althusser (*see below* of the encounter); as biological, 9, 287; and consciousness, 12; and Delgado, 249; as dialectical (historical), 10, 287–90; of the encounter, 13, 28, 47–53, 56–57, 105, 289–90; and horror, 255; as new, 1, 8–13, 48, 53, 111, 226; as neuroscientific, 12, 26; and psychoanalysis, 17–20; as reasonable, 12, 247; as teleological, 49, 290

Maturana, Humberto, 77, 85, 317, 318

Mbembe, Achille, 197, 222, 318

Melville, Herman, 192

Merry, Sally, 223, 318

Metamorphosis, 2, 3–4, 6, 14–15, 18, 28, 30, 92, 107, 140, 164, 165–67, 177, 209–10, 227–38, 254, 257; and biological conservation, 210; and destructive plasticity, 18, 254, 257; and insects, 165–67; and Marx, 30; and plasticity, 4, 107, 166–67, 238, 254; and resistance, 15

Metaphysics, 4, 28, 64, 97; and alterity, 4; and capitalism, 93–94, 287–88; and deconstruction, 291; and destruction, 288; and exchange, 288; and form, 7; and law, 69; and ontology, 18, 238; as political, 14–15, 227; and primitivism, 226; and speculation, 247; of subjectivity, 92

Mitropoulos, Angela, 271, 318

Mode of coming, 289–90

Money, 57, 74, 93–102, 106, 108, 198, 288

Monod, Jacques, 105–6, 108

Morrison, Toni, 281, 284

Motor scheme, 13, 16, 160, 192
Mourning, 6, 17–18, 30, 134–35, 137, 141–42, 155, 257, 272

Negri, Antonio, 154, 319
Neoliberalism, 1, 2, 8, 10, 13, 20, 91, 93, 244, 287
Networks, 36, 104–5, 152, 170, 180, 197, 240, 243, 252–54, 256
Neuropolitics, 235, 242, 255, 259, 262
Neuroscience, 1, 3, 4, 8–9, 12–15, 111, 113, 117, 123–24, 140, 235, 253; and cerebrality, 116, 118; and cybernetics, 242; and dystopia, 26; as ideology, 10, 11, 13, 103, 105, 152, 164, 193, 237, 256; and materialism, 12, 26, 107, 128; and plasticity, 9, 14, 15, 43, 116; and politics, 164, 235, 242, 250, 255, 299; and psychoanalysis, 118, 128; and trauma, 18, 117
New materialism, 8–13, 28, 48, 50, 57, 111, 129, 226; and Althusser, 53; and indigeneity, 226
New Wounded, the, 19, 112–19, 124, 127–28
Nietzsche, Friedrich, 6, 56, 62, 66–69, 111, 140, 141, 297, 319; and active forgetting, 66; and new materialism, 8, 48; and repetition, 67
Nora, Pierre, 296, 319

O'Sullivan, Simon, 198–99, 319
Ontology, 27, 48, 56, 93, 134, 152, 161, 167, 237, 238; and the accident, 24; and capitalism, 93, 97, 99, 101–3, 106, 288; and closure, 20, 220; and colonialism, 22; and cybernetics, 240; and the encounter, 55; and environment, 80; and Hegel, 22, 91, 92, 220; and Heidegger, 288, 289; and the human, 173, 180; and justice, 22; and life, 167, 172; and money, 98; and neuroscience, 12, 14; as ontological combustion, 161–62, 182; and plasticity, 1, 4, 15, 20, 25, 161
Oppenheimer, J. Robert, 233
Originary, 13, 15, 27, 44, 58–59, 93, 97–98, 101, 229, 269–70, 276, 290
Ovid, 3

Passeron, Jean-Claude, 55, 303
Persona, conceptual, 16, 194, 198
Philip, M. NourbeSe, 271, 273
Philo of Alexandria, 271
Philopoesis, 190–92
Plasticity, 2, 6–8, 18, 20, 23, 24; and aesthetics, 3, 16, 18, 136, 145; and alea, 238; and Althusser, 53; as age, era, or epoch, 13, 25, 139, 141, 160; and archive, 16, 202, 205; and Bakhtin, 193–94; and Benjamin, 202; and Bergson, 178–79, 182; and biology, 40, 43, 50, 53, 75, 77, 105, 160, 193; and brain, 8–10, 27, 40, 103, 116–19, 193, 240, 242, 282, 298; and capital, 91, 102, 104, 105; and consciousness, 10, 11, 193, 251; and control, 239, 247, 252, 254, 256; and cybernetics, 103, 239, 241, 298; and Darwin, 50, 53; and deconstruction, 27, 45, 135, 136, 146, 152; and Delgado, 246–50; as destructive, 2, 6–7, 18, 20, 23, 24, 116, 117–19, 238–40, 242, 248, 251, 254, 256–58; and discipline, 239; and dystopia, 26, 159, 161, 180; as emancipatory, 2, 6, 16, 24, 26, 44, 115, 160, 214, 295; and epigenetics, 43, 75, 77, 284; and ethics, 91, 250; and evolution, 50; as fluidity, 51, 137; and form, 4, 9, 17, 18, 19, 26, 27, 49, 50, 91, 107, 108, 111, 116, 133, 135, 139, 141, 146, 160, 161, 177, 194, 236, 238, 241; and forms

336 Index

of life, 161; and Freud, 126; and genetics, 247; and genre, 193; and Hegelian dialectic, 11, 21, 45, 91, 133, 135, 137, 139, 220; and horror, 234, 238, 240, 242, 256–57; and imagination, 192–93, 279; and insects, 161, 163–64, 177; and Luhmann, 85; as motor scheme, 13, 16, 160, 192; as mourning, 17; and narrative, 16; and neurons, 8–9, 11, 13, 26, 43, 111, 112, 160, 177, 235, 241, 247, 252, 256, 291; as itself plastic, 25, 75, 160, 167; as play 44; as poiesis, 77; as political vitality, 176, 179; as psychoanalytic, 18, 112; as reading, 5, 16, 17, 28, 139, 143, 145, 151, 161, 295; as repair, 20, 29, 71, 117, 119; and resistance, 16, 18, 108, 151, 177, 186, 212, 226, 239; and subjectivity, 17, 119, 295; and symbolic, 10, 58; and temporality, 5, 6, 16, 133, 135, 137–38, 177, 193, 202, 205, 219; as thought experiment, 234; and voir venir (to see what is coming), 135, 137, 138, 140, 146, 151; as zone of concepts, 192

Plastics, 159–60
Posthumanism, 27, 65, 66, 154, 181, 249
Pound, Ezra, 199
Primitive, the, 45, 64, 209–12, 218–19, 221–22, 224–26, 228
Psychic event, 19, 114, 116–20
Psychoanalysis, 1, 10, 17–19, 112–14, 116, 118, 122, 123–24, 128, 234, 237
Psychoneurology, 112
Pynchon, Thomas, 199

Race, 11, 204–5, 219, 222, 225, 270, 279, 283, 295, 298; and critical race theory 21, 161; and music, 205; and property, 218–19

Raffles, Hugh, 163
Rancière, Jacques, 194, 320
Reading, plastic. *See* Plasticity
Recognition, 2, 10–11, 14, 20–22, 27, 162–63, 192, 275; and colonialism, 212–22, 228; and Hegel, 64, 218–20; and law, 14, 69, 212–22, 228; and plasticity, 11, 21, 27, 214, 220–21
Reconciliation, 21, 212–13, 216, 218. *See also* Reparation
Reparation, 69, 149, 273, 275–76
Repetition, 11, 29, 62–63, 65–71, 97, 115, 120–23, 125–26, 243
Revolution, 5, 57, 94, 157, 219, 242, 270, 285, 286; French, 37, 91; as movements, 11, 16–17, 37, 107, 136, 150–51; as scientific, 70, 73–77, 291, 292; as technical, 241, 247, 252, 270
Ricoeur, Paul, 63
Rilke, Rainer Maria, 98–100, 102, 321
Riviere, Joan, 122
Rousseau, Jean Jacques, 48, 54, 56

Sacrifice, 23, 41, 64, 138–39, 282, 294
Said, Edward, 210–11, 297, 321
Santner, Eric, 39, 280, 321
Sartre, Jean-Paul, 62–63, 71
Seneca, 86, 265
Sexuality, 2, 11, 14, 21, 116–19, 124–25, 223, 225; as alternative to cerebrality, 19, 116, 118; as Freudian regime, 116, 119; as sexual identity/difference, 14, 20, 122
Shakespeare, William, 101–2, 153
Silva, Noenoe, 223, 311
Simondon, Gilbert, 260, 322
Sirhan Sirhan, 250
Skafish, Peter, 29, 299
Slavery, 101–2, 205, 269, 274–75; as master/slave dialectic, 64, 220
Sohn-Rethel, Alfred, 94–98, 322

Solms, Mark, 113
Sovereignty, 1, 2, 4, 13–15, 18, 20–27, 35–45, 58, 85–87, 93, 209–29, 254, 255, 258, 270, 271, 278–84, 292–94, 298
Species, 23, 37, 49, 248, 254; as alien, 227, 232; and accident, 23; and alienation, 138; and biopolitics, 174, 254; and biopower, 171; as collaborative, 170; and colonialism, 174; as companion, 162, 168, 169, 182; and competition between, 77; and control, 256, 260; and development, 178; as differentiation, 25, 162, 165, 245–46; and diversity, 163, 227; as endangered, 224, 245; and environment, 79, 163; and extinction, 167; as killable, expendable, 161, 162; and plasticity, 50, 59, 167, 177, 256; and survival, 246; and variability, mutability, 50
Species-being, 99, 287; as species-nature, 102
Spillers, Hortense, 281–82, 284, 322
Spinoza, Baruch, 48, 128, 251, 291; and ethics, 203
Spivak, Gayatri Chakravorty, 283, 304
Stoicism, 25, 82, 84
Stoler, Ann, 225, 322
Stora, Benjamin, 296, 322
Structuralism, 1, 29, 42, 210, 211, 254
Subjectivity, 1, 2, 6, 8, 11, 13–17, 20, 28, 42, 63, 81, 92, 94, 106, 113–14, 116, 119, 127, 130, 134, 138, 141, 144–45, 151, 155, 193, 196, 199, 206, 295 aboriginal, 214, 228; as aesthetic subjectivity, 16; and Hegel, 138; and mutability, 193; as new wounded, 128; and neurochemical alteration, 248; as political subjectivity, 11, 106, 145, 199, 206;

and psychoanalysis, 20, 113–14, 119, 127, 129
Symbolic, the, 9–10, 19, 23–25, 28, 39–42, 44–45, 85–86, 212, 222, 225, 228, 280–83, 291

Technologies of the self, 81–82, 86, 266
Telos, 5, 49, 51, 53, 54, 63–64, 68, 138, 165–66, 178, 244, 257, 278, 290
Temporality, 5–7, 16, 17, 18, 22, 29, 50, 52, 68–69, 95–96, 126, 135–36, 138–39, 141, 143, 151, 153, 190, 193–94, 202, 216, 219, 220, 266; and colonial recognition, 216, 226; and Derrida, 135, 141, 181, 193, 194; and Bakhtin, 193–94; and Benjamin, 202; and ethics, 202; and Freud, 18, 126; and Hegel, 5, 137, 138–39, 140, 151, 152, 220, 270; and Nietzsche, 69; and Ricoeur, 29; as spatiotemporality, 190
Thacker, Eugene, 186, 244, 252, 257, 310, 322–23
Tillich, Paul, 245
Trace, the, 31, 134, 142, 145, 149
Trauma, 3, 7, 18–19, 112–23, 28, 130, 140, 238, 296
Turing, Alan, 270

Uexküll, Jakob von, 79, 323

Varela, Francisco, 77, 317, 318
Vitalism, 8, 26, 171–72, 177

Waddington, Conrad, 43, 323
Walker, David, 204, 323
Walter, W. Grey, 241
War, 26, 111, 115, 130, 149–50, 161, 168, 172–73, 175, 189, 197, 199, 242, 243, 245, 248, 254, 280, 296; crimes, 189, 201, 203; as entomol-

ogy, 168–69, 171; and Freud 121; and terror, 26, 111, 161, 168, 170, 173, 175–77, 182, 184
Watson, James, 260
Weber, Max, 291
Wiener, Norbert, 240, 243–44, 246, 260, 270, 324

Wolfe, Patrick, 211, 324
Writing, 16–17, 21, 44, 83, 86, 88, 133–36, 140, 145, 192, 194, 237, 283

Žižek, Slavoj, 19, 116, 152, 237, 324; and jouissance 123; and the subject, 127

www.ingramcontent.com/pod-product-compliance
Lightning Source LLC
Chambersburg PA
CBHW070745020526
44116CB00032B/1978